Comprehensive ENT

Series Editor
Cemal Cingi, Department of Otorhinolaryngology,
Medical Faculty, Eskişehir Osmangazi University, Eskisehir, Türkiye

As technology progresses, there are continuous advances in every medical subspeciality, and otorhinolaryngology/ENT is a particularly outstanding example of this. ENT lends itself well to the development of innovative and sophisticated solutions, including those affecting the vital area of airway management. Rhinoplasty and related cosmetic procedures are now a well-established part of ENT practice, and make major contributions to patient well-being, quality of life and social function. The series also covers the key principles involved in the use of social media for advertising and sharing cosmetic outcomes, from minor procedures to full-scale surgical operations. The series gathers ENT and related sub-specialty experts from across the globe and translates their knowledge into easily accessible, well-structured summaries of the current state of knowledge, with accompanying illustrations, diagrams and summary tables. Each volume is under the leadership of editors who are thoroughly familiar with the area covered and understands exactly which information is of most relevance and interest to those entering the field for the first time or seeking to update their existing knowledge. The series both outlines precisely the current state of the art in each area of ENT practice and shows where the future of the feld may lie. The fundamental scientifc basis of various disorders is covered, including molecular and cellular aspects, as well as diagnostic practice and the appropriate use of investigations. Historical aspects will be covered where they cast light on the general direction of the specialty. The latest developments in clinical management, disease prevention and public health aspects are described. The series shows how these multiple scientifc and clinical aspects can be best understood in supporting an individual, personalized approach to patient care that fts the patient-centered ethos of twenty-frst century ENT healthcare.

Aslı Elif Tanuğur Samanci
Nuray Bayar Muluk • Taylan Samanci
Cemal Cingi

Propolis: Prevention and Healing Effects in Otorhinolaryngology

Springer

Aslı Elif Tanuğur Samanci
Bee&You R&D Center
Istanbul, Türkiye

Taylan Samanci
SBS Scientific Bio Solutions Co.
Istanbul, Türkiye

Nuray Bayar Muluk
Kırıkkale University, Faculty of Medicine
Otorhinolaryngology Department
Kırıkkale, Türkiye

Cemal Cingi
Eskisehir Osmangazi University, Faculty of Medicine, Otorhinolaryngology Department
Eskişehir, Türkiye

ISSN 2731-6742 ISSN 2731-6750 (electronic)
Comprehensive ENT
ISBN 978-3-031-68545-3 ISBN 978-3-031-68546-0 (eBook)
https://doi.org/10.1007/978-3-031-68546-0

This Springer imprint is published by the registered company Springer Nature Switzerland AG
The registered company address is: Gewerbestrasse 11, 6330 Cham, Switzerland

Preface

Welcome to our book, **"Propolis: Prevention and Healing Effects in Otorhinolaryngology."**

This tutorial explores propolis's exceptional characteristics and its significant influence on the health of the ears, nose, and throat. It also explores the therapeutic potential of this natural wonder in maintaining and restoring wellness in the field of otorhinolaryngology, from its ancient origins to its present applications.

Bees and honey possess considerable symbolism and religious importance in diverse civilizations. In the context of Christianity, honey is seen as a symbol of pleasantness and abundance, frequently linked to the Promised Land. Honey has great significance in Islam as a therapeutic substance, explicitly referenced in the Quran as a symbol of divine benevolence. Moreover, bees are occasionally regarded as emblems of industriousness and communal spirit. Honey holds significance in Hinduism as it is utilized in religious ceremonies and symbolizes purity and sacrifices to the deities. Honey was of sacred importance in ancient civilizations such as the Egyptians and Greeks, and it was used in religious rituals and to make gifts to the gods. Bees and honey frequently hold significant spiritual and metaphorical connotations in various religious and cultural contexts.

Propolis, a sticky material gathered by bees from different plants, is highly esteemed for its wide range of healing powers. Furthermore, Anatolian propolis obtains its ideal blend from the virgin Anatolian highlands, which serve as the habitat for 12,000 distinct plant species and are recognized as one of the most biodiverse areas globally. The field of otorhinolaryngology is increasingly acknowledging and researching its potential for prevention and healing. We aimed to investigate the diverse role of propolis in enhancing the health of the ear, nose, and throat.

Propolis demonstrates strong antibacterial properties, making it a great asset in fighting ear, nose, and throat infections. The extensive range of its antimicrobial activity against bacteria, viruses, and fungi has been thoroughly documented in several investigations. Propolis can hinder the growth of harmful microorganisms, which can aid in the prevention of common diseases such as otitis media, sinusitis, and tonsillitis.

Additionally, propolis has anti-inflammatory characteristics that are essential in relieving symptoms related to inflammatory diseases of the otorhinolaryngological system. Propolis can modulate the immune response and decrease tissue inflammation, resulting in pain relief, edema reduction, and congestion alleviation. This ultimately enhances patient comfort and facilitates a quicker recovery process. Moreover, propolis demonstrates exceptional antioxidant properties, which can be linked to its abundant concentration of flavonoids, phenolic acids, and other bioactive substances. The antioxidant activity of this substance aids in counteracting detrimental free radicals, which are involved in the development of many otorhinolaryngological illnesses, such as chronic rhinosinusitis and otitis externa. Propolis aids in the protection of vulnerable tissues from oxidative harm by scavenging free radicals, as well as promoting their regeneration and repair.

Studies have demonstrated that propolis can improve the process of wound healing in the otorhinolaryngological tract. Its capacity to enhance collagen synthesis, facilitate tissue regrowth, and expedite the healing of surface layers makes it an indispensable tool in treating severe injuries, surgical incisions, and persistent sores that impact the ear, nose, and throat.

Cooperation is a fundamental principle that applies to different areas of life, such as social, economic, and biological domains. Collaboration enables individuals to accomplish more excellent outcomes collectively by utilizing various skills, viewpoints, and resources.

This book is the outcome of collaborating with my very productive and skillful colleague **Nuray Bayar Muluk** in cooperation with **Asli Elif Tanugur Samancı** and **Taylan Samancı**, who are both related to the scientific and production aspects of bee products. I thank them for their energetic, collective, and cooperative efforts.

I anticipate that this book will illuminate the field and generate novel research concepts.

Eskişehir, Türkiye
4.4.2024

Cemal Cingi

Contents

Bee: Overview

1

1.1 Introduction

Insects belonging to the suborder Apocrita (order Hymenoptera) comprise about 20,000 species, including the well-known honeybee (*Apis*) and bumblebee (*Bombus* and *Psithyrus*) and thousands of other beelike wasps and flylike insects. There is a wide size range for adults, from around 2 mm to 4 cm, or 0.08–1.6 inches [1].

Bees and wasps share a common ancestry, but the main biological distinction is that wasps need insects or spiders to stock their nests or feed their young, while bees (apart from parasitic bees) use pollen and honey. Bees have a few branched or feathered hairs that pollen commonly attaches to, while wasps are coated with unbranched hairs; this is the most fundamental anatomical difference that goes along with their different feeding preferences [1].

Typically, male bees need to stay around longer to harvest pollen or take on other roles related to raising offspring. Female bees construct and provide the nest entirely, and they often have specialized anatomy that helps them transport pollen. Most bees collect pollen from a broad range of flower types; this trait is known as collectivity. Nevertheless, several species of bees are specialized for gathering pollen from specific flower families, while others are color-blind. Oligolectic bees collect pollen from only a few closely related flower species. Different flowers appear to have evolved distinct mouthpieces for bees, which serve as pollen collectors and carriers [1].

The vast majority of bees prefer to live alone and avoid human interaction. The female of these species constructs and supplies her nest, which is typically a burrow. Those bees do not belong to any particular caste. When making their nests, solitary bees can use various materials, including wood, pith of trees or canes, or even turrets or chimneys. Adult solitary bees typically only make it a little. A few weeks of the year may be all that certain species spend flying around, while the rest of the year is spent in their cells as eggs, larvae, pupae, and young adults [1].

A. E. Tanuğur Samanci et al., *Propolis: Prevention and Healing Effects in Otorhinolaryngology*, Comprehensive ENT,
https://doi.org/10.1007/978-3-031-68546-0_1

When the cells are sealed, the larvae get all the nourishment they need from solitary bees. Some bees, like honeybees and bumblebees, feed their young in stages [1].

1.2 Bees' Heritage

Wasps are the ancestors of bees. The majority of wasps' diet consists of insects and spiders, as these creatures provide a significant source of protein for the wasps' offspring. When the first flowering plants appeared around 125 million years ago, certain wasps shifted their feeding habits from hunting to collecting pollen to feed their young. They may have been prowling for pollinating insects, which feast on flowers, drink their nectar, or eat some pollen. It did not take long to realize that eating pollen was better than hunting. Bees likely became vegetarians since pollen is a good source of protein and does not defend itself. Adaptations distinct from those of hunters were necessary for pollen and nectar collection. Therefore, they began to transform and evolve into bees. There are still bees that look a lot like wasps. Some bees, like wasps, have almost no hair, and, like wasps, only the females of the species possess stingers. Physical appearance is just the beginning of the parallels. Some species of bees and wasps live alone and care for their young, while others are gregarious and help each other out.

Consider bumblebees and yellow jacket wasps for social behavior and yearly colony formation. An overwintered queen emerges in the spring of both species. Along with laying eggs, the queen constructs a nest and gathers nourishment. New queens emerge, mate, and hibernate; in the fall, the female workers hatch and continue feeding and caring for the colony until the cycle starts again in the spring [2].

1.3 Native Bees

The native bee [3] population is a valuable resource. Bees can be found in every flower-filled North American forest, from alpine meadows in the Rocky Mountains National Forest to the Sonoran Desert in Arizona's Coronado National Forest and from Alaska's Tongass National Forest to Florida's Ocala National Forest. With 4000 native bee species ranging from the small Perdita minimum to the enormous carpenter bee, the United States is home to various habitats, including woods, farms, towns, and wildlands. Many people do not know this, but the United States did not have honeybees when European settlers brought hives from Europe. These cunning creatures took little time to break free of domestication. Honeybees swarmed into hollow trees to build nests, just as they had for thousands of years in Asia and Europe. Long before honeybees arrived, native pollinators—bees other than honeybees—were pollinating the continent's flowering plants. Most pollination, particularly for native plants, is still done by them, even in today's much-changed settings.

It is impressive though that honeybees are clueless when pollinating eggplant or tomato blossoms. Pumpkins, cherries, blueberries, and cranberries are native plants that struggle to pollinate compared to native bees [2].

The size, shape, and color of native bees can vary greatly. They differ in the places they spend most of their time, the kinds of nests they construct, the types of flowers they visit, and the times of year they are active. No one pays any attention to them or even knows what they are. Despite this, pollination is an essential ecological function that they perform for 80% of blooming plants. Imagine a world devoid of the splendor of blossoming trees, bushes, and wildflowers. How many of us know that bees are responsible for pollinating over three-quarters of our nation's fruits, nuts, and veggies? Honeybees are masters of foraging. For instance, in the brief time that the southeastern blueberry bee, *Habropoda*, is laborious and spends in the field, she can visit up to 50,000 blueberry blooms and pollinate enough of them to provide over 6000 ripe blueberries. You may expect to pay at least $20 for those 6000 blueberries on the market. Even if not every bee you see buzzing around has a monetary value of $20, their collective efforts ensure that blossoming plants continue to thrive. Bees are essential to the survival of our planet because they pollinate the 250,000 species of flowering plants [2].

1.4 The Apoidea

As a group, the Apoidea comprises seven families: five or six subfamilies, 45 genera, and 3000 species make up the Colletidae, a prehistoric wasplike bee family; Andrenidae, which include some parasitic species, are solitary mining bees of medium to large size; family Halictidae consists of the well-known "sweat bees" (*Dialictus zephyrus*) and other "mining" or "burrowing" bees that feed on human sweat; bees of the Melittidae family serve as a bridge between the lower and upper bee hierarchy; Megachilidae bees are known for their complex nest constructions; and Apidae (including bumblebees, honeybees, carpenter bees, cuckoo bees, and digger or mining bees) and Stenotritidae are a tiny family of bees native to Australia [1].

1.5 Killer Bee

The so-called killer bee is a cross between two honeybee subspecies, one from Africa and one from Europe. The Africanized honeybee came from a crossbreeding between native European honeybees and those from Africa in 1957 due to an unintentional release in Brazil. Its European counterpart is not more poisonous, but this species responds considerably faster to dangers to the colony, launches more attacks, pursues longer and farther, and takes longer to calm down. Hundreds of deaths are allegedly attributable to them [1].

1.6 Honeybee (Tribe Apini)

The term "honeybee" (Figs. 1.1 and 1.2) refers to any member of the Apini tribe of insects, a subfamily of the Apidae family in the Hymenoptera order. Though technically there are seven species of bees in the genus *Apis*, the everyday use of the term "honeybee" refers exclusively to *Apis mellifera*, the typical domestic bee. You may hear this species called the western honeybee or the European honeybee [1].

Since they are all social insects, honeybees always choose to live in hives or nests. Among the most fascinating things about honeybees is the way they dance within the hive to signal to one another the proximity, size, quality, and location of food sources in the vicinity [1].

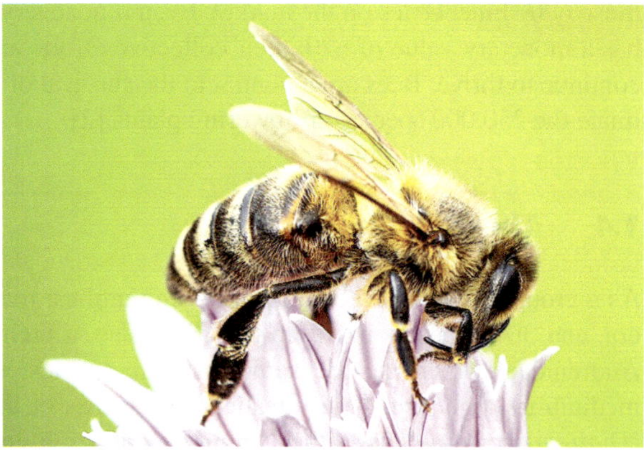

Fig. 1.1 Anatolian honeybee (Yozgat region). (*Courtesy of* **Ali Ihsan Gokcen**)

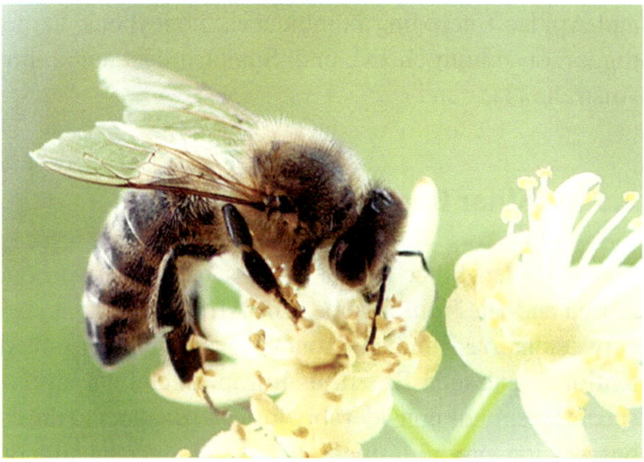

Fig. 1.2 Anatolian honeybee (Black Sea region). (*Courtesy of* **Ali Ihsan Gokcen**)

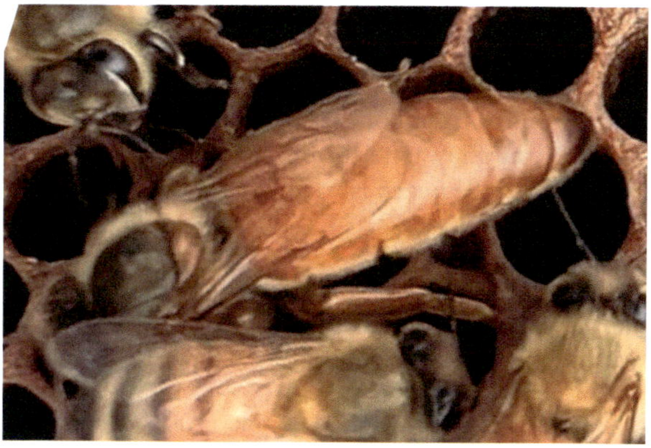

Fig. 1.3 Queen bee (*Apis mellifera* carnica). (*Courtesy of* **Taylan Samancı**)

1.6.1 *Apis* Species

All *Apis* species, except *A. mellifera*, are found only in some southern or southeastern Asian areas (Fig. 1.3). In South Asia, you can find the tiny honeybee, or *A. florea*, which makes its homes in shrubs and trees. The black dwarf honeybee, or *A. andreniformis*, is a resident of the wooded regions of Southeast Asia. Southeastern Asia is also home to *A. dorsata*, the gigantic honeybee, which may occasionally produce combs that are approximately 3 m (about 9 feet) in diameter. Originally from southern and southeastern Asia, the Eastern honeybee (*A. cerana*) has been domesticated in certain regions. Similar to the Koschevnikov's bee (*A. koschevnikovi*), it is endemic to Borneo and a few other Southeast Asian islands as well as the Malay Peninsula. The islands of Mindanao in the Philippines and Indonesia are the original habitats of *A. nigrocincta*. *Apis* is a species that includes many subspecies and strains [1].

The average length of *A. mellifera* is 1.2 cm, or around 0.5 inch, though different strains of this species can vary in size. The color of the head and thorax (the middle region) runs with the strain and is rather bristly. On top of the head, you will find two big compound eyes and three little ones called ocelli. In addition to excellent eyesight, it has two very sensitive antennae that can sense odors [1].

1.6.2 Honeybee Sexes and Castes

The honeybee [4] is bisexual, with two distinct female castes. The females of the species are classified into two groups: the workers, who do not reach sexual maturity, and the queens, who are more significant than the workers. Only in early June can you see the bigger males, also called drones, instead of the more minor workers. Stingers are present on the workers and queens but not the drones [1].

To regulate fertilization, queen honeybees keep sperm in a special chamber called the spermatheca. Queens can lay unfertilized or fertilized eggs. Drones are the offspring of fertilized eggs, while workers or virgin queens are the offspring of fertilized eggs. The honeycomb's vertical, larger-than-average cells, known as queen cells, are where the eggs of future queens are laid. The virgin queens are given royal jelly made by the workers' salivary glands after they hatch. Virgin queens transform into workers when their diet is not restricted to only royal jelly. Workers may lay unfertilized eggs during the swarming season, giving birth to drones [1] if the queen is weak or absent.

References

1. Bee. Britannica. Last Updated: Dec 1, 2023. https://www.britannica.com/animal/honeybee. Accessed 8 Dec 2023.
2. Moisset B, Buchmann S. Bee Basics. An Introduction to Our Native Bees. United States Department of Agriculture. https://efotg.sc.egov.usda.gov/references/public/SC/Bee_Basics_North_American_Bee_ID.pdf. Accessed 8 Dec 2023.
3. How many species of native bees are in the United States? USGS. https://www.usgs.gov/faqs/how-many-species-native-bees-are-united-states. Accessed 21 June 2024.
4. The Wildlife Trusts. https://www.wildlifetrusts.org/wildlife-explorer/invertebrates/bees-and-wasps/honey-bee. Accessed 21 June 2024.

Anatomy and Life Cycle

2

2.1 Bee Anatomy or Morphology

Bees, like all insects, have a thorax, an abdomen, and a head. Not only that, but they are also wingless and have six legs. The head is equipped with the following parts: • two touch- and smell-sensitive antennae; • two pairs of compound eyes and three pairs of simple eyes; • and the jaws, or mandibles, that are utilized for biting, working pollen and wax "loaves," burrowing, and so on. Two sets of flight-supporting membranous wings joined by tiny hooks and three sets of legs make up the thorax. The abdomen has six or seven segments depending on the species, internal wax glands in some bees (like honeybees and bumblebees), a stinger (a modified ovipositor) at the tip (in females only), and plumose hairs (branched) in other parts of the body. Scopae, which some females use to transfer pollen, are formed of stiff hairs and can be found on the underbelly or the hind legs. To transmit pollen grains from their bodies to their transport mechanism, bees often brush themselves, collecting them from their feathery hairs [1].

The ecologically significant proboscides, or relative length of mouthpart segments within the tongue, allow bees to be classified into two main categories. Honey is collected using both the long and short tongues. While bees of the Apidae and Megachilidae families are more likely to gather nectar from open, flat blooms, those of deeper blossoms with longer throats are also acceptable. Shorter beaks and a narrower range of flower preferences characterize the remaining bee families. They can only feed on flowers with shallow petals, such as carrot, daisy, and aster families. There may be some overlap in size between male and female bees, but generally, the females are bigger [1].

A. E. Tanuğur Samanci et al., *Propolis: Prevention and Healing Effects in Otorhinolaryngology*, Comprehensive ENT,
https://doi.org/10.1007/978-3-031-68546-0_2

2.2 Life Cycle

After laying eggs, the three species of honeybees spend the next 3 days turning into grubs, the larvae's common name. While all grubs are initially given royal jelly, this diet is only maintained for the queens-to-be. When they reach maturity, the grubs change into pupae. On average, workers emerge after 21 days, drones after 24 days, and queens after 16 days. The queens struggle among themselves after emerging from the hive until just one is left. When the young queens come out of the hive, the old queen and most of her workers have usually fled. Swarming is a common reproductive strategy, and the swarm may split into two or more colonies depending on where they lay their eggs [2].

2.3 Nesting

Some kinds of bees are more suited to raising young than others; these bees construct nests [3] and provide food for their young. However, there are parasitic species in the Apidae, Halictidae, and Megachilidae families. The term "cuckoo" now describes them, just as it does birds. Cuckoo bees, like cuckoo birds (such as cowbirds), use other people's nests to hatch their young. A few bee species are used as nests by most cuckoo bee species. Some kinds of cuckoo bees are so specific that they will only attack the nests of other species. Before laying her egg, the female of some cuckoo bee species kills the host's larva. Cuckoo bee larvae, on the other hand, mostly eat stored food and the poor hosts' larvae. Cuckoo bees have lost a lot of hair and pollen baskets, so they do not collect pollen anymore. Wasps and cuckoo bees are frequently confused at first sight. Sure enough, cuckoo bees will stop by flowers to suck the nectar [1].

Except for cuckoo bees, every kind of bee builds a nest, which they then fill with pollen, nectar, and saliva; deposit their eggs in; and finally seal to keep the larvae safe. To nourish their offspring, bees often combine dry pollen with nectar and knead the mixture into a pollen loaf. They add saliva to this concoction. It is believed that saliva is a key component that prevents fungal and bacterial infections [1].

A few species of native bees construct their nests underground, while others use beetle holes or hollow stems, and others use their strong jaws to carve out holes in wood. In any case, they begin constructing their nest by picking out the ideal piece of land; if that is not the case, they keep looking. It would not be right if their houses were too big, too little, flooded, or did not get enough sunshine. The female of a single bee colony will supply her larvae with all the food they need to mature into adults, except bumble and honeybees. Mass provisioning is the term used to describe this [1].

2.3.1 Miners

Apidae [4], Andrenidae, Halictidae, Megachilidae, and Colletidae are among the bigger families that include ground nesters. It can take them several days of digging, but they find a dry, sunny site with little chance of flooding and get to work. They carve out a lengthy passageway just slightly broader than they are. Not everyone gets along with neighbors; some only like being near members of their species, regardless of whether they are related or not. Each bee builds her own home and provides for her brood; thus, even though these groups build their nests together, they are still solitary. Other bees exhibit varying degrees of cooperation, splitting up the work of building the nest and gathering food. Subterranean tunnels can reach depths of one foot or more. Halfway through or toward the conclusion, it could twist. The female bee constructs a wider chamber, or brood cell, at the tunnel's terminus. A single larva will be cared for in a brood cell. The mother bee supplies the brood cell with nectar and pollen for a single bee to mature from an egg to an adult. After that, she shuts the compartment and lays an egg within. At the end of each branch that she attaches to the tunnel, there will be another brood cell that is adequately supplied with pollen and nectar and has one egg [1].

2.3.2 Hole Nesters: Masons and Leafcutters

Members of many families exploit preexisting vulnerabilities. These bees use hollow stems or holes bored into dead wood by beetles or insects. Some bee species build their nests in cracks or cavities in rocks, while others choose smooth surfaces. There, they build rows of brood cells and fill them one by one with larvae, pupae, and young adults to use as nurseries and growth chambers [1].

Mason and leafcutter bees are mostly groundless hole nesters that alter their nest chambers with specific materials. Some build thicker plugs to seal the nest entrance from parasites and mud to separate chambers. The name for these bees is mason bees. For the same reason, some bees—known as leafcutter bees—cut circular bits of leaf to line the inside walls of their nest burrow. Perhaps you have noticed the meticulously cut circles from the leaves of your prized rose plants. You should not hold it against these working mothers that they have access to this housing material. Bees rely on more than just pollen and honey; they also need to gather materials for their nests and locate good places to dwell and forage, just as birds [1].

2.3.3 Carpenters

A few species of bees are capable of digging their tunnels. Their mandibles, or powerful jaws, allow them to bore holes in wood. It is a good thing they favor pliable wood and despise hard finishes. Simple measures, such as painting or staining the wood, can protect wood buildings from their destructive potential. You have probably seen carpenter bees and their job; they are small but powerful insects. You can normally find a mound of sawdust beneath the hole's entrance at the beginning of the nesting and burrowing seasons. The bees make spiral barriers that resemble "particle boards" between neighboring cells. Spiral partition cell closures are more commonly built by bees than wasps [1].

2.3.4 Floral Specialization

Pollen from a broad range of flowering plants is used by some bees, who are considered generalists. From the time the queen bee emerges in early spring until the colony dies out in late summer or early fall, the bees rely on a succession of flowering plants, making them generalists. Some bee species are more specialized than others in pollination; these bees often only collect pollen from a few plant groups. Redundancy in floral visits is already built into plant reproduction, which is a blessing. Coevolutionary partnerships between flowering plant species and pollinators like bees and other insects are common. When foraging for nectar, bees often visit more flower types than when pollinating. Bees specializing in pollinating cucurbit plants (squash, pumpkin, and zucchini) are an example of floral specialization.

Additionally, cactus, blueberry, and globe mallow bees are experts at pollinating flowers. While foraging, certain species of bees are only active for a short period in each growing season and rely on food sources within a few flowering plant groups. The larvae of bees belonging to the genus *Macropis* eat pollen and oil collected from loosestrife flowers (*Lysimachia*). Bees of the genus *Macropis* need to visit other flowers to satisfy their nectar needs, as loosestrife blooms do not have any. *Anthemurgus passiflorae* is one example of a highly specialized bee. We know that this bee exclusively feeds on yellow passionflower, scientifically called as *Passiflora lutea* [1].

During the day, the majority of blooming plants blossom. The majority of their nectar production occurs at these times. Thus, the fact that the majority of bee species adhere to a consistent routine should be familiar. Nevertheless, a few species within the major bee groups engage in foraging exclusively during the early morning or late evening hours. They are, of course, pollinating plants that put their blooms on during specific periods. They are known as crepuscular bees or matinal bees. Even bees that only work at night and follow the moonlight exist in the tropics! [1].

2.3.5 Females and Males

The norm is that beehive females sleep in their nests when they are not busy working. Contrarily, male bees do not help with nest construction or provisioning. Therefore, they seek out alternative areas to relax and slumber. Occasionally, you can see a swarm of male bees clinging to flowers, branches, or twigs with their mandibles. It is common to see slumbering male gourd and squash bees within squash blooms. When the squash flowers wilt in the garden due to the sun's heat, you should look for them [1].

2.4 Polyandry

The term used when a queen mates with more than one drone is polyandry. A colony's fitness and survival are both enhanced by polyandry, which enhances genetic variety within the colony. Expanded population size, foraging activity, and food supply are among the traits shared by genetically diverse colonies that encourage the development of new queens and colonies [2].

References

1. Moisset B, Buchmann S. Bee basics. An introduction to our native bees. United States Department of Agriculture. https://efotg.sc.egov.usda.gov/references/public/SC/Bee_Basics_North_American_Bee_ID.pdf. Accessed 8 Dec 2023.
2. Bee. Britannica. Last Updated: Dec 1, 2023. https://www.britannica.com/animal/honeybee. Accessed 8 Dec 2023.
3. Ground Nesting Bees. The bee conservancy. https://thebeeconservancy.org/ground-nesting-bees/. Accessed 21 June 2024.
4. Honey Bees, Bumble Bees, and Allies (Family Apidae). https://www.inaturalist.org/taxa/47221-Apidae. Accessed 21 June 2024.

3 Hives

3.1 Introduction

The combs that comprise the hive are two layers of six-sided chambers constructed from wax that the bees make and secrete. The cells contain food from honey, nectar from plants, and pollen bread, also known as bee bread. Honey, made by bees from blossom nectar, was the only easily accessible sugar for humans until the modern era. That is why people have been bringing honeybees into their homes for generations. Beekeeping is the practice of maintaining honeybee colonies. Honeybees are vital to farming for more than just their honey production; they pollinate many domesticated plants [1].

3.2 Hive Life

To raise their young, several species of honeybees (genus *Apis*) reside in enclosed structures known as beehives. While the term "beehive" can refer to the nest of any colony of bees (Figs. 3.1, 3.2, and 3.3), the term "nest" is used more specifically in scholarly and professional writings. In this context, "nest" refers to a colony that makes its home in an exposed or man-made cavity or even in a hanging basket. An artificial or man-made structure used to house honeybee nests is called a hive. As a colony animal, *Apis* is home to multiple species. *Apis mellifera*, the western honeybee, and *Apis cerana*, the eastern honey bee, are the two most common species in hives for honey production [2–4].

The honeycomb-like structure inside the nest is a collection of closely packed hexagonal prismatic cells made of beeswax. Honey and pollen are stored in the cells, and the bees' brood—eggs, larvae, and pupae—is also housed in the cells [2].

A. E. Tanuğur Samanci et al., *Propolis: Prevention and Healing Effects in Otorhinolaryngology*, Comprehensive ENT,
https://doi.org/10.1007/978-3-031-68546-0_3

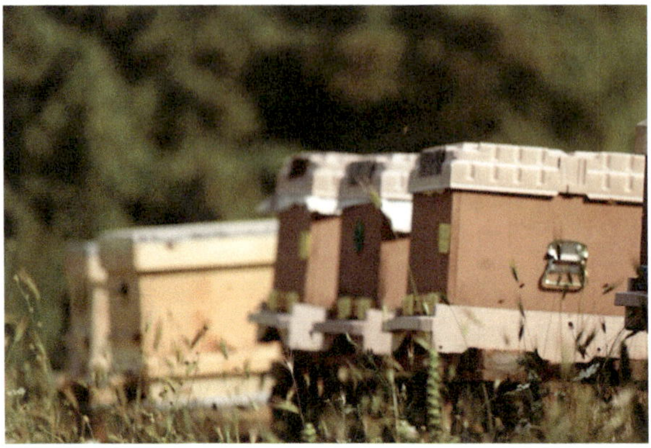

Fig. 3.1 Beehives: Toros Mountain. (*Courtesy of* **Ali Ihsan Gokcen**)

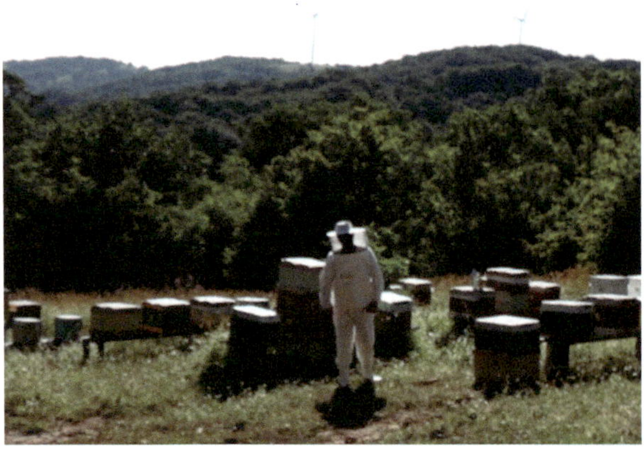

Fig. 3.2 Beehives: Istranca region/Kırklareli/Turkey. (*Courtesy of* **Ali Ihsan Gokcen**)

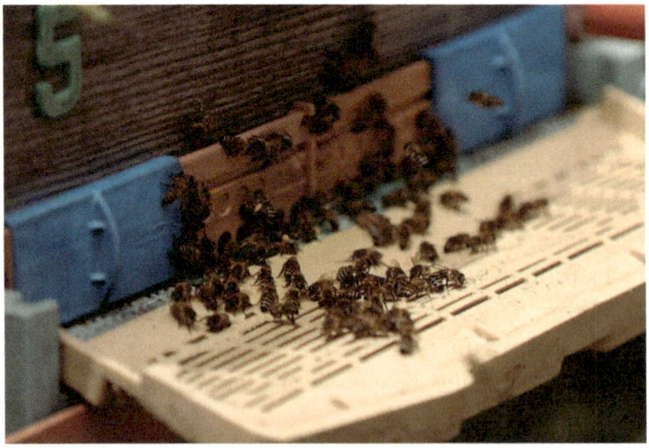

Fig. 3.3 Entry and exit to the beehive/Istanbul/Turkey. (*Courtesy of* ***Taylan Samancı***)

A beehive has multiple functions. Beekeeping serves several purposes, such as making honey, pollinating crops in the area, providing bees for apitherapy, and reducing the impact of colony collapse disorder. Beekeepers often move their hives to help pollinate crops in other parts of the United States [2, 5, 6, 7].

3.3 Honeybee Nests in Several Locations

Cavities in rocks, trees, and caverns are ideal places for honeybees to lay their eggs. While other subgenera's species sport exposed aerial combs, these birds in warmer regions may construct nests that dangle from the branches. The bees have a relatively consistent amount of room to move around in a hive with multiple parallel honeycombs. In most cases, it only has one door. Western honeybees will not build in cavities that are less than 10 or more than 100 liters in volume, and they will only use about 45 liters in volume. Among the several nest-site preferences shown by western honeybees are the following: a height above ground between 1 and 5 meters (3.3 and 16 feet), an entrance facing downward, an equatorial orientation, and a distance of more than 300 meters (980 feet) from the main colony. The majority of bees spend many years in their nests [2].

The bees will polish the bark around the nest entrance and apply a thin layer of propolis, a hardened plant resin, to the walls of the nest chamber. While honeycombs are affixed to the walls of the cavity on all sides, the bees create pathways around the edges of the combs. Honeybee nests are identical in design; on top of the comb is where the honey is kept, and below it are rows of cells that store pollen, workers, and drones. It is common practice to construct the peanut-shaped queen cells near the comb's base [2].

3.3.1 Ancient Hives

The ancient Egyptians maintained beehives constructed by humans. The Fifth Dynasty wall murals at the Egyptian sun temple of Nyuserre Ini show beekeepers removing honeycombs from hives while puffing smoke into the air. These paintings predate 2422 BC. The tomb of Pabasa, which dates back to the 26th Dynasty (c. 650 BC), contains inscriptions that explain the manufacturing of honey. The inscriptions describe the storage of honey in jars and cylindrical hives [2].

In the remains of Rehov, which had 2000 inhabitants in 900 BC—both Israelites and Canaanites—archaeologist Amihai Mazar lists 30 complete hives. These findings point to the existence of a sophisticated honey industry in Israel some 4000 years ago. Straw and unbaked clay made up the 150 beehives, many of which were shattered. Their arrangement seemed quite logical. According to the University of Haifa professor Ezra Marcus, the find shed light on ancient beekeeping depicted in Near Eastern art and literature. The presence of an altar adorned with fertility symbols near the hives suggests a possible religious significance of beekeeping. Although beekeeping has been around longer than these ruins, this apiary is the oldest one that has been found [2].

3.3.2 The Traditional Hives

Beehives, the classic housing for beehives, kept the colony contained. Since the bees were not given any interior structures, they made their honeycomb within the hives. It is often impossible to move the comb without damaging it because of the cross-attachments. The difference between this and the modern movable-frame hives is that the former is sometimes referred to as a fixed-frame hive. Most hives were destroyed during harvest, but some adapted by placing top baskets that bees could remove when they were full of honey. Over time, more contemporary apparatus, including box hives of varied sizes and with or without frames, superseded them [2].

In the past, bees would smash the wax honeycomb to extract honey from the hive. This harvesting method meant that conventional beehives produced more beeswax than contemporary ones but much less honey [2].

Bee gums, skeps, clay/tile hives, and mud hives are the four main types of traditional beehives [2].

3.3.3 Mud Hives

Mud hives are still used in Egypt and Siberia. They are long cylinders constructed from unfired mud, straw, and manure [2].

3.3.4 Clay Hives

Traditional beehives in the eastern Mediterranean were constructed from clay tiles. Throughout antiquity, people in Egypt, the Middle East, Greece, Italy, and Malta utilized long cylindrical forms of baked clay. They were sometimes used alone, but more commonly arranged in rows to offer shade, at least for the ones not directly above. As beekeepers collected honey, they would light a cigarette at one end to lure the bees to the other [2].

For almost 2000 years, bees have made their homes in skeps, just baskets laid end over end. Constructed initially from wicker that had been coated with mud and manure, they are thought to have originated in Ireland. However, during the Middle Ages, straw replaced wicker in nearly all of them. Coils of straw or grass were used to make skeps throughout western and northern Europe. One entry at the skep's base is required for its basic form. Once again, the bees must construct their honeycomb to attach to the inside of the skep since no internal framework is given. Skeps in the early modern period were roughly 36 liters in volume, two pecks, or 18 liters [2].

When using a skeptic, the beekeeper cannot check the comb for pests and diseases, and removing the honey is a tedious and sometimes disastrous process that wipes out the entire colony. Beekeepers would expel the bees from the skep or try to construct a comb with solely honey by employing an eke, the bottom extension, or a cap, the top extension. To remove the honeycomb, it was common practice to kill the bees, sometimes with lit sulfur. Another method to obtain honey from skeps is to squeeze them in a vise [2].

As of 1998 [2], most US states outlawed keeping beehives that could not be examined visually for signs of disease or parasites.

A smaller woven basket, or cap, would sit above a tiny hole in the main skep in later forms. They used this cover as a makeshift super to reduce the amount of honey that had to be removed from the hives while minimizing harm to the bees and their young. A ring of four or five straw coils set under a straw beehive in England was known as an eke, imp, or nadir, and it provided additional space for brood development. To "eke" out a little extra space, builders would use an eke; to add a full story below, they would use a nadir, a greater extension [2].

A "basket" in Old Norse is where the word "skeppa" comes from. A "skepper" is a surname that is still used today in Western countries to describe someone who manufactured these woven beehives. In England, a "girth" made of leather or cow horn was used to manage the thickness of the straw coil, and briar strips were used to sew the coils together. Artworks, sculptures, and ancient texts often feature depictions of skeps. Signs using the skep frequently denote activity ("the busy bee") [2].

More elaborate skeps with pierced hardwood lids that could hold glass jars emerged in the latter half of the eighteenth century. Adding the comb to the glass jars would make the designs more appealing to potential customers [2].

3.4 The Bee Gums

Until the turn of the twentieth century, hollow tree parts were utilized throughout the eastern United States, particularly in the Southeast. Black gum (*Nyssa sylvatica*) trees were a common source, thus the name "gums" [2].

Apiaries or "bee yards" were used to prop up parts of the hollow trees. As an attachment for the honeycomb, sticks or crossed sticks were occasionally inserted under a board cover. The honey collection from these, like that from skeps, decimated the colony. Before even entering the beehive, the harvester would often kill the bees. To do this, a metal container containing sulfur gas was inserted into the gum [2].

In the past, beekeepers in Central Europe frequently used both naturally occurring tree hollows and man-made tree trunks with hollows cut into them. In Poland, for instance, a barć was a type of beehive that was shielded from predators, including forest dormice, pine martens, bears, and severe weather conditions like cold. The bees were temporarily calmed by using smoke and removing a protective piece of wood from the aperture, so harvesting honey from them did not harm the colony [2].

Honey producers can set themselves apart from competitors and charge a premium price for their wares, thanks in part to the continued usage of bee gums. Even though they are called log hives in Europe, bee gums are still used in Mont Lozère, France. These log hives are hollowed out artificially and cut to a specified size; their length is shorter than that of bee gums [2].

Although beehive designs underwent several iterations of improvement beginning in the eighteenth century, the first distinctly modern designs only emerged in the nineteenth century [2].

Thomas Wildman, writing between 1768 and 1770, documented the middle phases of hive design. He detailed improvements over the harmful old skep-based beekeeping methods, which allowed for harvesting honey without killing the bees. For instance, in a 10-inch-diameter (250 mm) hive, Wildman would place a parallel array of wooden bars over the top of a straw hive or skep "so that there are in all seven bars of the deal" [to which the bees set their combs]. A separate straw top will be attached later. In a manner reminiscent of modern supers, he also detailed the use of such hives in a multistory configuration. At the appropriate times, he would add straw hives below, and when they were empty of brood and honey, he would remove them from above. This allowed him to preserve the bees separately for the following season's harvest. A subsequent improvement, foreshadowed by contemporary applications of movable-comb hives, was also detailed by Wildman: hives equipped with "sliding frames" against which the bees could construct their comb. Wildman recognized the contributions of Swammerdam, Maraldi, and de Reaumur to our understanding of bees; he translated Reaumur's account of bees' natural history and included it in his work. He also detailed the efforts of others to design harvesting hives in a way that protected bee life, referencing, for example, reports from Brittany from the 1750s by Comte de la Bourdonnaye [2].

Ukrainian commercial beekeeper Petro Prokopovych made honey harvesting easier in 1814 by inventing one of the earliest beehive frames [2].

In 1845, Jan Dzierżon stated that one and a half inches from the center of one top bar to the center of the next one was the ideal space between combs for comfortable beehive operations. Instead of using wood strips for shifting top bars, Dzierżon installed grooves into the side walls of the hive in 1848. The bee gap was later used to describe the grooves, which were 8 mm x 8 mm (0.31 in × 0.31 in). August Adolph von Berlepsch of Thuringia (Bienenzeitung, May 1852) and L.L. Langstroth of the United States (October 1852) developed their movable-frame hives using the abovementioned dimensions. Nevertheless, Langstroth recommended leaving "about 3/8 inch" of space between the beehive body and the frames and "about 1/2 inch" above the top bars of the frames [2].

Beehives can stand on end or lay flat. These days, you are likely to see one of the three distinct kinds of modern hives:

- The Langstroth hive.
- The top-bar hive.
- The Warre hive.

The majority of beehives have been fine-tuned to attract honeybees and cormorants. Some hives are specifically made for certain species of meliponines, including *Melipona beecheii*. The UTOB hive and the Nogueira-Neto hive are two types of such hives [2].

References

1. Bee. Britannica. Last Updated: Dec 1, 2023. https://www.britannica.com/animal/honeybee. Accessed 8 Dec 2023.
2. Beehive. Wikipedia. https://en.wikipedia.org/wiki/Beehive. Accessed 8 Dec 2023.
3. Apis cerana. University of Florida. http://entnemdept.ufl.edu/creatures/misc/bees/Apis_cerana.htm. Accessed 8 Dec 2023.
4. Apis mellifera. University of Florida. http://entnemdept.ufl.edu/creatures/MISC/BEES/euro_honey_bee.htm Accessed 8 Dec 2023.
5. Honey. USDA Research Facilities. https://web.archive.org/web/20170705151257/http://www.fpl.fs.fed.us/documnts/usda/agib666/aib66610.pdf. Accessed 8 Dec 2023.
6. Honey Bees, Bumble Bees, and Allies (Family Apidae). https://www.inaturalist.org/taxa/47221-Apidae. Accessed 21 June 2024.
7. Honey Bees on the Move: From Pollination to Honey Production and Back. https://www.ers.usda.gov/publications/pub-details?pubid=101475. Accessed 21 June 2024.

4 Bee Families

4.1 Introduction

The United States is home to 4000 different kinds of native bees. From cold, icy Canada to hot, sunny Mexico, you can find bees belonging to the five most common families: Apidae, Halictidae, Andrenidae, Megachilidae, and Colletidae. You can find them in forests, deserts, backyards, and even the National Mall in the middle of our nation's capital. Up in the highlands, you could find a solitary beehive [2].

For bees, there are seven distinct families. All families have a common evolutionary past and a unique collection of characteristics. As a further subdivision, these seven families include 28 subfamilies. Each subfamily's distinctive and fascinating anatomical and biological characteristics are as follows [1]:

Even the Arctic bumblebee, a little but tenacious insect, makes its home in the Arctic. The fledgling queen starts caring for her first brood in the persistent frost. Occasionally, she will protect and warm her young by pressing her flying muscles on her brood cells and vibrating them for hours. Also, like other birds, she has a brood patch—a naked area on her belly—that she uses to warm her young. Larvae grow more quickly due to this exercise and the heat it generates, which warms the waxen brood cells. Some insects, like bumblebees, have a similar internal temperature to that of mammals. Rapid flexing of their flying muscles may turn them into energy powerhouses. Because of the high energy expenditure of this activity, they rely on the early-flowering maples and willows for an abundance of nectar. After spending many hours caring for her first brood, the young queen must finally leave the nest to get food and water for her family [2].

A. E. Tanuğur Samanci et al., *Propolis: Prevention and Healing Effects in Otorhinolaryngology*, Comprehensive ENT,
https://doi.org/10.1007/978-3-031-68546-0_4

4.2 Family Melittidae

With 201 species, Melittidae is the second smallest bee family. The first remains of melittid bees were discovered around 53 million years ago, during the Eocene Epoch. Melittid bees are ground-dwelling, solitary insects adapted to feed only on a few closely related plant species. The arid regions of southern Africa are their preferred habitat [1].

For instance, an oil bee species, *Macropis nuda*, would only forage for oils in the blossoms of yellow loosestrife (*Lysimachia*) plants. Most of their use is as a larval food supply and to coat egg cells with these floral oils [1].

4.3 Family Apidae

With around 6000 species, the Apidae family is the most enormous bee family. Among its members is the earliest fossil bee, which dates back around 115–95 million years. The honeybee and 300 distinct species of bumblebee are also members of the Apidae family. Bees are an essential part of agriculture, but the Apidae family is interesting for more than just the sociable and solitary species [1].

Example: the enormous, solitary, and swiftly flying "Dawson's burrowing bee" (*Amegilla dawsoni*). In Western Australia, where they are endemic, female burrowing bees construct enormous underwater nests. The size of the male burrowing bee determines how he mates [1].

The Apidae family is the most prominent bee family, comprising many native species and the introduced honeybee. The Latin word for honeybee, *Apis*, is the family name's origin. The family encompasses every kind of bumblebee, several species of cuckoo bee, and carpenter bees. In addition to stingless bees, this family includes orchid bees native to tropical regions [2].

4.3.1 Bumblebees

Bumblebees [3] may be found in over 50 species in North America. Bumblebees are well-known to many. Their coats are thick with fur and have a predominantly black color scheme accented by white, bright orange, or yellow bands. In common with honeybees, bumblebees are more gregarious than the majority of native bee species and often live in large colonies with a single queen and several workers. Colonies of bumblebees, on the other hand, are seldom as large or persistent as honeybees. Most bumblebees build their nests underground, but occasionally, you will see them partially aboveground, covered in thatch. Finding an abandoned mouse nest or a similar burrow is the first thing a young queen does in the spring since the chambers they require for their nests are more significant than those of solitary bees. After that, she begins to get it ready for her young. After constructing a giant cell for her brood, she fills several wax pots with pollen and honey. After she has stocked up on food, the queen will lay her eggs, initially only laying six. All of these firstborn females are employed as laborers. After her brood has matured, the queen spends most of her time within the nest, where she lays eggs, and the workers tend to the nest inside and outside [2].

A few hundred workers may be found in the colony as it expands at a rapid pace. In most cases, the queen is larger than the workers. You will not often see giant bumblebees foraging after a queen has her first brood. As summer draws closer, the queen deposits male and female eggs. Soon after emerging from the nest, the females transform into queens rather than sterile workers and quickly mate with the males. At summer's end, the elderly queen, all the male bees, and the workers in the bumble beehive die. Only the newly minted queens, who have mated, have managed to stay alive. They retire for the winter to a remote location. The queens emerge and establish new colonies when the seasons change from winter to spring and willows bloom. Pollen baskets, or corbiculae, are found on both honey and bumblebees' rear legs. Comparatively, other bees' pollen baskets, known as scopae, are less specialized. Bees of the honeybee and bumblebee species have a flattened tibial segment on the back of their legs and rows of solid, long hairs running along their margins. Instead of having pollen grains attach to the hairs of other species' scopae, these bees can compress pollen, along with some nectar and saliva, into a compact mass known as a corbicular pellet because of the form of their baskets. A small number of bumblebee species have evolved into cuckoos and lay their eggs in the nests of other species. They can get along without pollen baskets or workers [2].

Large greenhouses utilize buzz pollination services provided by bees to grow tomatoes successfully all year round. Because tomatoes yield a lot of pollen but little nectar, you only need a queen, a nesting box, and some sugar water. While the bumblebees are not restricted in their movement, they spend most of their time within the greenhouse. The pollination services provided by bumblebees are an essential part of farming. Forage crops for cattle rely on them as pollinators of some clovers [2].

4.3.2 Carpenter Bees

Usually, carpenter bees are giant and dark colored. If it were not for one defining characteristic, you may mistake a carpenter bee for a bumblebee. Carpenter bees are nearly hairless and glossy on the upper abdomen, but bumblebees are fuzzy throughout. Rather than preparing to set up a home, men begin their search for potential courting and mating venues in the early spring. This is done because they are aware that these locations will attract females. They aggressively guard the region, driving away other males who dare to get too close. Surprisingly, they will frighten away almost everything that moves, even human gardeners. The good news is that they are venomless (the stingers are found only in females), so you may safely ignore them. Carpenter bees get their popular name because females utilize strong mandibles to create extensive tunnel networks to construct their nests. Not all carpenter bees are good pollinators.

When nectar is stored in a flower but is inaccessible due to a lengthy throat, the carpenter bee will occasionally use her beak-like mouthparts to cut a hole at the base of the bloom. She then consumes the nectar while avoiding the stigma and anthers responsible for dispersing the pollen from the flower. That said, carpenter bees might be considered nectar thieves, as they take nectar from flowers without helping them. Even bumblebees may steal flowers. Look at your garden's trumpet honeysuckles, horse mints, and abelias. Flowers whose throats have been slashed by thirsty carpenter bees are a clear indicator of these attacks. Although their size disparity makes confusing them with their bigger cousins impossible, the genus *Ceratina* includes little carpenter bees. They do not dig their nests but instead use poisonous stems like roses or blackberry brambles [2].

The pollination of cucurbit blossoms is carried out by squash bees (*Peponapis* and *Xenoglossa*). Pollen from cucurbits is the sole food source for *Peponapis* squash bees. Like honeybees, squash bees are small and brownish in appearance. When you see their distinct actions around the blossoms of these crops, you will know that they are different. Regarding the daily cycles of cucurbit blossoms, squash bees are highly attuned. When these vital crop plants' blossoms are opening just before daybreak, they start their work shift [2].

4.4 Megachilidae Family

The Megachilidae [4] are the third most numerous bee family with more than 4000 species. While Antarctica is the only continent without bees in this family, you may find them in various settings, from tropical woods to arid wastelands. Their ingenuity and variety are truly remarkable. The building materials utilized by megachilid bees for their nests can range from flower petals and mud to leaves and plant resin, as well as dirt, gravel, and even plastic bags. Walls, live plants, tree branches, stones, empty bug nests, snail shells, and termite nests are all suitable dwelling places for these creatures [1].

The giant bee on the planet, Wallace's enormous bee, or *Megachile pluto*, is a member of the Megachilidae family. In 1859, Alfred Russel Wallace, a co-discoverer of natural selection, first met Wallace's enormous bee. *Megachile pluto* is a considerable butterfly; females may grow to be 1.5 inches long and 2.5 inches wide, although it was just discovered again in 1981 [1].

It was not until 2019 that scientists realized that Wallace's enormous bee was still alive and well! Scientists flocked to the North Molucca islands off the coast of Indonesia when a strange new species surfaced in an Internet auction. This bee is notoriously hard to spot since it makes its home in abandoned termite nests high in trees. Researchers searched the tropical jungle for 5 days before discovering a solitary *Megachile pluto*. After filming and photographing her, they let her go [1].

There is still a chance that *Megachile pluto* might go extinct. These "huge" bees were in danger due to deforestation and the demand for ivory [1].

Bees that cut leaves and build mansions are members of this family. The females build the nest using mud and leaves. Although some of these bees lay their eggs in the ground, most develop their nests in hollow trees or logs. A few species in this family are not initially from the United States but have made accidental or deliberate introductions to our nation. This family of bees is unique in that pollen is carried on the underside of the abdomen rather than the back legs [2].

You may identify a megachilid bee by looking for a bee that is approximately the size of a honey bee and has a yellow belly covered with pollen. On rare occasions, the pollen may be white. Yet, while arriving at their nests, certain megachilid bees resemble flying "Cheetos" snacks due to their enormous yellow and orange pollen loads. The blue orchard bee, scientifically known as *Osmia lignaria*, is a controlled pest in the West that helps pollinate fruit trees, particularly those that produce almonds and sweet cherries. As a kind of nesting material, farmers are supplying drilled boards. Even though it has yet to be tested nationally, it is already showing great promise as a substitute for the struggling honeybee (Figs. 4.1 and 4.2). We still need to learn a lot about how to quickly raise and employ this lovely blue bee [2].

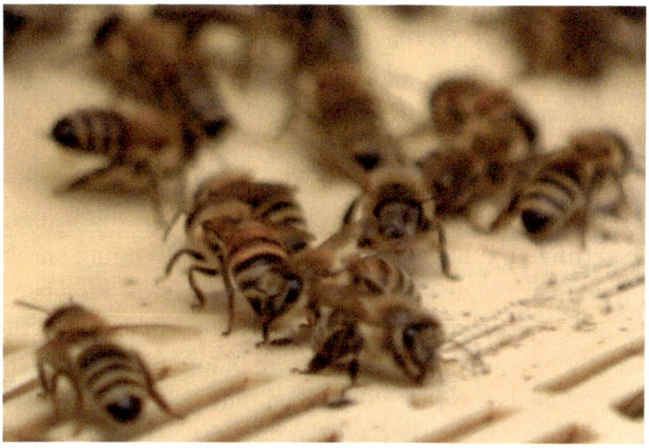

Fig. 4.1 Anatolian honeybee (Istanbul region). (*Courtesy of* **Taylan Samancı**)

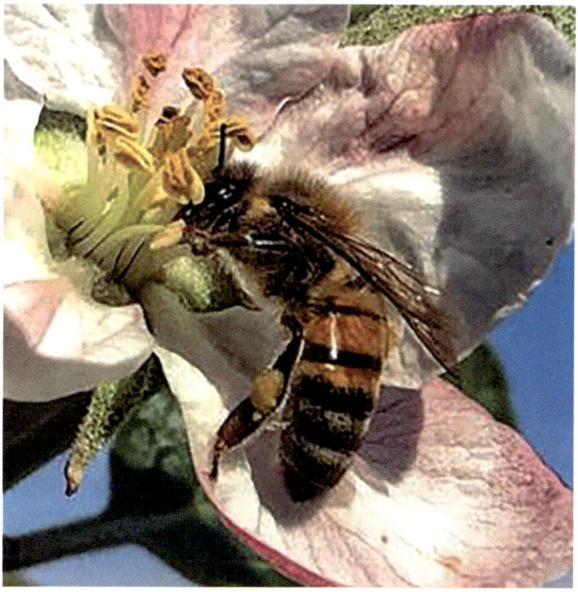

Fig. 4.2 Anatolian honeybee (Ordu region). (*Courtesy of* **Ali Fuat Varol**)

4.5 Andrenidae Family

Nearly 3000 species of solitary bees that nest on the ground make up the Andrenidae family. Many andrenid bees have evolved to feed only on certain blooming plants. They are primarily found in arid regions in the western hemispheres of the Americas, Europe, and Africa. The earliest known fossils of andrenid bees were found 32 million years ago, during the Oligocene Epoch [1].

The image above shows *Andrena crataegi* as an example. *Andrena crataegi* first appears at the beginning of spring. This bee pollinates fruit trees in the East of the United States. When it comes to pollinating apple trees, they shine. Indulge in a delicious New York apple, and be grateful to the *Andrena crataegi*! [1].

The colloquial moniker "miner bees" comes from all andrenid bees being ground nesters. Although they often appear reddish, black, or dark, they may also be yellow, metallic blue, or a combination. Bees of medium to big size are usually reserved. Unlike other bees, they have velvety patches (foveae) on their faces, in the space between their eyes and the base of their antennae; nevertheless, you may need a microscope to see these patches. A lot of them only do something in the spring. After spending the summer, fall, and winter underground, the following generation will emerge in the spring, just in time for their favorite flowers to bloom [2].

Without azaleas, what would the eastern woods look like? Honeybees are unable to fertilize the blossoms of this native blooming shrub. Unlike other flowers, they retain their pollen within the anthers and wait for a bee with the right talent to shake it like a saltshaker. Additionally, sticky threads bind the pollen clusters together. A variety of solitary bees, including bumblebees, are adept in pollinating azalea blossoms. One is the dark-colored, skinny bee found in the eastern United States, called the Cornell azalea bee (Andrena Cornell). Because azalea pollen is its preferred diet, it always ventures close to azaleas. Her pollen baskets are uniquely suited to the size and shape of the pollen clusters produced by these blooms, with their long, widely spread hairs. The andrenid family of bees is known for its early spring arrival. They frequent spring blooms such as violets, willows, maples, and other early bloomers. When pollinating apple blooms, some andrenid bees are top dogs [2].

4.6 Halictidae Family

The Halictidae family includes about 4500 species, making it the second biggest bee family. An estimated 96–75 million years have passed since the family's beginning. Amber from the Dominican Republic and the Baltic Region is a common place where fossils from this family can be found [1].

Phobite algirus is one such example. When it comes to pollen, halictid bees are fine. The hedge nettle *Stachys* plant is the only food source for this bee species. Bees of the species *Rophites algirus* have a unique way of collecting pollen from hedge nettles. They insert their heads inside the bloom and then use their flying muscles to vibrate. After the bee has pollinated her entire face, she will put the pollen on her rear legs and return to the nest by flying [1].

This family includes some of the most stunning bee species. These bees will win your heart with their shimmery, glittering bodies. The majority are metallic green. However, others can be any blue, copper, gold, or black hue. Underground is where the majority of them lay their eggs. Some share the entrance to their nests, while others are solitary. They are often somewhat reclusive and only disclose that. However, certain sweat bees go above and beyond by dividing up tasks like protecting their nests' entrances and caring for their offspring. Typically, they are identical twins who share a nest. Species of sweat bees that practice actual social behavior include those whose mothers and founders divide up the job of building the colony among their daughters. The Americas are home to several species of halictids, including the green-, yellow-, and black-striped *Agapostemon*. *Augochlora pura*, meaning "the pure magnificent green bee," is a beautiful halictid bee native to the eastern United States. Its unique behavior includes constructing its nest beneath the bark of a decaying wood. She constructs a home from the discarded, partially decomposed material, lining it with her saliva and secretions to protect her eggs and pollen. Before laying an egg and closing the cell, she kneads the pollen into several loaves shaped like tiles. She then plasters on the inner wall of the brood chamber. Foraging ants and other predators hide under loose bark; thus, this protection is required. The alkali bee, or *Nomia melanderi*, is a fascinating and economically significant halictid bee native to the western United States. The alkali bee is named because it is most commonly found at home on naturally alkaline soils. It is not uncommon for hundreds of thousands of humans to live close to one another. Although it coexists peacefully with other alkali bees, it could be more sociable since each queen builds her own nest and cares for her offspring. Some farmers use the alkali bee's nesting habits to control this species to a certain degree since it is an excellent pollinator of alfalfa. They provide the ideal habitat for alkali bees in areas close to alfalfa fields. Farmers will even go to extreme lengths to artificially produce nesting beds by laying down a tarp, coating it with clay, and watering it as required. Once set up, these alkali bee beds may keep going strong for decades. A few species of cuckoo bees are also found in this family; these bees share the characteristics of their hairless and somewhat wasplike relatives. A vivid crimson abdomen is seen in some [2].

4.7 The Stenotritidae Family

The Stenotritidae family is the smallest of the seven bee families, with only 21 species. The stenotritids have the most restricted distribution of all the bee families, occurring just in Australia. Although no stenotritid fossils have been found, it is believed that this family branched off from Colletidae more than 92 million years ago. The solitary bees known as stenotritids are swift and extensive and love the beach. They may lay eggs as deep as 10 feet below the surface! [1].

Take *Ctenocolletes nigricans* as an example. The sandy ground is ideal for these bees' solitary ground nesting habits. The gum trees (*Eucalyptus*) and other members of the Myrtaceae family, prominent in Australia, have become food sources for this species [1].

4.8 Colletidae Family

The Colletidae family is home to 2600 species, most native to South America and Australia. Almost every species of colletid lives alone. Although colletid bees do possess a forked tongue, contemporary bees do not. This beetle's tongue form developed independently within the family to aid in painting a cellophane-like lining within the nest, even though it has similarities with its ancient wasp forebears [1].

An example is the "Yarrow's fork-tongue" beetle, or *Caupolicana yarrowi*. This beetle produces a fermented mixture of pollen, nectar, and yeast to nourish its young. The "bee beer" is confined within the brood cells because the bees coat them with a cellophane-like substance. The larvae consume protein-rich "beer" while swimming in the sloppy mixture [1].

References

1. Bee Diversity and Taxonomy. https://www.museumoftheearth.org/bees/diversity. Accessed 8 Dec 2023.
2. Moisset B, Buchmann S. Bee basics. An introduction to our native Bees. United States Department of Agriculture. https://efotg.sc.egov.usda.gov/references/public/SC/Bee_Basics_North_American_Bee_ID.pdf. Accessed 8 Dec 2023.
3. Honey Bees, Bumble Bees, and Allies (Family Apidae). https://www.inaturalist.org/taxa/47221-Apidae. Accessed 21 June 2024.
4. Güler Y, Dikmen F, Töre D, Aytekin AM. Türkiye'nin Akdeniz Bölgesi'ndeki Megachilidae faunası çeşitliliğindeki mevcut bilgilere katkılar (contributions to existing knowledge on the diversity of Megachilidae fauna in the Mediterranean region of Turkey). TED. 2014;38:255–78.

Honey: Overview

5

5.1 Introduction

The healing properties of honey have made it a popular natural remedy. According to reports, it contains over 200 different chemicals. Fructose and glucose make up the bulk of honey, but it also includes fructo-oligosaccharides [1], many enzymes, vitamins, minerals, and amino acids [2]. Depending on the plants that bees feed on, honey can have a wide range of compositions. A wide variety of substances can be found in honey, including flavonoids, phenolic acids, ascorbic acid, tocopherols, catalase, superoxide dismutase, reduced glutathione, Maillard reaction products, and peptides. Nearly all honey naturally occurs and contains these substances. An antioxidant effect is produced by a synergistic interaction between most of these compounds [3–8].

5.2 What Exactly Is Honey?

Honey is a natural product formed from the nectar of flowers by honeybees (*Apis mellifera*; family: Apidae) [9, 10] (Figs. 5.1, 5.2, and 5.3). Honey has been used by humans since ancient times, nearly 5500 years ago [11]. Most ancient populations, including the Greeks, Chinese, Egyptians, Romans, Mayans, and Babylonians, consumed honey for nutritional and medicinal purposes [11, 12]. Honey is the only insect-derived natural product with nutritional, cosmetic, therapeutic, and industrial values [13, 14]. Honey is reviewed as a balanced diet and is equally famous for males and females of all ages [15]. Honey does not need to be refrigerated; it never spoils and can be stored unopened at room temperature in a dry place [16, 17]. The honey's water activity (WA) is between 0.56 and 0.62, and its pH value is almost 3.9 [16, 17]. Honey has been utilized as a natural sweetener since the ancient period

A. E. Tanuğur Samanci et al., *Propolis: Prevention and Healing Effects in Otorhinolaryngology*, Comprehensive ENT,
https://doi.org/10.1007/978-3-031-68546-0_5

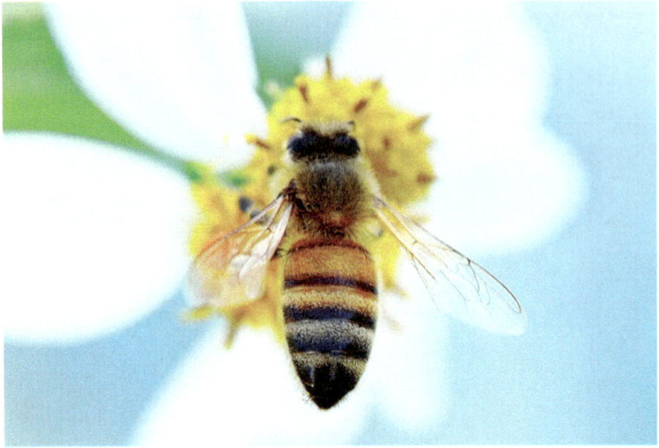

Fig. 5.1 Anatolian honeybee (Toros region). (*Courtesy of* **Ali Ihsan Gokcen**)

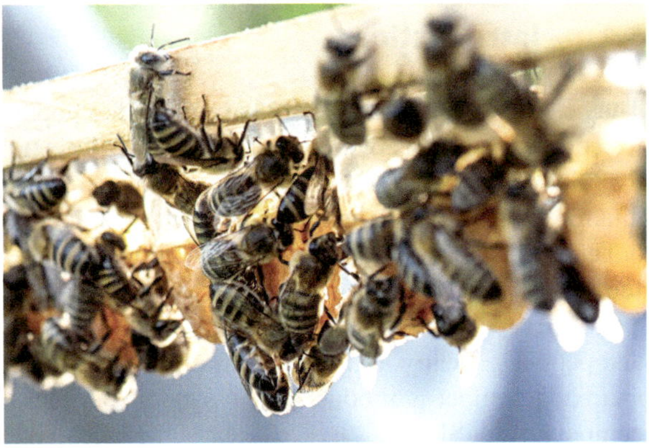

Fig. 5.2 Honeycomb production/Tekirdag/Turkey. (*Courtesy of* **Taylan Samancı**)

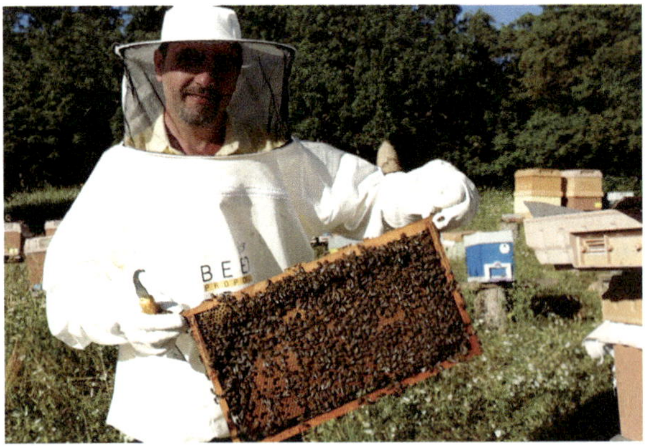

Fig. 5.3 Honeybee brood comb/Toros/Turkey. (*Courtesy of* **Taylan Samancı**)

since it has a high level of fructose (honey is 25% sweeter than table sugar) [17, 19]. Moreover, using honey in beverages is also increasingly popular [17]. Nowadays, information on the usage of honey to cure many human diseases can be found in general magazines, journals, and leaflets about natural products, and it suggests a wide variety of unknown activities [20]. Evidence indicates that honey can exert several health-beneficial effects, including antioxidant [21], anti-inflammatory [22], antibacterial [23], antidiabetic [24], respiratory, gastrointestinal [25], cardiovascular, and nervous system [26] protective effects.

5.2.1 Chemical Composition of Natural Honey

Although sugar and water comprise most of the natural honey, it also includes over 200 other components, such as enzymes, vitamins, minerals, and amino acids. Nearly all of the honey's dry weight is sugar. Honey is mainly composed of fructose (32.56–32.8%) and glucose (28.56–31.3%), the two most abundant sugars in the fruit, accounting for 85–95% of the total sugars absorbed by the body [8, 27, 28].

Maltose, sucrose, isomaltose, turanose, nigerose, melibiose, panose, maltotriose, and melezitose are among the other sugars that fall under the disaccharide category. The presence of a few oligosaccharides is also noted. As probiotic agents, the fructo-oligosaccharides found in honey range from 4% to 5% [1, 28]. Among honey's many essential ingredients, water ranks second. Gluconic acid, a byproduct of the enzymatic breakdown of glucose, is one of the organic acids that make up 0.57% of honey. The organic acids imparted the unique flavor and acidity of honey [29]. Mineral compound concentrations vary between 0.1% and 1%. The most abundant metals are potassium, magnesium, calcium, sodium, sulfur, and phosphorus. Some examples of trace elements include manganese, iron, copper, and zinc [30–32].

There are also nitrogenous molecules, vitamins C and B1 (thiamine), and B2 complex vitamins, such as riboflavin, nicotinic acid, pantothenic acid, and B6 [29]. Honey's protein content is quite low, ranging from 0.1% to 0.5% [33, 34]. According to a new study [35], some protein amounts vary depending on the honeybee's country of origin.

Among the many enzymes found in honey are oxidases, invertases, amylases, catalases, and many more. Glucose oxidase, invertase (saccharase), and diastase (amylase) are the primary enzymes found in honey. When bees produce honey, they play a crucial function [29]. To aid calcium absorption, the enzyme glucose oxidase converts glucose into hydrogen peroxide and gluconic acid. Hydrogen peroxide has antibacterial characteristics. Saccharose is broken down into glucose and fructose by invertase. The amylase enzyme breaks down lengthy strands of starch into dextrin and maltose. Hydrogen peroxide may be converted into oxygen and water with catalase [36].

5.2.2 The Physical Characteristics of Raw Honey

Honey is valuable for more than just its flavor and composition. Honey that has just been extracted has a thick consistency. Its composition, especially its water content, determines its viscosity, which depends on a wide range of components. Honey also has the potential to absorb and retain moisture from its surroundings, which is called hygroscopicity. Honey with 18.8% water or less will soak up moisture from the air that is more humid than 60%. Colloidal particles likely cause the surface tension of honey, which varies depending on where the honey is made. It contributes to honey's foaming properties and high viscosity [29].

From nearly colorless (like water) to almost black, the hue of liquid honey can range from transparent to deep amber. Most honey hues fall somewhere between amber and yellow. Transparency or clarity is determined by the number of suspended particles, including pollen, whereas color changes with botanical source, age, and storage circumstances [29]. Rare honey varieties include sunflower, which is a bright yellow; chestnut, which has reddish overtones; eucalyptus, which is grayish; and honeydew, which is greenish. Because glucose crystals are white when they crystallize, honey takes on a lighter hue after they do. The honey's composition and storage conditions determine the amount, shape, size, and quality of the monohydrate glucose crystals that develop during crystallization. The rate of crystallization increases as the glucose content of honey decreases and the water content increases [29].

5.3 Traditional Uses of Natural Honey

Artifacts from the Stone Age show that people began using honey 8000 years ago [36]. Greeks, Romans, Egyptians, and Assyrians all used honey to remedy intestinal illnesses and wounds [37]. This chapter provides a brief overview of how honey has helped people from ancient civilizations.

5.3.1 Honey Within the Ayurvedic Tradition of India

The term Ayurveda originated from the Sanskrit roots âyus, meaning "life" or "life principle," and Veda, meaning "a system of knowledge." The two words together form the composite word. Therefore, "Ayurveda" means "knowledge of life" in a nutshell [38]. According to the ancient Vedic society, one of nature's greatest gifts to humanity was honey. Ayurvedic literature states that honey helps those whose digestive systems are not robust.

Additionally, it has been highlighted that honey is an excellent remedy for a bothersome cough. Ayurvedic practitioners hold honey in high esteem for its beneficial effects on oral hygiene [39]. Because of its hypnotic effects, it has been used to cure insomnia for ages. Traditional Ayurvedic practitioners also advise using honey topically for various medical conditions, including burns and other skin ailments, heart palpitations and pains, lung imbalances, and anemia. In Ayurvedic medicine, honey has a lengthy treatment history for ocular conditions. It enhances eyesight when applied to the eyes daily. Additionally, honey is thought to help the ward fight cataracts [8, 39].

5.3.2 Honey in Ancient Egypt

In 900 different cures, honey was referenced 500 times, making it the most prevalent Egyptian medication [37]. A mixture of mrht (grease), byt (honey), and ftt (lint/fiber) as transliterated from hieroglyphic symbols is prescribed for a typical wound salve in the Smith papyrus. This Egyptian book dates from 2600 to 2200 BC [40]. In addition to wine and milk, honey was a common component in Egyptian medicine. As an offering to their gods, the ancient Egyptians would sometimes bring honey [41]. As a further method of embalming, they made use of honey. The antimicrobial qualities of honey aided in the healing of infected wounds. Additionally, honey was used topically as an ointment [42].

5.3.3 Honey in Ancient Greeks

Honey and unfermented grape juice make up the ancient Greek drink oenomel. Some people use it as a natural treatment for gout and other neurological conditions [42]. When it came to discomfort, the famous Greek physician Hippocrates recommended honey in the form of oxymel (vinegar and honey), hydromel (water and honey) to quench thirst, and a combination of honey, water, and other therapeutic ingredients for severe fevers [40]. He also used honey as a laxative; as a method of preventing and treating baldness, a wound, a sore throat, and an eye ailment; as a topical antiseptic; and for the prevention and treatment of scars [36].

5.4 Biological Activities of Honey

5.4.1 Antioxidant Activity

Oxidants, like oxygen, may play a role in damage prevention and are found in foods and the human body. While the exact role of natural antioxidants in the human body is still not completely understood, studies have shown that honey can have an antioxidant effect on aging and the production of reactive oxygen species (ROS) and free radicals. These substances interact with DNA, enzymes, cellular lipids and proteins, and cell membranes. Several illnesses can develop as a result of these harmful interactions. Thankfully, antioxidants prevent free radicals from causing harm by capturing them before they can. Protective antioxidants include both enzymatic and nonenzymatic substances [43]. Honey's capacity for antioxidant characteristics is inversely proportional to its brightness, so darker honey has a higher antioxidant value. Since the concentration of phenolic compounds correlates with honey's radical absorbance activity values, it has been demonstrated that these compounds are the primary drivers of honey's antioxidant activity. Other studies have shown that honey's antioxidant activity is due to the synergy of its many active compounds. This means honey can serve as an antioxidant in the food you eat. The scientific literature suggests that honey, on its own or in conjunction with traditional treatment methods, may be an effective antioxidant in reducing oxidative stress [44]. Based on the results of most of these studies, it is crucial to investigate the antioxidant effects of honey on various human diseases [9].

5.4.2 Antimicrobial Activity

The primary causes of honey's antimicrobial properties can be traced back to its enzymatic glucose oxidation reaction and specific physical properties. Still, other factors such as low water activity (WA), acidity of the surrounding environment (low pH), protein content (low), carbon-to-nitrogen ratio (high), redox potential (low) from the abundance of reducing sugars, honey's viscosity (limiting dissolved oxygen), and other chemical agents and phytochemicals can also play a role. Honey inhibits the growth of yeast and bacteria due to its properties, such as low WA and water acidity, glucose oxidase, and hydrogen peroxide [45]. Honey's low antibacterial level is due to a combination of several compounds, including terpenes, pinocembrin, benzyl alcohol, 3,5-dimethoxy-4-hydroxybenzoic acid (syringic acid), methyl-3,5-dimethoxy-4-hydroxybenzoate (methyl syringate), 2-hydroxy-3-phenylpropionic acid, 2-hydroxybenzoic acid, 3,4,5-trimethoxybenzoic acid, and 1,4-dihydroxybenzene.

5.4.3 Apoptotic Activity

Cancer cells are characterized by inadequate apoptotic turnover and uncontrolled cellular proliferation [46]. Chemicals that are applied for cancer treatment are apoptosis inducers [47]. Honey makes apoptosis in many cancer cells through depolarization of the mitochondrial membrane [47, 48]. Honey increases caspase-3 activation and poly (ADP-ribose) polymerase (PARP) cleavage in human colon cancer cell lines, which is related to its high phenolic component [49]. Moreover, it causes apoptosis by modulating the expression of pro- and anti-apoptotic proteins in colon cancer [50]. Honey induces the expression of p53, caspase-3, and pro-apoptotic protein Bax and also downregulates the expression of anti-apoptotic protein Bcl2 [49]. Honey produces ROS, leading to the activation of p53 and p53, which, in turn, modulates the expression of pro- and anti-apoptotic proteins such as Bcl-2 and Bax [49]. Oral administration of honey increases the expression of the pro-apoptotic protein Bax and also reduces the anti-apoptotic protein Bcl-2 expression in tumor tissue of Wistar rats [51]. Intravenous injection of manuka honey shows its apoptotic effect on cancer cell lines through the involvement of caspase-9, which in turn activates caspase-3, the executor protein. Because many of the chemotherapeutics used today are apoptosis inducer agents, manuka honey has the potential to be a natural anticancer agent due to its apoptotic characteristics, which include DNA fragmentation, loss of Bcl-2 expression, and PARP activation.

Anti-inflammatory and immunomodulatory actions: Damage to tissues caused by chronic inflammation can impede recovery. Animal models, cell cultures, and clinical trials have all shown that honey can reduce inflammatory responses. The anti-inflammatory effect of honey is due to its phenolic content, which suppresses the pro-inflammatory activities of cyclooxygenase-2 (COX-2) and inducible nitric oxide synthase (iNOS). Honey and its ingredients may also regulate proteins like iNOS, ornithine decarboxylase, tyrosine kinase, and COX-2. Various kinds of honey have been found to stimulate the production of tumor necrosis factor-alpha, interleukin-1 beta (IL-1β), and IL-6. Honey also boosts the generation of antibodies, eosinophils, neutrophils, monocytes, and natural killer cells in both primary and secondary immune responses in tissue culture.

5.4.4 Wound Healing

The healing of wounds is one of honey's most studied and beneficial applications [18]. During World War I, the Russians utilized honey to speed up the healing process and avoid wound infections. The Germans mixed cod liver oil with honey to remedy burns, ulcers, fistulas, and boils [36]. Honey is effective in treating a wide variety of wounds, including those caused by abrasions, abscesses, amputations, burns, chilblains, diabetes, malignancy, leprosy, or wounds of the abdominal wall or perineum. Using honey as a wound dressing speeds up the healing process and eliminates infections more effectively. In addition to reducing inflammation and stimulating tissue regeneration, honey has a cleaning effect on wounds. A nonadhesive tissue bandage can be made from pads impregnated with honey [36, 52, 53].

It is still unclear as to what precise chemical process allows honey to promote wound healing. However, the use of honey as a wound dressing is subject to several suggestions. The effectiveness will be influenced by the kind of wound and how bad it is. If you want the honey to stay there when mixed with wound exudates, you must use enough of the right kind. It needs to go beyond the wound's edges and cover it completely. Applying it on a dressing rather than a wound has better outcomes. Honey should be carefully packed into all the crevices, and an occlusive dressing should be placed over the incision to stop any bleeding [36, 54, 55]. It provides a calming effect at first and then speeds up the healing process for burns. As a wound barrier, it prevents tumor implantation during laparoscopic cancer surgery. Applying honey to exposed wounds has not been associated with any infections. It may play a therapeutic function in resolving periodontal disease and gingivitis [56]. In one of cases was knee amputation in a young boy, which was heavily infected with Pseudomonas and Staphylococcus aureus. Ten weeks after using sterile active manuka honey dressing pads to treat *Staphylococcus aureus*, which had not responded to standard treatment methods, the patient fully recovered [57]. Burns also produce similar outcomes. Applying a honey dressing to a wound helps it heal faster, prevents infection, and lessens discomfort [58]. Reducing edema and discharge, speeding up regeneration with little scarring, effectively debriding wounds, and decreasing mortality were all seen in studies with Fournier's gangrene [59].

Ulcerations caused by varicose veins and breast cancer treated with severe surgery can be effectively alleviated with honey. Furthermore, it is utilized after radical surgery for vulvar cancer to produce an infection-free wound with minor debridement of the wound and duration of hospital stay [60]. Patients who experience postoperative wound infections after hysterectomies or cesarean sections can find relief by applying topical honey to the affected region. This helps to reduce the need for antibiotics and hospital stays, speeds up the healing process, and minimizes the creation of scars [53]. It works well on decubitus ulcers and bed sores [61].

Clinical trials compare different burn dressings, such as honey, amniotic membrane, silver sulfadiazine, and boiling potato peel. Compared to other dressings, honey promoted faster healing, less contracture, and less scarring in these patients [36, 62]. Skin grafts treated with honey have also shown good histological retention [63] (Noornejad, Motalleb). Applying natural honey is an excellent way to manage radiation-induced mucositis, according to Motallebnejad, et al. [64].

Unusual as it may seem, honey was sometimes used to confirm the early stages of measles. The eruptions, which supposedly develop worse the next day after being rubbed with honey, must be kept applying honey until they completely disappear [62].

5.5 The Healing Power of Honey

For thousands of years, people have consumed honey made by bees from blossom nectar. The ancient Chinese, Romans, Egyptians, and Greeks all employed honey topically for medical reasons [65, 66]. Most of its content consists of sugars (such as fructose, sucrose, glucose, and other sugars), with little water, proteins, hydrogen peroxide, and gluconic acid rounding out the composition. When used topically, honey not only cleans and debrides but also forms a protective barrier against infection. Both in vitro and in vivo investigations have characterized and verified its antibacterial activities as a topical treatment, and evidence supports its effectiveness in wound healing [66–80]. Honey has recently been studied for its potential benefits in treating burns, skin grafts, Fournier's gangrene, radiation-induced mucositis, and dermatologic conditions like dermatitis and seborrhea. DM, hypercholesterolemia, hypertension, and gastroenteritis have also been studied when taken orally.

Honey is thought to have antibacterial qualities due to its high sugar and low moisture content, acidity of gluconic acid, and antiseptic effects of hydrogen peroxide. Honey's ability to influence LDL cholesterol levels when taken orally is likely due to its flavonoid content and antioxidant properties. According to certain studies, darker honey may contain more antioxidants than lighter ones [73, 80–88].

5.6 Uses of Topical Honey

More data from well-conducted clinical trials are needed to demonstrate the usefulness of honey for specific illnesses despite its anti-inflammatory, anti-glycemic, antioxidant, and antibacterial characteristics. In 2001, a comprehensive review was conducted that found honey to help control postoperative wound healing, maintain sterility, and eradicate infections. However, the review did conclude that more extensive randomized trials were necessary to confirm these findings. Earlier research suggested that honey could be helpful in wound care for cesarean sections, nonhealing wounds that do not respond to other treatments, and chronic, surgical, and traumatic wounds. The results showed that honey improved healing, decreased healing times, decreased edema, allowed more effortless dressing, and reduced infection [89–95].

Nevertheless, it is essential to exercise care when interpreting the research results that have examined honey's effects on burns and acute traumatic wounds. A recent Cochrane systematic review indicated that most of these studies needed to be of higher quality. However, the analysis found that honey is supported by the most significant evidence for the treatment of venous leg ulcers [65, 74, 79, 93].

Further research on the potential benefits of topical honey for diabetic foot ulcer therapy is ongoing, with a double-masked, randomized controlled study investigating the use of honey dressings as a treatment for diabetic foot ulcers [75]. According to a 2008 review [76] by the same researchers, when it comes to self-applying honey to treat diabetic foot ulcers, it is essential to make sure that there is enough blood flow (check for foot pulses and an average arterial-brachial index), that antimicrobial agents are used appropriately to treat infections, and that the patient is willing to do it.

References

1. Chow J. Probiotics and prebiotics: a brief overview. J Ren Nutr. 2002;12:76–86.
2. White JW. Composition of honey. In: Crane E, editor. Honey: a comprehensive survey. London: Heinemann; 1979. p. 157–92.
3. Alvarez-Suarez JM, Tulipani S, Romandini S, Bertoli E, Battino M. Contribution of honey in nutrition and human health: a review. Mediterr J Nutr Metab. 2010;3:15–23.
4. Johnston JE, Sepe HA, Miano CL, Brannan RG, Alderton AL. Honey inhibits lipid oxidation in ready-to-eat ground beef patties. Meat Sci. 2005;70:627–31.
5. Turkmen N, Sari F, Poyrazoglu ES, Velioglu YS. Effects of prolonged heating on antioxidant activity and colour of honey. Food Chem. 2006;95:653–7.
6. Rakha MK, Nabil ZI, Hussein AA. Cardioactive and vasoactive effects of natural wild honey against cardiac malperformance induced by hyperadrenergic activity. J Med Food. 2008;11:91–8.
7. Al-Mamary M, Al-Meeri A, Al-Habori M. Antioxidant activities and total phenolics of different types of honey. Nutr Res. 2002;22:1041–7.
8. Eteraf-Oskouei T, Najafi M. Traditional and modern uses of natural honey in human diseases: a review. Iran J Basic Med Sci. 2013;16(6):731–42. PMID: 23997898; PMCID: PMC3758027

9. Samarghandian S, Farkhondeh T, Samini F. Honey and health: a review of recent clinical research. Pharm Res. 2017;9(2):121–7. https://doi.org/10.4103/0974-8490.204647. PMID: 28539734; PMCID: PMC5424551
10. Dashora N, Sodde V, Bhagat J, Kirti SP, Labo R. Antitumor activity of Dendrophoe falcate against Ehrlich ascites carcinoma in Swiss albino mice. Pharm Crops. 2011;7:1.
11. Adebolu TT. Effect of natural honey on local isolates of diarrhea causing bacteria in southwestern Nigeria. Afr J Biotechnol. 2005;4:1172–4.
12. Ashrafi S, Mastronikolas S, Wu CD. Use of honey in treatment of Aphthous ulcers IADR/AADR/CADR 83rd general session. Baltimore; 2005. p. 9–12.
13. James H. Papyrus Harris, donation to the temple of re at Heliopolis. In: Birch S, editor. Breasted ancient records of Egypt part four pSalt 825, Egyptian magical text. 1876.
14. Bansal V, Medhi B, Pandhi P. Honey—a remedy rediscovered and its therapeutic utility. Kathmandu Univ Med J (KUMJ). 2005a;3:305–9.
15. Bell SG. The therapeutic use of honey. Neonatal Netw. 2007;26:247–51.
16. Hassapidou M, Fotiadou E, Maglara E, Papadopoulou SK. Energy intake, diet composition, energy expenditure, and body fatness of adolescents in northern Greece. Obesity (Silver Spring). 2006;14:855–62.
17. Babacan S, Rand AG. Characterization of honey amylase. J Food Sci. 2007;72:C050–5.
18. Medhi B, Puri A, Upadhyay S, Kaman L. Topical application of honey in the treatment of wound healing: a meta analysis. JK Sci. 2008;10:166–9.
19. Pataca LC, Borges Neto W, Marcucci MC, Poppi RJ. Determination of apparent reducing sugars, moisture and acidity in honey by attenuated total reflectance-Fourier transform infrared spectrometry. Talanta. 2007;71:1926–31.
20. Inglett GE. A history of sweeteners—natural and synthetic. J Toxicol Environ Health. 1976;2:207–14.
21. Ahmed S, Othman NH. Honey as a potential natural anticancer agent: a review of its mechanisms. Evid Based Complement Alternat Med. 2013;2013:829070.
22. Khalil I, Moniruzzaman M, Boukraâ L, Benhanifia M, Islam A, Islam N, et al. Physicochemical and antioxidant properties of Algerian honey. Molecules. 2012;17:11199–215.
23. Attia WY, Gabry MS, El-Shaikh KA, Othman GA. The anti-tumor effect of bee honey in Ehrlich ascite tumor model of mice is coincided with stimulation of the immune cells. J Egypt Public Health Assoc. 2008;15:169–83.
24. Estevinho L, Pereira AP, Moreira L, Dias LG, Pereira E. Antioxidant and antimicrobial effects of phenolic compounds extracts of Northeast Portugal honey. Food Chem Toxicol. 2008;46:3774–9.
25. Abdulrhman M, El-Hefnawy M, Ali R, El-Goud AA. Honey and type 1 diabetes mellitus. In: Liu CP, editor. Type diabetes—complications, pathogenesis, and alternative treatments. Croatia: In Tech; 2008.
26. Ghosh S, Playford RJ. Bioactive natural compounds for the treatment of gastrointestinal disorders. Clin Sci (Lond). 2003;104:547–56.
27. Moundoi MA, Padila-Zakour OI, Worobo RW. Antimicrobial activity of honey against food pathogens and food spoilage microorganisms. NYSAES. 2001;1:61–71.
28. Ezz El-Arab AM, Girgis SM, Hegazy ME, Abd El-Khalek AB. Effect of dietary honey on intestinal microflora and toxicity of mycotoxins in mice. BMC Complement Altern Med. 2006;6:1–13.
29. Olaitan PB, Adeleke EO, Ola OI. Honey: a reservoir for microorganisms and an inhibitory agent for microbes. Afr Health Sci. 2007;7:159–65.
30. Sampath Kumar KP, Bhowmik D, Chiranjib B, Chandira MR. Medicinal uses and health benefits of honey: an overview. J Chem Pharm Res. 2010;2:385–95.
31. Rashed MN, Soltan ME. Major and trace elements in different types of Egyptian mono-floral and non-floral bee honeys. J Food Compos Anal. 2004;17:725–35.
32. Lachman J, Kolihová D, Miholová D, Košata J, Titěra D, Kult K. Analysis of minority honey components: possible use for the evaluation of honey quality. Food Chem. 2007;101:973–9.

33. Lee DC, Lee SY, Cha SH, Choi YS, Rhee HI. Discrimination of native bee-honey and foreign bee-honey by SDS–PAGE. Korean J Food Sci. 1998;30:1–5.
34. Jagdish T, Joseph I. Quantification of saccharides in multiple floral honeys using fourier transform infrared microattenuated total reflectance spectroscopy. J Agri Food Chem. 2004;52:3237–43.
35. Won S-R, Li C-Y, Kim J-W, Rhee H-I. Immunological characterization of honey major protein and its application. Food Chem. 2009;113:1334–8.
36. Bansal V, Medhi B, Pandhi P. Honey—a remedy rediscovered and its therapeutic utility. Kathmandu Univ Med J. 2005b;3:305–9.
37. Al-Jabri AA. Honey, milk and antibiotics. Afr J Biotechnol. 2005;4:1580–7.
38. Telles S, Puthige R, Visweswaraiah NK. An Ayurvedic basis for using honey to treat herpes. Med Sci Monit. 2007;13:LE17–17.
39. Honey in history. 23 October 2008. http://www.mapi.com/newsletters/maharishi_ayurveda/august_2008.
40. Zumla A, Lulat A. Honey –a remedy rediscovered. J Royal Soc Med. 1989;82:384–5. (PMC free article) (PubMed)
41. Honey—Egypt. 26 June 2012. http://www.honey-health.com/honey-34.shtml
42. Honey. 26 June 2012. http://en.wikipedia.org/wiki/Honey
43. Pérez RA, Iglesias MT, Pueyo E, Gonzalez M, de Lorenzo C. Amino acid composition and antioxidant capacity of Spanish honeys. J Agric Food Chem. 2007;55:360–5.
44. Gheldof N, Wang XH, Engeseth NJ. Buckwheat honey increases serum antioxidant capacity in humans. J Agric Food Chem. 2003;51:1500–5.
45. Patton T, Barrett J, Brennan J, Moran N. Use of a spectrophotometric bioassay for determination of microbial sensitivity to manuka honey. J Microbiol Methods. 2006;64:84–95.
46. Boukraa L, Niar A. Sahara honey shows higher potency against *Pseudomonas aeruginosa* compared to north Algerian types of honey. J Med Food. 2007;10:712–4.
47. Nicholson DW. From bench to clinic with apoptosis-based therapeutic agents. Nature. 2000;407:810–6.
48. Earnshaw WC. Nuclear changes in apoptosis. Curr Opin Cell Biol. 1995;7:337–43.
49. Fauzi AN, Norazmi MN, Yaacob NS. Tualang honey induces apoptosis and disrupts the mitochondrial membrane potential of human breast and cervical cancer cell lines. Food Chem Toxicol. 2011;49:871–8.
50. Viuda-Martos M, Ruiz-Navajas Y, Fernández-López J, Pérez-Alvarez JA. Functional properties of honey, propolis, and royal jelly. J Food Sci. 2008;73:R117–24.
51. Jaganathan SK, Mandal M. Honey constituents and their apoptotic effect in colon cancer cells. J ApiProduct ApiMedical Sci. 2009;1:29–36.
52. Efem SEE. Clinical observations on the wound healing properties of honey. Br J Surg. 1988;75:679–81.
53. Al-Waili NS. Mixture of honey, bees wax and olive oil inhibits growth of staphylococcus aureus and candida albicans. Arch Med Res. 2005;36:10–3.
54. Molan PC. A brief review of the use of honey as a clinical dressing. Primary Intention. 1998;6:148–58.
55. Molan PC, Brett M. Honey has potential as a dressing for wounds infected with MRSA. The second Australian wound management association conference. Brisbane; 1998.
56. Khan FR, Ul Abadin Z, Rauf N. Honey: nutritional and medicinal value. Inte J Clin Pract. 2007a;61:1705–7.
57. Dunford C, Cooper R, Molan PC. Using honey as a dressing for infected skin lesions. Nurs Times. 2000;96:7–9.
58. Subrahmanyam M. Topical application of honey in treatment of burns. Br J Surg. 1991;78:497–8.
59. Gurdal M, Yucebas E, Tekin A, Beysel M, Aslan R, Sengor F. Predisposing factors and treatment outcome in Fournier's gangrene. Analysis of 28 cases. Urol Int. 2003;70:286–90.
60. Cavanagh D, Beazley J, Ostapowicz F. Radical operation for carcinoma of the vulva. A new approach to wound healing. J Obstet Gynaecol Br Commonw. 1970;77:1037–40.

61. Van der Weyden EA. The use of honey for the treatment of two patients with pressure ulcers. Br J Community Nurs. 2003;8:S14–20.
62. Meda A, Lamien EC, Millogo J, Romito M, Nacoulma OG. Ethnopharmacological communication therapeutic uses of honey and honeybee larvae in Central Burkina Faso. J Ethnopharmacol. 2004;95:103–7.
63. Subrahmanyam M. Storage of skin grafts in honey. Lancet. 1993;341:63–4.
64. Motallebnejad M, Akram S, Moghadamnia A, Moulana Z, Omodi S. The effect of topical application of pure honey on radiation-induced mucositis: a randomized clinical trial. J Contemp Dent Pract. 2008;9:1–9.
65. Lee D. Honey of a Remedy for Nonhealing Wounds. Medscape General Surgery. April 30, 2009. https://www.medscape.com/viewarticle/702071_2. Accessed 9 Dec 2023.
66. Natural Standard Database Monograph. Food, herbs & supplements: honey. By subscription at: https://www.naturalstandard.com/monographs/herbssupplements/honey
67. Davis C. The use of Australian honey in moist wound management: a report for the Rural Industries Research and Development Corporation. October 2005. https://rirdc.infoservices.com.au/downloads/05-159.pdf. Accessed 23 Apr 2009.
68. Lusby PE, Coombes AL, Wilkinson JM. Bactericidal activity of different honeys against pathogenic bacteria. Arch Med Res. 2005;36:464–7.
69. Armon PJ. The use of honey in the treatment of infected wounds. Trop Dr. 1980;10:91.
70. Ndayisaba G, Bazira L, Habonimana E, et al. Clinical and bacteriological results in wounds treated with honey. J Orthop Surg. 1993;7:202–4.
71. Molan PC. The role of honey in the management of wounds. J Wound Care. 1999;8:415–8.
72. Cooper RA, Halas E, Molan PC. The efficacy of honey in inhibiting strains of Pseudomonas aeruginosa from infected burns. J Burn Care Rehabil. 2002;23:366–70.
73. Gethin G, Cowman S. Manuka honey vs hydrogel: a prospective, open label, multicentre randomized controlled trial to compare desloughing efficacy and healing outcomes in venous ulcers. Medscape Today. February 2009. https://www.medscape.com/medline/abstract/18752540?cid=med&src=nlbest. Accessed 16 Apr 2009.
74. Jull AB, Rodgers A, Walker N. Honey as a topical treatment for wounds. Cochrane Database Syst Rev. 2008;(4):Article No.:CD005083.
75. Eddy JJ, Gideonsen MD. Observations from practice: topical honey for diabetic foot ulcers. J Fam Pract. 2005;54:533–5.
76. Eddy JJ, Gideonsen MD, Mack PM. Practical considerations of using topical honey for neuropathic diabetic foot ulcers: a review. Wis Med J. 2008;197:187–90. https://store.wisconsinmedicalsociety.org/_WMS/publications/wmj/issues/wmj_v107n4/107no4_eddy.pdf. Accessed 23 Apr 2009.
77. Han DH, Denison MS, Tachibana H, Yamada K. Relationship between estrogen receptor-binding and estrogenic activities of environmental estrogens and suppression by flavonoids. Biosci Biotechnol Biochem. 2002;66:1479–87.
78. Beretta G, Orioli M, Facino RM. Antioxidant and radical scavenging activity of honey in endothelial cell cultures (EA. hy926). Planta Med. 2007;73:1182–9.
79. Cushnie TP, Lamb AJ. Antimicrobial activity of flavonoids. Int J Antimicrob Agents. 2005;26:343–56.
80. Obi CL, Ugoji EO, Edun SA, Lawal SF, Anyiwo CE. The antibacterial effect of honey on diarrhoea causing bacterial agents isolated in Lagos, Nigeria. Afr J Med Med Sci. 1994;23:257–60.
81. Tomasin R, Gomes-Marcondes MC. Oral administration of *Aloe vera* and honey reduces Walker tumour growth by decreasing cell proliferation and increasing apoptosis in tumour tissue. Phytother Res. 2011;25:619–23.
82. Fernandez-Cabezudo MJ, El-Kharrag R, Torab F, Bashir G, George JA, El-Taji H, et al. Intravenous administration of manuka honey inhibits tumor growth and improves host survival when used in combination with chemotherapy in a melanoma mouse model. PLoS One. 2013;8:e55993.

83. Candiracci M, Piatti E, Dominguez-Barragán M, García-Antrás D, Morgado B, Ruano D, et al. Anti-inflammatory activity of a honey flavonoid extract on lipopolysaccharide-activated N13 microglial cells. J Agric Food Chem. 2012;60:12304–11.
84. Bilsel Y, Bugra D, Yamaner S, Bulut T, Cevikbas U, Turkoglu U. Could honey have a place in colitis therapy? Effects of honey, prednisolone, and disulfiram on inflammation, nitric oxide, and free radical formation. Dig Surg. 2002;19:306–11.
85. Leong AG, Herst PM, Harper JL. Indigenous New Zealand honeys exhibit multiple anti-inflammatory activities. Innate Immun. 2012;18:459–66.
86. Al-Waili NS, Boni NS. Natural honey lowers plasma prostaglandin concentrations in normal individuals. J Med Food. 2003;6:129–33.
87. Cho H, Yun CW, Park WK, Kong JY, Kim KS, Park Y, et al. Modulation of the activity of pro-inflammatory enzymes, COX-2 and iNOS, by chrysin derivatives. Pharmacol Res. 2004;49:37–43.
88. Araâjo JR, Gonçalves P, Martel F. Chemopreventive effect of dietary polyphenols in colorectal cancer cell lines. Nutr Res. 2011;31:77–87.
89. Hussein SZ, Mohd Yusoff K, Makpol S, Mohd Yusof YA. Gelam honey inhibits the production of proinflammatory, mediators NO, PGE (2), TNF-a, and IL-6 in carrageenan-induced acute paw edema in rats. Evid Based Complement Alternat Med. 2012;2012:109636.
90. Timm M, Bartelt S, Hansen EW. Immunomodulatory effects of honey cannot be distinguished from endotoxin. Cytokine. 2008;42:113–20.
91. Khan FR, Abadin UI, Rauf N. Honey: nutritional and medicinal value. Medscape Today November 21, 2007b. https://www.medscape.com/viewarticle/565913. Accessed 16 Apr 2009.
92. Moore OA, Smith LA, Campbell F, Seers K, McQuay HJ, Moore RA. Systematic review of the use of honey as a wound dressing. BMC Complement Altern Med. 2001;1:2.
93. Al Waili NS, Saloom KY. Effects of topical honey on post-operative wound infections due to gram positive and gram negative bacteria following caesarean sections and hysterectomies. Eur J Med Res. 1999;4:126–30.
94. Stephen-Haynes J. Evaluation of a honey-impregnated tulle dressing in primary care. Br J Community Nurs. 2004;9(Suppl):S21–7.
95. Ahmed AK, Hoekstra MJ, Hage JJ, et al. Honey-medicated dressing: transformation of an ancient remedy into modern therapy. Ann Plast Surg. 2003;50:143–7.

Propolis: Overview

6

6.1 Introduction

Honey, propolis, pollen, royal jelly, and even bee venom (apitoxin) are all part of apitherapy, an alternative medicine practice that uses bee products to treat and prevent illness (Figs. 6.1 and 6.2). Their usage has been documented in traditional medicines for a long time, reaching back to Galen and Hippocrates in Greece, Egypt, Russia, Korea, and China. The Bible and the Quran, among other holy writings, refer to their usage [1].

In the past, people have used bee products for various purposes. Honey, for instance, served as both a food source and an offering in religious ceremonies; propolis served as an adhesive; pollen was used for agricultural purposes and plant breeding; and beeswax was used for casting metals and incendiary weapons [2]. Atherosclerosis, hypertension, myocardial infarction, ischemia-reperfusion damage, and other cardiovascular diseases (CVDs) have recently been shown to have potential advantages in the prevention and treatment of these conditions [3–7]. This discovery carries excellent significance since myocardial infarction (MI) is a leading global killer and disability-inducing event, and it frequently serves as the initial indicator of coronary artery disease. Patients with established illness may also experience it several times [8, 9].

Heart disease risk factors, both internal and external, like high cholesterol, obesity, oxidative stress, and blood platelet hyperactivation, significantly raise the probability of CVD [10, 11]. Nevertheless, certain dietary elements, like polyunsaturated fatty acids and phytosterols like β-sitosterol, may provide some protection. Additionally, phenolic substances can lower the risk of cardiovascular diseases. To be more precise, there is an inverse association between mortality from CVDs and intake of phenolic chemicals, particularly flavonoids [12].

Certain bee products may lower the risk of cardiovascular diseases because of their antioxidant [13] and antiplatelet [7] characteristics. As an example, honey's

A. E. Tanuğur Samanci et al., *Propolis: Prevention and Healing Effects in Otorhinolaryngology*, Comprehensive ENT,
https://doi.org/10.1007/978-3-031-68546-0_6

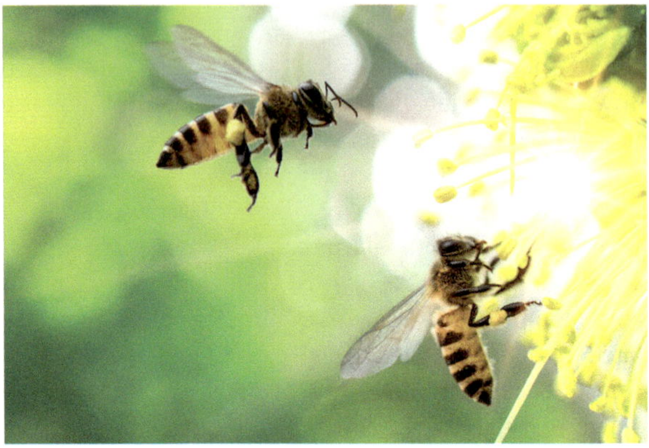

Fig. 6.1 The bees carrying the collected pollen to the hive. (*Courtesy of* **Ali İhsan Gokcen**)

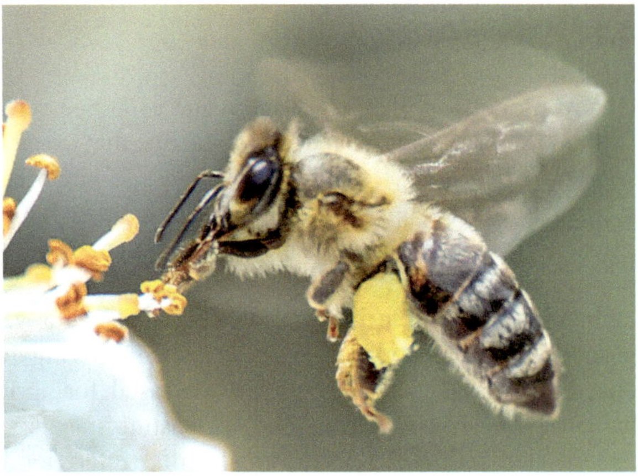

Fig. 6.2 The bees carrying the collected pollen to the hive. (*Courtesy of* **Ali İhsan Gokcen**)

chemical composition includes phenolic substances such as chrysin, quercetin, luteolin, and pinocembrin [7, 14, 15], which have anti-inflammatory, antioxidant, and antiplatelet effects, among other cardioprotective qualities. Although these have been seen in animal and in vitro studies, there is a single in vivo investigation with a human model. This was done on individuals who were in good health. The benefits of honey and its active ingredients on cardiovascular diseases have already been well studied and documented elsewhere [7]. Further, it is still being determined if honey or its pure phenolic components are superior for preventing and treating CVDs.

6.2 Propolis

Bees use materials derived from various plant parts, buds, and exudates to create propolis, a resinous combination that is naturally occurring (Figs. 6.3 and 6.4). The waxy and mechanical properties of propolis allow bees to utilize it in building and

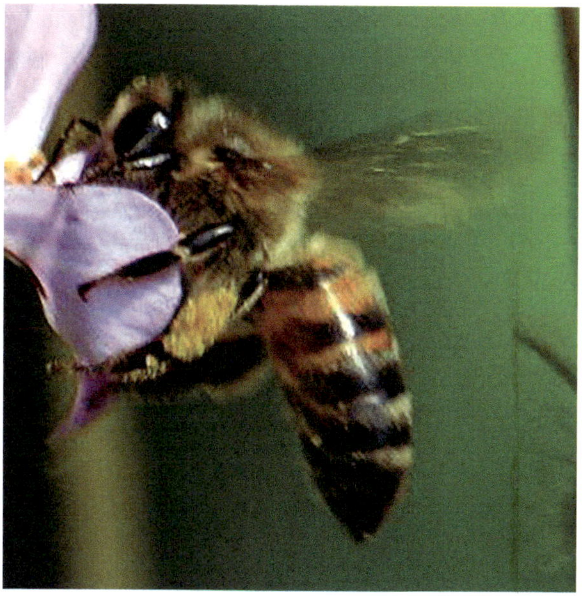

Fig. 6.3 The bee collecting propolis, Ordu region. (*Courtesy of* **Ali Fuat Varol**)

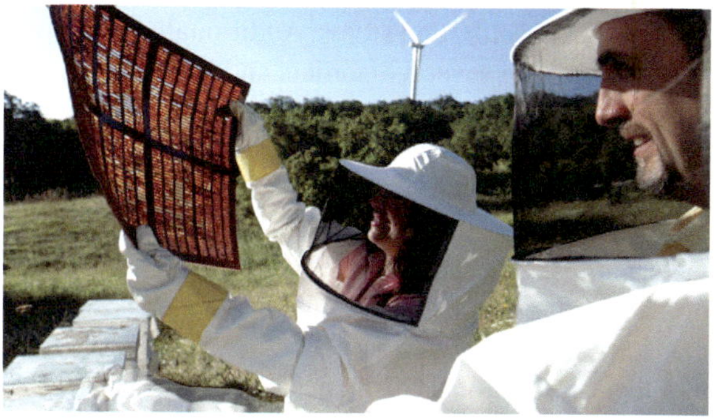

Fig. 6.4 Propolis production trap/Istranca region/Kırklareli/Turkey. (*Courtesy of* **Taylan Samancı**)

repairing their hives. It protects against weathering threats like wind and rain and external invaders like snakes and lizards. Bees also use it to seal holes and cracks and smooth out the inside walls. Bees collect propolis from various plants, the most common of which is the poplar tree in regions with a moderate environment. Propolis is now used in antimicrobial formulations for conditions such as cold syndrome, burns, wound healing, herpes simplex, genitals, neurodermatitis, and upper respiratory tract infections [16].

Honeybees create propolis, a resinous combination, using materials gathered from various plant parts, buds, and exudates. The Greek roots of the English term "propolis"—"at the entrance to" and "community" or "city"—indicate that this natural substance is employed for hive defense. Bee glue is another name for propolis. As a result of its waxy texture and mechanical characteristics, bees utilize propolis to build and repair their hives. This includes sealing holes and cracks, smoothing the inside walls [17, 18], and creating a barrier against weather elements and potential predators like snakes and lizards. Bees in various temperate climate zones collect propolis from multiple plants [16].

Honey and propolis have a positive impact on human health. People have used propolis since ancient times, most notably in folk medicine, to treat multiple illnesses. The Egyptians understood fully that bee glue had putrefactive characteristics, so they used it to embalm their corpses. The Incas used propolis as a remedy for fever. It was recommended topically for treating cutaneous and mucosal wounds by Greek and Roman doctors as a wound disinfectant, antiseptic, and healing substance [18]. The seventeenth-century London pharmacopeias included propolis as an approved medicine. From the seventeenth to the twentieth centuries, propolis was popular in Europe due to its antibacterial properties. Stradivari applied beeswax as a varnish on his violins in Italy [19]. The curative effects of propolis were well documented at the turn of the nineteenth century. Throughout World War II, it was utilized in several Soviet facilities to treat TB, with positive results such as reduced lung issues and improved appetite. Wounds, burns, sore throats, and stomach ulcers were treated with propolis in the Balkan states [20]. An article detailing propolis's chemical composition and characteristics was published for the first time in 1908 and subsequently indexed in the chemical abstract [16, 21].

These days, you may get many topical formulations of propolis, a natural medicine, at most health food stores. Additionally, it is a popular alternative medicine for self-treatment of several disorders and is utilized in cosmetics. Propolis is now used in cold syndrome (infections of the upper respiratory tract, common cold, and flu-like illnesses) formulations, burn treatments, acne treatments, neurodermatitis, herpes simplex and genitals, and wound healing preparations for the skin. Toothpaste and mouthwashes formulated with propolis help reduce the risk of cavities and alleviate gum disease and stomatitis symptoms. Its application in healthy meals and drinks is extensive and also found in cosmetics. You may find it in many clean items that have had the wax removed and in pills, creams, throat tablets, powder, and mouthwash solutions. Cosmetics, pharmacy, and veterinary medicine use it because of its antioxidant, antiviral, and antibacterial qualities [16].

6.3 Features

Initially cold and brittle, propolis transforms into a soft, malleable, gooey, and sticky substance when subjected to heat [22]. Its hue ranges from yellow-green to red to dark brown, and its perfume is distinctive and pleasant; the exact shade depends on its age and origin [18–23]. The resins' sources also determine the color, ranging from light yellow to deep brown. However, transparent propolis reports have also been made [16].

6.4 Composition

Compounds found in propolis come from both plants and bees. A variety of organic substances make up 5% of raw propolis, along with pollen, essential oils, waxes, resins, and other components [17, 24, 25]. During the chemical identification of novel varieties of propolis, more than 300 components have been found in various samples [23–26], and new ones are continually being discovered [18, 27, 28]. The location and timing of collecting determine the relative amounts of the different chemicals found in the propolis [16].

Various analytical techniques have been employed to isolate and identify the components of propolis. The chemicals that have been discovered are classified into the following classes of chemically related substances: substances that contain polyphenols, benzoic acids, cinnamic acid, sesquiterpene and triterpene hydrocarbons, benzaldehyde, various acids and their derivatives, alcohols, ketones, heteroaromatic compounds, terpene and sesquiterpene alcohols, aliphatic hydrocarbons, minerals, sterols, steroid hydrocarbons, sugars, and amino acids [29]. Low concentrations of volatile chemicals (made by the plants used as sources) are not surprising [26]. It is believed that sugars are unintentionally delivered as bees travel over the resin or when they elaborate propolis. All propolis samples have a core set of chemicals that define their unique qualities [16].

Different types of propolis include unique components. Several components appear in multiple samples from various locations, and a few can be found in samples taken from certain plants [30].

The biological activity of propolis samples from different regions is affected by the varying climates in those regions [31]. Polyphenols, aromatic acids, and diterpenic acids are the primary bioactive chemicals in propolis; however, there is slight variation across the many varieties of propolis in terms of these molecules. Variations in raw material treatments and regional flora can also affect the final composition [16].

6.5 Melting Point

From 25 to 45 degrees Celsius, propolis becomes a sticky, flexible, and soft substance. When frozen, it becomes rigid and brittle. Even when heated to greater degrees, the treated material retains its brittleness. As the temperature rises beyond 45 °C, it gets sticky and gooey. Typically, propolis has a melting point of 60–70 °C, although it can reach 100 °C for some samples [16].

6.6 Propolis Solubility

Due to its complicated structure, propolis is not suitable for direct usage. A commercial solvent is used to extract propolis. Examples of typical extraction solvents are water, acetone, chloroform, methanol, ethanol, dichloromethane, and ether.

Since many bactericidal components are soluble in alcohol or water, it should be possible to isolate the active ingredients and keep them inert [32]. The composition of propolis varies depending on two factors: first, the extraction process [23], and second, the solvent used [33].

6.7 Research on Propolis

The chemical composition of propolis varies with the plant species and its place of origin, but it is known to include over 2000 components. Bee propolis is a functional food that has gained popularity. The following chemicals make up 45–55% of the total: phenolic compounds (including phenolic acid and its esters and flavonoids), essential oils making up 10%, waxes and fatty acids making up 25–35%, pollen containing amino acids accounting for 5%, and a variety of other substances, including sugars, vitamins, and minerals, making up 5% [34, 5].

A propolis water solution inhibits mitochondrial respiration, as pointed out by Majiene et al. [36].

In their study, Zhang et al. [37] discovered that, when tested in vitro against several platelet agonists, including 10 μM ADP, 5 μg/mL collagen, and 50 μM thrombin receptor activator peptide (TRAP), the aqueous extract of propolis (25–300 mg/L) inhibited human blood platelet aggregation. In platelet-rich plasma, turbidimetry was used to quantify platelet aggregation.

According to Bojic et al. [35], the anti-aggregatory activities were seen in vitro at doses ranging from 5 μM to 10.4 mM in propolis ethanol extract, which had a total phenolic component content of 136.14 mg/g and a total flavonoid content of 19.28 mg/g. Ten healthy individuals had their total blood samples tested using an impendence analyzer after being given ADP to stimulate platelet aggregation. Since flavonoids are the primary components of propolis, Bojic et al. [35, 38], Hubbard et al. [39], and Faggio et al. [40] suggest that they are the ones responsible for propolis's antiplatelet characteristics. They can stop blood platelet aggregation caused by thrombin, ADP, and collagen by blocking cyclooxygenase, phospholipase C A2, and other enzymes in intracellular signaling pathways. The oxidative burst and NO production may both be mitigated by flavonoids.

It is worth noting that several writers have pointed to the cardioprotective properties of propolis in vivo [34, 40]. Total flavonoids of propolis (25 and 50 mg/kg/day) protected mice against pathological ventricular hypertrophy and heart failure, according to He et al. [41]. The AKT/phosphoinositide 3-kinase (PI3-K) signaling pathway was a part of the studied propolis' protective action. Neointimal development in a rabbit carotid artery balloon-induced damage model with hypercholesterolemia was recently reported by Chao et al. [42] recently reported. For 6 weeks following surgery, the rabbits (n = 24) were orally administered propolis at doses of 125 mg/kg and 250 mg/kg, and they were also given a 1% high-cholesterol diet. Propolis was seen to decrease rabbit body weight and blood lipid level at both of the dosages administered. In addition to reducing oxidative stress, lipid deposition, and collagen fiber, propolis decreased neointimal hyperplasia and carotid stenosis in these mice. Several indicators, such as plasma nitric oxide and superoxide dismutase activity, were used to ascertain the impact of propolis on oxidative stress. It is worth noting that propolis has been seen to suppress the production of Toll-like receptor 4 (TLR4), nuclear factor-κB (NF-κB), and tumor necrosis factor-α (TNF-α). The authors propose that this action of propolis may enhance the degree of vascular inflammation using the TLR4/NFκB pathway. This study's findings provide promising evidence that propolis might be the subject of future research into preventing and treating vascular restenosis.

It was found by Wang et al. [43] that the total flavonoids of propolis suppress the apoptosis of cardiac cells triggered by adriamycin in rats with chronic heart failure. In addition, the phosphorylation state of Cx43 may be regulated by employing a propolis preparation.

Caffeic acid phenethyl ester, composed of 2-phenylethyl 3-(3,4-dihydroxyphenyl)-2-propenoate, is one of the most potent components of propolis. Its molecular formula is C17H16O4. There are several ways to extract CAPE from propolis, which was initially discovered as an ingredient in propolis. This compound's wide range of pharmacological effects was detailed in a review by Tolba et al. [34]. To illustrate, CAPE showed signs of antioxidant activity and even protected against ischemia-reperfusion damage, which can affect many different organs (e.g., the colon, brain, liver, and heart).

References

1. Olas B. Bee products as interesting natural agents for the prevention and treatment of common cardiovascular diseases. Nutrients. 2022;14(11):2267. https://doi.org/10.3390/nu14112267.
2. Fratellone PM, Tsimis F, Fratellone G. Apitherapy products for medicinal use. J Altern Complement Med. 2016;22:1020–2.
3. Khalil M, Sulaiman SA. The potential role of honey and its polyphenols in preventing heart disease: a review. Afr J Tradit Complement Altern Med. 2010;7:315–21.
4. Alvarez-Suarez JM, Giampieri F, Battino M. Honey as a source of dietary antioxidants: structures, bioavailability and evidence of protective effects against human chronic diseases. Curr Med Chem. 2013;20:621–38.
5. Eteraf-Oskouei T, Najafi M. Traditional and modern uses of natural honey in human diseases: a review. Iran J Basic Med Sci. 2013;16:731–42.
6. Wehbe R, Frangieh J, Rima M, El Obeid D, Sabatier JM, Fajloun Z. Bee venom: overview of main compounds and bioactivities for therapeutic interests. Molecules. 2019;24:2997.
7. Olas B. Honey and its phenolic compounds as an effective natural medicine for cardiovascular diseases in humans? Nutrients. 2020;12:283.
8. Kapoor S, Jain MK, Nayak L. Thrombosis. In: Lazarys HM, Schmaier A, editors. Concise guide to hematology. Berlin/Heidelberg: Springer; 2019. p. 149–61.
9. Shen Z, Geng Q, Huang H, Yao H, Du T, Chen L, Wu Z, Miao X, Shi P. Antioxidative and cardioprotective effects of *Schisandra chinensis* bee pollen extract on isoprenaline-induced myocardial infarction in rats. Molecules. 2019;24:1090.
10. Flora GD, Nayak MK. A brief review of cardiovascular diseases, associated risk factors and current treatment regimes. Curr Pharm Des. 2019;25:4063–84.
11. Shibata K, Hashimoto T, Miyazaki T, Miyazaki A, Nobe K. Thrombolytic therapy for acute ischemic stroke: past and future. Curr Pharm Des. 2019;25:242–50.

12. Zampelas A, Magriplis E. Dietary patterns and risk of cardiovascular diseases: a review of the evidence. Proc Nutr Soc. 2019;79:68–75.
13. Samarghandian S, Farkhondeh T, Samini F. Honey and health: a review of recent clinical research. Pharm Res. 2017;9:121–7.
14. Cianciosi D, Forbes-Hernández TY, Afrin S, Gasparrini M, Reboredo-Rodriguez P, Manna PP, Zhang J, Bravo Lamas L, Martínez Flórez S, Agudo Toyos P, et al. Phenolic compounds in honey and their associated health benefits: a review. Molecules. 2018;23:2322.
15. Nguyen HTL, Panyoyai N, Kasapis S, Pang E, Mantri N. Honey and its role in relieving multiple facets of atherosclerosis. Nutrients. 2019;11:167.
16. Wagh VD. Propolis: a wonder bees product and its pharmacological potentials. Adv Pharmacol Sci. 2013;2013:308249. https://doi.org/10.1155/2013/308249. Epub 2013 Dec 9. PMID: 24382957; PMCID: PMC3872021
17. Burdock GA. Review of the biological properties and toxicity of bee propolis (propolis). Food Chem Toxicol. 1998;36(4):347–63.
18. Bankova VS, De Castro SL, Marcucci MC. Propolis: recent advances in chemistry and plant origin. Apidologie. 2000;31(1):3–15.
19. Monti M, Berti E, Carminati G, Cusini M. Occupational and cosmetic dermatitis from propolis. Contact Derm. 1983;9(2):163.
20. Wollenweber E, Hausen BM, Greenaway W. Phenolic constituents and sensitizing properties of propolis, poplar balsam and balsam of Peru. Bull Liaison—Groupe Polyphenols. 1990;15:112–20.
21. Helfenberg KD. The analysis of beeswax and propolis. Chemiker-Zeitung. 1908;31:987–98.
22. Hausen BM, Wollenweber E, Senff H, Post B. Propolis allergy. (II). The sensitizing properties of 1,1-dimethylallyl caffeic acid ester. Contact Derm. 1987;17(3):171–7.
23. Marcucci M. Propolis: chemical composition, biological properties and therapeutic activity. Apidologie. 1995;26(2):83–99.
24. Park YK, Alencar SM, Aguiar CL. Botanical origin and chemical composition of Brazilian propolis. J Agric Food Chem. 2002;50(9):2502–6.
25. Pietta PG, Gardana C, Pietta AM. Analytical methods for quality control of propolis. Fitoterapia. 2002;73(1):S7–S20.
26. De Castro SL. Propolis: biological and pharmacological activities. Therapeutic uses of this bee-product. Annu Rev Biomed Sci. 2001;3:49–83.
27. Banskota AH, Tezuka Y, Prasain JK, Matsushige K, Saiki I, Kadota S. Chemical constituents of Brazilian propolis and their cytotoxic activities. J Nat Prod. 1998;61(7):896–900.
28. Alencar SM, Oldoni TLC, Castro ML, et al. Chemical composition and biological activity of a new type of Brazilian propolis: red propolis. J Ethnopharmacol. 2007;113(2):278–83.
29. Walker P, Crane E. Constituents of propolis. Apidologie. 1987;18:327–34.
30. Ghisalberti EL. Propolis: a review. Bee World. 1979;60:59–84.
31. Kujumgiev A, Tsvetkova I, Serkedjieva Y, Bankova V, Christov R, Popov S. Antibacterial, antifungal and antiviral activity of propolis of different geographic origin. J Ethnopharmacol. 1999;64(3):235–40.
32. Kumar N, Ahmad MKK, Dang R, Husain A. Antioxidant and antimicrobial activity of propolis from Tamil Nadu zone. Journal of Medicinal Plants Research. 2008;2(12):361–4.
33. Cowan MM. Plant products as antimicrobial agents. Clin Microbiol Rev. 1999;12(4):564–82.
34. Tolba MF, Omar H, Azab SS, Khalifa A, Abdel-Naim AB, Abdel-Rahman SZ. Caffeic acid Phenethyl Ester: a review of its antioxidant activity, protective effects against ischemia-reperfusion injury and drug adverse reactions. Crit Rev Food Sci Nutr. 2014;56:2183–90.
35. Bojic M, Antolic A, Tomicic M, Debeljak Z, Males Z. Propolis ethanolic extracts reduce adenosine diphospate induced platelet aggregation determined on whole blood. Nutr J. 2018;17:52.
36. Majiene D, Trumbeckaite S, Savickas A, Toleikis A. Influence of propolis water solution on heart mitochondrial function. J Pharm Pharmacol. 2006;58:709–13.
37. Zhang YX, Yang TT, Zhang WF, Wang JF, Wu YP. Inhibitory effect of propolis on platelet aggregation in vitro. J Healthc Eng. 2017;10:3050895.

38. Bojic M, Debeljak Z, Medic-Saric M, Tomicic M. Interference of selected flavonoid aglycons in platelet aggregation assays. Clin Chem Lab Med. 2012;50:1403–8.
39. Hubbard GP, Wolfram S, Lovegrove JA, Gibbins JM. Ingestion of quercetin inhibits platelet aggregation and essential components of the collagen-stimulated platelet activation pathway in humans. J Thromb Haemost. 2004;2:2138–45.
40. Faggio C, Sureda A, Morabito S, Sanches-Silva A, Mocan A, Nabavi SF, Nabavi SM. Flavonoids and platelet aggregation: a brief review. Eur J Pharmacol. 2017;807:91–101.
41. He T, Sui X, Sun W, Yang P, Sui D, Cui H, Wang W, Wang X, Liu Y, Sun G. The protective effects and mechanism of total flavonoids of propolis on pathological cardiac hypertrophy and heart failure in mice. J Am Coll Cardiol. 2018;72:C161.
42. Chao J, Yongming P, Songtao X, Chen Y, Jian J, Minli C, Fuliang H. Propolis ameliorates restenosis in hypercholesterolemia rabbits with carotid balloon injury by inhibiting lipid accumulation, oxidative stress, and TLR4/NF-κB pathway. J Food Biochem. 2021;45:e13577.
43. Wang HH, Zeng J, Wang HZ, Jiang YX, Wang J, Zhou PP. Effects of total flavonoids of propolis on apoptosis of myocardial cells of chronic heart failure and its possible mechanism in rats. Chin J Appl Physiol. 2015;31:201–6.

Propolis as an Antiseptic

7

7.1 Introduction

Numerous topical and hard-surface uses necessitate the widespread use of disinfectants and antiseptics in healthcare facilities. Alcohols, phenols, iodine, and chlorine are just a few of the biocides included in these goods. Many of these agents have a long history of usage. More information on these active compounds' mechanism of action than antibiotics is needed. However, the majority of them show broad-spectrum antibacterial activity [1].

7.2 Antiseptics

Numerous topical and hard-surface uses necessitate the widespread use of disinfectants and antiseptics in healthcare facilities. Specifically, they help prevent nosocomial infections and are integral to infection control procedures [2, 3]. People use more antiseptics and disinfectants because they worry about microbial contamination and illness hazards in food and other consumer goods. Antisepsis, disinfection, and preservation have long made use of the various active chemical agents (or "biocides") included in these goods [4]. Regardless, compared to antibiotics, more needs to be understood regarding the mechanism of action of these active medicines. Typically, biocides are more versatile than antibiotics, and unlike antibiotics, which often target particular intracellular locations, biocides can potentially target several places simultaneously. Some have speculated that microbial resistance, especially cross-resistance to antibiotics, may develop due to the extensive use of disinfection and antiseptic products. Whenever feasible, this review aims to connect the dots between the present state of knowledge and the clinical setting by considering what is known about the mechanisms of microbial resistance to antiseptics and disinfectants and their modes of action [1].

A. E. Tanuğur Samanci et al., *Propolis: Prevention and Healing Effects in Otorhinolaryngology*, Comprehensive ENT,
https://doi.org/10.1007/978-3-031-68546-0_7

A "biocide" is a chemical agent that kills microbes; these agents are often broad spectrum. For example, "-static" can be used to describe agents that inhibit growth (e.g., bacteriostatic, fungistatic, and prostatic) or "-cidal" can be used to describe agents that kill the target organism (e.g., sporicidal, virucidal, and bactericidal), depending on the biocide's antimicrobial activity. The following terms are used in this review: antibiotics, antiseptics, and disinfectants. Antiseptics are defined as organic substances that either occur naturally or are synthesized. They inhibit or destroy certain microorganisms, usually at low concentrations. On the other hand, disinfectants are biocides that kill or inhibit the growth of microorganisms on inanimate objects or surfaces. Although disinfectants are not always sporicidal, they can be sporostatic [1].

7.3 Mechanisms

Our knowledge of how antiseptics and disinfectants work to kill germs has come a long way [5–7]. The mechanisms of their activity against viruses [10, 11], protozoa [12], and fungi [8, 9] have, in contrast, been under very little investigation. Only a little is also understood regarding how these substances render prions inactive [13].

Likely, a standard series of processes occurs regardless of the kind of microbial cell (or entity). One way to think about it is that the antiseptic or disinfectant comes into contact with the cell surface, penetrates it, and finally acts at the designated site(s). Different cell types (or entities) have distinct surface characteristics and compositions, which might change due to environmental factors [14, 15]. Most antimicrobial drugs seem to work intracellularly [6, 18]. However, interactions at the cell surface might significantly impact viability (e.g., with glutaraldehyde) [16, 17]. It is disheartening that so little is known about the penetration of antimicrobial drugs into various bacteria, as the outermost layers of microbial cells can significantly influence their sensitivity (or lack thereof) to these substances [1].

7.4 Propolis Formulations

The emulsification and solvent evaporation process created ethanolic extract (PE) microparticles containing propolis. The dry residue (DR) value of ethyl cellulose was examined in three different ratios to that of PE: 1:0.25, 1:4, and 1:10. In addition, either 1.0 or 1.5% w/w of polysorbate 80 was utilized as an emulsifier in the exterior phase. The only way to get particles with regular morphology and no amorphous or sticky properties was to employ a 1:0.25 ethyl cellulose:DR ratio with a 1.0% polysorbate 80 content. In terms of diameter, the microparticles averaged 85.83 μm. Approximately 62.9 ± 0.52% of the microparticles' propolis could be trapped. Creating propolis aqueous dosage forms using these ethyl cellulose microparticles would be beneficial since they avoid PE's harsh and disagreeable taste, aromatic odor, and high ethanol content [19, 20].

Pharmaceutical formulations used to treat oral mucosal illnesses included gelatin, ethanolic propolis extract (PE), poloxamer 407, or carbopol 934P. Specific gravity, pH, weight of dry residue, and total flavonoid content were used to evaluate the quality of the generated PE. We created mono-polymeric and binary polymeric formulations and examined their mucoadhesion, pH, gelling temperature (Tsol/gel), and continuous flow rheology. Information gathered about these formulations suggests that they might help treat illnesses affecting the oral mucosa [21].

7.5 Antibacterial and Antiseptic Properties of Propolis

The disc diffusion approach stands out among the many prominent techniques used to test antibacterial activity. To test for antimicrobial activity, agar plates are infected with a suspension of a sensitive indicator microbe by spreading it evenly over the surface. Then, blank paper discs holding the sample are put on top. Measurements of the circumference of growth inhibition zones in the agar layer surrounding the disc assess antibacterial activity following an incubation period at the ideal temperature [22]. According to these authors, the solubility and, by extension, the diffusivity of the individual components in agar make this laborious method a poor choice for comparing bioactivities. Instead, they recommend the dilution method, which is widely used for the same purpose and yields more reliable results. Using a variety of concentrations, propolis samples are diluted twofold sequentially and then introduced to a set amount of liquid or solid media. Every experimental condition is supplemented with bacterial inoculums, and after incubation under ideal circumstances, the presence of growth is examined. When comparing propolis extracts, broth microdilution is an appropriate approach since it allows for the quick and simultaneous screening of several samples and produces more consistent findings.

Furthermore, it enables the calculation of the minimal bactericidal concentration (MBC) and the minimal inhibitory concentration (MIC), which are the concentrations at which bacteria can be seen to proliferate and die, respectively [19, 22–27]. The microbe whose sensitivity will be evaluated is coated with agar solutions on top of the thin-layer chromatography plates from which the propolis samples were eluted. After incubation, the antibacterial activity may be seen as distinct patches [28].

Research on the antibacterial effects of propolis has shown that it mainly kills Gram-positive bacteria, with only weak or nonexistent effects against Gram-negative bacteria when tested in low concentrations [29–35]. Based on their testing of propolis samples from various geographic locations (both tropical and temperate zones) against *Staphylococcus aureus* and *Escherichia coli*, Kujumgiev et al. [36] found similar findings. The 12 samples examined had the same impact, and all had strong antibacterial properties against *S. aureus* but no effect against *E. coli*. It is worth noting that the samples came from diverse places.

7.5.1 Anti-inflammatory Activity

Various viruses, damaged cells, irritants, free radicals, and other potentially damaging stimuli can trigger the intricate biological reaction known as inflammation in vascular tissues. The host defense system's principal effect is anti-inflammatory action. Almeida and Menezes evaluated the research on propolis's anti-inflammatory effects. Propolis inhibits the activity of many enzymes found in guinea pig mast cells, including myeloperoxidase, NADPH-oxidase, ornithine decarboxylase, tyrosine-protein-kinase, and hyaluronidase. Flavonoids and cinnamic acid derivatives, which are active, are responsible for this anti-inflammatory action. The first group comprises acacetin, quercetin, and naringenin; the second includes CA and CA phenyl ester [37]. Typical components of poplar propolis, such as CAPE and galangin, have anti-inflammatory properties and have been shown to considerably reduce inflammations caused by carrageenan in rats, including edema, pleurisy, and adjuvant arthritis [38, 39]. In laboratory and animal studies, an ethanol extract of propolis reduced the production of prostaglandins and leukotrienes by zymosan-induced acute peritoneal inflammation and peritoneal macrophages from mice. During inflammation in vivo, dietary propolis significantly inhibited the lipoxygenase pathway of arachidonic acid metabolism. Among the three compounds tested, CAPE had the most significant impact on arachidonic acid metabolism [40].

7.5.2 Impact on Immunomodulation

A water-soluble propolis derivative (WSD) was studied for its immunomodulatory effects. Experimental infections in mice with bacterial (*Klebsiella pneumoniae*, *Staphylococcus aureus*) and fungal (*Candida albicans*) pathogens were found to be facilitated by WSD, whether administered orally or intravenously. Even *Klebsiella pneumoniae* infections caused by cyclophosphamide therapy showed signs of enhanced resistance. In vitro, interleukin-1 production by peritoneal macrophages was boosted by the WSD, which was correlated with their increased total protein secretion. Furthermore, the popliteal lymph node test showed that WSD did not induce lymphocyte proliferation. As a means to enhance the host's nonspecific defenses, the WSD was proposed to activate macrophages [41].

7.5.3 Dental Care

The agar dilution method was used to determine the minimum inhibitory concentrations (MICs) and minimum bactericidal concentrations (MBCs) of EEP on the growth of test microorganisms. Five propolis samples were collected from four regions in Turkey and Brazil and tested for their antimicrobial activity against nine anaerobic strains. The MIC values for propolis activity varied from 4 to 512 mg/mL, and all strains were sensitive. The tested microorganisms had the most effective MIC values when exposed to propolis from Kazan-Ankara. Kazan-Ankara EEP samples had MBC values between 8 and 512 mg/mL. Within 4 h of incubation, *Peptostreptococcus* anaerobic and micros, *Lactobacillus acidophilus*, and *Actinomyces naeslundii* died; *Prevotella oralis*, *Prevotella melaninogenica*, and *Porphyromonas gingivalis* died 8 hours later; *Fusobacterium nucleatum* died 12 hours later; and *Veillonella parvula* died 16 hours later. Research has demonstrated that propolis samples more effectively targeted Gram-positive anaerobic bacteria than Gram-negative ones. As shown by GC-MS analysis, propolis includes aromatic acids such as caffeic acid as well as flavonoids including pinobanksin, quercetin, naringenin, galangin, and chrysin, which are utilized in the treatment of oral cavity illnesses [42].

The infectious condition known as dental caries is a significant issue in public health across the globe. *Streptococcus mutans*, *Streptococcus sobrinus*, and members of the *Actinomyces* and *Lactobacillus* genera are among the bacteria that cause this disease. As antibiotic resistance increases, the pharmaceutical industry is refocusing its efforts on finding new antibacterial drugs. The researchers looked at how the bacterium *Lactobacillus fermentum* responded to ethanolic propolis extracts. Following growing microbiological samples from cavities of patients diagnosed with dental caries and with indications of tooth extraction, this bacterium was isolated following its identification by polymerase chain reaction using species-specific primers. The presence of *L. fermentum* was identified in 9 out of 40 cases, or 22%. The microplate dilution susceptibility test revealed that the ethanolic propolis extract has antibacterial action. The results indicated that these polyphenols varied from 9 ± 0.3 to 85 ± 2.1 mg/mL. The following compounds were identified by chromatographic analysis: caffeic acid, myricetin, quercetin, kaempferol, apigenin, pinocembrin, galangin, and caffeic acid phenethyl ester [43].

References

1. McDonnell G, Russell AD. Antiseptics and disinfectants: activity, action, and resistance. Clin Microbiol Rev. 1999;12(1):147–79. https://doi.org/10.1128/CMR.12.1.147. Erratum in: Clin Microbiol Rev 2001 Jan;14(1):227. PMID: 9880479; PMCID: PMC88911.
2. Larson EL. Antiseptics. In: Olmstad RN, editor. APIC infection control & applied epidemiology: principles & practices. St. Louis: Mosby-Year Book, Inc.; 1996. p. 19-1–19-7, G1–G17.
3. Rutala WA. APIC guidelines for selection and use of disinfectants. Am J Infect Control. 1995;23:313–42.
4. Block SS. Historical review. In: Block SS, editor. Disinfection, sterilization, and preservation. 4th ed. Philadelphia: Lea & Febiger; 1991. p. 3–17.
5. Hugo WB. Disinfection mechanisms. In: Russell AD, Hugo WB, Ayliffe GAJ, editors. Principles and practice of disinfection, preservation and sterilization. 3rd ed. Oxford: Blackwell Science; in press.
6. Russell AD, Chopra I. Understanding antibacterial action and resistance. 2nd ed. Chichester: Ellis Horwood; 1996.
7. Russell AD, Furr JR, Maillard J-Y. Microbial susceptibility and resistance to biocides. ASM News. 1997,63.481–7.
8. Russell AD. Antifungal activity of biocides. In: Russell AD, Hugo WB, Ayliffe GAJ, editors. Principles and practice of disinfection, preservation and sterilization. 3rd ed. Oxford: Blackwell Science; in press.

9. Russell AD, Furr JR. Biocides: mechanisms of antifungal action and fungal resistance. Sci Prog. 1996;79:27–48.
10. Maillard J-Y. Mechanisms of viricidal action. In: Russell AD, Hugo WB, Ayliffe GAJ, editors. Principles and practice of disinfection, preservation and sterilization. 3rd ed. Oxford: Blackwell Science; 1998. , in press.
11. Maillard J-Y, Russell AD. Viricidal activity and mechanisms of action of biocides. Sci Prog. 1997;80:287–315.
12. Furr, J. R. Sensitivity of protozoa to disinfection B. Acanthamoeba and contact lens solutions. *In* A. D. Russell, W. B. Hugo, and G. A. J. Ayliffe (ed.), Principles and practice of disinfection, preservation and sterilization, 3rd ed., in press. Blackwell Science, Oxford
13. Taylor, D. M. Inactivation of unconventional agents of the transmissible degenerative encephalopathies. In A. D. Russell, W. B. Hugo, and G. A. J. Ayliffe (ed.), Principles and practice of disinfection, preservation and sterilization, 3rd ed., in press. Blackwell Science, Oxford
14. Brown MRW, Gilbert P. Sensitivity of biofilms to antimicrobial agents. J Appl Bacteriol Symp Suppl. 1993;74:87S–97S.
15. Brown MRW, Williams P. The influence of environment on envelope properties affecting survival of bacteria in infections. Annu Rev Microbial. 1985;39:527–56.
16. Power EGM. Aldehydes as biocides. Prog Med Chem. 1995;34:149–201.
17. Russell AD. Glutaraldehyde: current status and uses. Infect Control Hosp Epidemiol. 1994;15:724–33.
18. Russell AD, Russell NJ. Biocides: activity, action and resistance. Symp Soc Gen Microbiol. 1995;53:327–65.
19. Wagh VD. Propolis: a wonder bees product and its pharmacological potentials. Adv Pharmacol Sci. 2013;2013:308249. https://doi.org/10.1155/2013/308249. Epub 2013 Dec 9. PMID: 24382957; PMCID: PMC3872021
20. Avanço GB, Braschi ML. Preparation and characterization of ethylcellulose microparticles containing propolis. J Basic Appl Sci. 2008;29(2):129–34.
21. Hirata AN, Bruschi ML. Development and characterization of semisolid systems to deliver propolis in the oral cavity. J Basic Appl Sci. 2010;31(1):33–9.
22. Kujumgiev A, Tsvetkova I, Serkedjieva Y, Bankova V, Christov R, Popov S. Antibacterial, antifungal and antiviral activity of propolis of different geographic origin. J Ethnopharmacol. 1999;64(3):235–40.
23. Kumar N, Ahmad MKK, Dang R, Husain A. Antioxidant and antimicrobial activity of propolis from Tamil Nadu zone. J Med Plants Res. 2008;2(12):361–4.
24. Cowan MM. Plant products as antimicrobial agents. Clin Microbiol Rev. 1999;12(4):564–82.
25. Laskar RA, Sk I, Roy N, Begum NA. Antioxidant activity of Indian propolis and its chemical constituents. Food Chem. 2010;122(1):233–7.
26. Roy N, Mondal S, Laskar RA, Basu S, Mandal D, Begum NA. Biogenic synthesis of au and ag nanoparticles by Indian propolis and its constituents. Colloids Surf B. 2010;76(1):317–25.
27. Ugur A, Arslan T. An *in vitro* study on antimicrobial activity of propolis from Mugla province of Turkey. J Med Food. 2004;7(1):90–4.
28. Yaghoubi MJ, Ghorbani G, Soleimanian Zad S, Satari R. Antimicrobial activity of Iranian propolis and its chemical composition. Daru. 2007;15(1):45–8.
29. Marcucci M. Propolis: chemical composition, biological properties and therapeutic activity. Apidologie. 1995;26(2):83–99.
30. Drago L, Mombelli B, De Vecchi E, Fassina MC, Tocalli L, Gismondo MR. *In vitro* antimicrobial activity of propolis dry extract. J Chemother. 2000;12(5):390–5.
31. Sforcin JM, Fernandes A Jr, Lopes CAM, Bankova V, Funari SRC. Seasonal effect on Brazilian propolis antibacterial activity. J Ethnopharmacol. 2000;73(1–2):243–9.
32. Kartal M, Yildiz S, Kaya S, Kurucu S, Topçu G. Antimicrobial activity of propolis samples from two different regions of Anatolia. J Ethnopharmacol. 2003;86(1):69–73.
33. Dobrowolski JW, Vohora SB, Sharma K, Shah SA, Naqvi SAH, Dandiya PC. Antibacterial, antifungal, antiamoebic, antiinflammatory and antipyretic studies on propolis bee products. J Ethnopharmacol. 1991;35(1):77–82.

34. El Fadaly H, El Badrawy EEY. Flavonoids of propolis and their antibacterial activities. *Pakistan journal biological*. Science. 2001;21:204–7.
35. Stepanović S, Antić N, Dakić I, Švabić-Vlahović M. *In vitro* antimicrobial activity of propolis and synergism between propolis and antimicrobial drugs. Microbiol Res. 2003;158(4):353–7.
36. Kujumgiev A, Tsvetkova I, Serkedjieva Y, Bankova V, Christov R, Popov S. Antibacterial, antifungal and antiviral activity of propolis of different geographic origin. J Ethnopharmacol. 1999;64(3):235–40. https://doi.org/10.1016/s0378-8741(98)00131-7.
37. Almeida ECD, Menezes H. Anti-inflammatory activity of propolis extracts: a review 2104. J Venomous Anim Toxin. 2002;8:191–212.
38. Borrelli F, Maffia P, Pinto L, et al. Phytochemical compounds involved in the anti-inflammatory effect of propolis extract. Fitoterapia. 2002;73(1):S53–63.
39. Du Toit K, Buthelezi S, Bodenstein J. Anti-inflammatory and antibacterial profiles of selected compounds found in south African Propolis. S Afr J Sci. 2009;105(11–12):470–2.
40. Mirzoeva OK, Calder PC. The effect of propolis and its components on eicosanoid production during the inflammatory response. Prostaglandins Leukot Essent Fat Acids. 1996;55(6):441–9.
41. Dimov V, Ivanovska N, Popov S, Bankova V. Immunomodulatory action of propolis: IV. Prophylactic activity against gram-negative infections and adjuvant effect of the water-soluble derivative. Vaccine. 1992;10(12):817–23.
42. Koru O, Toksoy F, Acikel CH, et al. *In vitro* antimicrobial activity of propolis samples from different geographical origins against certain oral pathogens. Anaerobe. 2007;13(3–4):140–5.
43. Saavedra N, Barrientos L, Herrera CL, Alvear M, Montenegro G, Salazar LA. Effect of Chilean propolis on cariogenic bacteria lactobacillus fermentum. Ciencia e Investigacion Agraria. 2011;38(1):117–25.

Propolis as an Antibacterial

8

8.1 Introduction

Two levels should be addressed when considering the antibacterial activity of propolis. Two aspects of this are associated: one directly impacting the microbe and the other with stimulation of the immune system, which activates the organism's innate defenses [1, 2]. Adenosine triphosphate (ATP) synthesis, disturbance of membrane potential, and decreased bacterial motility are all inferred effects of propolis based on its action method. It has been found that propolis has a more potent antibacterial effect against Gram-positive bacteria compared to Gram-negative bacteria. The synthesis of hydrolytic enzymes by Gram-negative bacteria and their species-specific outer membrane structure contribute to this phenomenon since they degrade the active components of propolis [3, 4]. One of the many phenolic chemicals in propolis is a prenyl derivative of p-coumaric acid. Brazilian researchers Veiga et al. found that artepillin C concentrations were greater in ethanolic propolis than in hexane extracts. The antimicrobial activity against MRSA *S. aureus* was similarly vigorous in these extracts [5]. Research has shown that artepillin C can inhibit the growth of the anaerobic bacteria *Porphyromonas gingivalis* through membrane blebbing [6]. Additionally, tefillin C has anti-inflammatory actions through nitric oxide [7] and prostaglandin E [2] inhibition and NF-kappaB regulation.

8.2 Antimicrobial Action

The disc diffusion approach stands out among the many prominent techniques used to test antibacterial activity. To test for antimicrobial activity, agar plates are infected with a suspension of a sensitive indicator microbe by spreading it evenly over the surface. Then, blank paper discs holding the sample are put on top. Finding the width of the growth inhibition zones in the agar layer surrounding the disc is one

A. E. Tanuğur Samanci et al., *Propolis: Prevention and Healing Effects in Otorhinolaryngology*, Comprehensive ENT,
https://doi.org/10.1007/978-3-031-68546-0_8

way to measure antibacterial activity after an incubation period at an ideal temperature [8, 9]. According to these authors, the solubility and, by extension, the diffusivity of the individual components in agar make this laborious method a poor choice for comparing bioactivities. Instead, they recommend the dilution method, which is widely used for the same purpose and yields more reliable results. Using a variety of concentrations, propolis samples are diluted twofold sequentially and then introduced to a set amount of liquid or solid media. Every experimental condition is supplemented with bacterial inoculums, and after incubation under ideal circumstances, the presence of growth is examined. When comparing propolis extracts, broth microdilution is an appropriate approach since it allows for the quick and simultaneous screening of several samples and produces more consistent findings.

It also lets you figure out the MIC, which is the lowest concentration that prevents bacteria from growing visibly, and the MBC, which is the lowest concentration that kills bacteria [8, 10–14]. In a nutshell, the microbe whose sensitivity is going to be evaluated is coated with agar solutions on top of the thin-layer chromatography plates from which the propolis samples were eluted. When incubation is done correctly, antibacterial activity is visible as regions of clear color [15].

8.3 Antimicrobial Properties of Propolis

Al-Museiab propolis ethanolic extract's (EEMP) anti-*E. coli* and *Staphylococcus aureus* were more sensitive to EEMP than other Gram-positive and Gram-negative bacteria. In contrast, standard *E. coli*, Salmonella typhi, *Listeria monocytogenes*, *Helicobacter pylori*, *Streptococcus pyogenes*, *Pseudomonas aeruginosa*, *Staphylococcus aureus*, *Klebsiella pneumonia*, and *Enterobacter aerogenes* were isolated using the disc diffusion and agar well diffusion methods. The coli strain exhibited a far higher sensitivity to EEMP than other Gram-negative bacteria. Findings from disc diffusion techniques using a 10% concentration of crude EEMP demonstrated that while *Staphylococcus aureus* showed high sensitivity to EEMP inhibition, *C. albicans* did not budge. At a 10% concentration, statistical analysis revealed significant differences ($P < 0.05$) between the disc and agar diffusion techniques of EEP; however, at 20% and 30% concentrations of extract, respectively, no significant differences ($p \leq 0.05$) were seen [16].

Ethanol extracts from propolis (EEP) halted the development of *S. aureus*, according to Furth Grange and Davey. *Staphylococcus aureus*, *Enterococcus* spp., *Bacillus cereus*, *Pseudomonas aeruginosa*, and *Escherichia coli*. E. coli development, but had no impact on *Klebsiella pneumoniae* [17]. It is believed that the synergistic action of phenolic and other chemicals in propolis, particularly the flavonoids pinocembrin, galangin, and pinobanksin [17, 18], is responsible for its antibacterial action. There was a more pronounced effect on the proliferation of Gram-positive bacteria [19]. The antimicrobial activity was seen in a variety of microorganisms, including *Staphylococcus aureus* [20, 21], *Streptococcus pyogenes* [22], *Candida* [23], *Streptococcus mutans* [24], anaerobic bacteria of the human oral cavity [25], *Salmonella* [26], and other miscellaneous microorganisms, including *Mycobacterium*

[27]. Screening studies were conducted at a dilution of 1:20 (3 mg of solid material per mL) in nutrient agar, suggesting a preferential inhibitory effect on cocci and Gram-positive rods [8, 28].

Similar antibacterial action is exhibited by other prenyl derivatives identified in propolis, including 3-prenyl-cinnamic acid allyl ester and 2-dimethyl-8-prenylchromene [29]. This means for treating skin infections caused by microorganisms like *S. aureus* [30] could cause kaempferide. Propolis ethanolic extract with high levels of kaempferide, artepillin C, drupanin, and p-coumaric acid has shown antibacterial and antioxidant properties against *S. aureus, S. saprophyticus, Listeria monocytogenes and E. faecalis* [31].

Pinocembrin and apigenin are two other flavonoids that may be found in propolis. In their investigation of Chilean propolis, Veloz et al. discovered that the antibacterial properties of these two compounds were more potent than those of a polyphenol mixture or chlorhexidine, with minimum inhibitory concentrations (MICs) of 1.4 μg/mL and 1.3 μg/mL, respectively, against *Streptococcus mutans* [32]. Isolated pinocembrin has shown antibacterial action against *S. mutans, S. sobrinus, S. aureus, E. faecalis, L. monocytogenes, Pseudomonas aeruginosa and K. pneumoniae* [33–36]. Isolated apigenin acts against Gram-negative bacteria: *P. aeruginosa, K. pneumoniae*, *Salmonella enterica* serotype Typhimurium, *Proteus mirabilis* and *Enterobacter aerogenes* [37]. It was also shown that apigenin and β-lactam antibiotics have a synergistic antibacterial activity when used against methicillin-resistant *S. aureus* (MRSA) [38] and ceftazidime-resistant *Enterobacter cloacae* [39] when combined with apigenin.

Aromatic carboxylic acids like cinnamic acid and its derivatives are abundant in nature, mostly in plants. You may find them in blooms and the verdant inside of plants. Being mostly plant secretions, propolis is an excellent source of cinnamic acid and esters. Numerous studies have shown that cinnamic acid is effective against various types of bacteria, including *Aeromonas* spp., *Vibrio* spp., *E. coli, L. monocytogenes, Mycobacterium tuberculosis, Bacillus* spp., *Staphylococcus* spp. *Streptococcus pyogenes, Micrococcus flavus, P. aeruginosa, S. enterica serotype Typhimurium, Enterobacter cloacae and Yersinia ruckeri* [40–42]. Cinnamic acid and its derivatives hinder bacterial growth by interfering with ATPases, cell division, and biofilm formation. Furthermore, they exhibited anti-quorum sensing properties [1, 43].

Among propolis's numerous intriguing components include terpenoid lupeol and flavonoids such as quercetin, chrysin, kaempferol, fisetin, and decanoic acids, namely 10-hydroxyl-2-decanoic acid [44]. Park et al. found that lipases effectively reduced fatty acid levels in propolis extract in their Korean study. Both the beeswax and the resins that make up propolis are naturally hydrophobic. Utilizing fat-degrading enzymes enhances the process of extracting and isolating beneficial chemicals in propolis, perhaps leading to increased use. The lysozyme TL IM response enhances the antimicrobial effect against *Propionibacterium acnes* and *Staphylococcus epidermldis* [45].

An alternate, nonalcoholic mixture of solvents, such as polyethylene glycol 400 (PEG), water, and olive oil, was used to generate propolis extracts, which Kubiliene et al. compared in terms of composition and biological activity. They found no significant changes when comparing the overall concentration of phenolic chemicals with ethanolic extracts. However, there needed to be more specificity in determining various chemicals. Naringenin, galangin, and kaempferol were observed in PEG-water solutions. The extraction of ferulic acid, caffeic acid, p-coumaric acid, quercetin, and artepillin C was made possible by adding PEG and exposing it to higher temperatures. A mixture of water, oil, and PEG generated a nonalcoholic propolis extract. This extract exhibited equal or greater antibacterial activity against *S. aureus*, *B. cereus*, *P. aeruginosa*, *E. coli*, and finally EEP [46].

The antibacterial activity of propolis extracts has recently been assessed by determining the total phenolic (TP) and flavonoid (FP) content. Antimicrobial activity in vitro is not necessarily accurately reflected by TP and FP assays, according to Bridi et al. The TP findings showed a clear correlation between the amount of flavonoids and antioxidant capabilities in the samples with the greatest and lowest concentrations. However, they were not crystal clear when it came to antibacterial action. When deciding on global quality standards for propolis, further tests like antibacterial and oxygen radical absorbance capacity (ORAC) should be considered [47].

If other bee products and propolis also have antibacterial properties, then using them together should make them much more potent. Such reliance was investigated by Al-Waili et al. utilizing a mixture of honey and propolis sourced from Saudi Arabia and Egypt. According to this study's results, the antibacterial action of propolis and honey is amplified for both *S. aureus* and *E. coli*. The impact on the MIC value was nearly double that of Saudi propolis, indicating a considerable effect. More activity in Egyptian raw materials needs to be done [48].

Few studies have examined how propolis affects anaerobic microorganisms. Nevertheless, the results of this study show that this bee product is highly effective against several types of bacteria, including *Clostridium*, *Bacteroides*, *Porphyromonas*, *Prevotella*, *Fusobacterium*, *Actinomyces*, and *Propionibacterium* [49–52]. Research out of Poland found that modest amounts of ethanolic extract from propolis (EEP) (0.01–0.06 mg/mL) were particularly effective against anaerobic bacteria belonging to the *Fusobacterium* group. On the other hand, at concentrations of 1–3 mg/mL, EEP was toxic to bacteria belonging to the genera *Actinomyces*, *Bacteroides*, *Clostridium*, *Peptococcus*, *Peptostreptococcus*, and *Propionibacterium* [53–55].

There is substantial evidence in the scientific literature that propolis has antibacterial characteristics [56]. A study of the data on the effects of propolis on about 600 aerobic and anaerobic bacterial strains (57 in total) was recently conducted by Przybyłek and Karpiński (2019). In that study, you may find information on specific bacterial species that are susceptible to propolis activity and values for the least inhibitory concentration (the concentration at which no microorganism growth is seen in the tests) [57]. According to many research, propolis has a stronger antibacterial effect against bacteria that are Gram-positive rather than Gram-negative [57–59]. One possible explanation for the discrepancy is that Gram-negative bacteria include bacterial hydrolytic enzymes in their outer membranes. These enzymes might break down the active components of propolis, making them less effective [60, 61].

The phenolic and flavonoid content of propolis is often believed to be responsible for its putative antibacterial capabilities. Antimicrobial activity in vitro is not always proportional to the concentration of those components, as demonstrated by Bridi et al. (2015) [62]. Hence, alternative methods of determining the biological activity of propolis should be considered. One of propolis's properties that helps prevent bacterial resistance from forming is its multitude of active components, which can be found in varied combinations and amounts [63].

Furthermore, it seems that propolis's antibacterial characteristics are influenced by its composition, which in turn is influenced by its geographical origin [64, 65]. Specifically, research has shown that Middle Eastern propolis is the most effective against Gram-positive and Gram-negative bacteria, whereas Korean, Irish, and German propolis is the least effective [57]. Propolis has an antibacterial effect and enhances the efficiency of conventional antibiotics and other natural products, such as honey, when used together [56, 66–68].

8.4 Antimicrobial Action Mechanisms of Propolis

In terms of how it kills bacteria, propolis can disrupt their ability to cause disease by making their cell membranes more permeable, reducing their mobility, disrupting their membrane potential, and preventing them from making RNA and DNA [57, 58]. The compositional complexity of propolis makes it impossible to pinpoint the exact mechanism that is responsible for each of its many effects. Research aims to compare the effects of various components or combinations of components to those of unfractionated propolis extracts by comparing the results. A wide variety of metabolic pathways may be responsible for propolis's antibacterial effects. Both the vast literature on the subject and more recent studies have provided summaries of these topics [57–59]. Consequently, this essay will center on research that showcases some fresh perspectives on the subject.

The biological activity of propolis can be attributed to both biochemical routes and physical mechanisms, according to a recent research [69]. Exclusion zone (EZ) water is the result of propolis being applied to a surface; this layer effectively blocks the passage of colloidal particles. Many chemical components of propolis contain negatively charged functional groups, which are essential to the electrokinetic mechanism upon which the phenomenon is founded [69, 70]. The colloid-excluding characteristic is thus highly general and is not particularly sensitive to the specifics of the propolis's composition or geography. Physically speaking, any bacterium or virus that is floating in a solution of water (such as in our own bodily fluids or on the mucosal lining) is considered a colloidal particle. A physical barrier in the shape of EZ may be created by propolis, which means that it can inhibit infections from entering surfaces (such as respiratory epithelium) [69].

Textiles functionalized with propolis have antibacterial qualities and have medicinal applications (e.g., as wound dressings) according to a small number of recent research [71–73]. When chemically attached to cotton fibers, propolis in one instance lasted after many washes [71]. The so-called disc diffusion approach allowed for the observation of a bacteria-free zone next to the propolis-functionalized fabric. Since this process does not need chemical (contact) interaction with bacteria, EZ might be produced even while the diffusion of constrained propolis components is highly unlikely. It was also proposed that other EZ-generating materials might serve as the initial barrier against surface-colonizing microbes, such as in healthcare settings [74].

Taking into account further physicochemical features of propolis, its chemical components include both mobile protons and fixed negative charges. Propolis gets its acidic pH [75] from the diffusible protons, which have positive charges. It is known that cationic drugs can decrease the negative charges on bacterial cells, increase the permeability of their membranes, and ultimately cause the cell death of the bacteria [76]. Due to their more receptive surface charge and greater sensitivity to mobile protons, Gram-positive bacteria may be more susceptible to the bactericidal effects of propolis than Gram-negative bacteria. Additional research is needed to validate this association, but it might be useful for screening and isolating propolis samples with stronger bactericidal action against Gram-negative bacteria [56].

References

1. Przybyłek I, Karpiński TM. Antibacterial properties of Propolis. Molecules. 2019a;24(11):2047. https://doi.org/10.3390/molecules24112047. PMID: 31146392; PMCID: PMC6600457.
2. Sforcin JM, Bankova V. Propolis: is there a potential for the development of new drugs? J Ethnopharmacol. 2011a;133:253–60. https://doi.org/10.1016/j.jep.2010.10.032.
3. Sforcin JM. Biological properties and therapeutic applications of propolis. Phytother Res. 2016;30:894–905. https://doi.org/10.1002/ptr.5605.
4. Kędzia B, Hołderna-Kędzia E. Aktywność antybiotyczna propolisu krajowego i europejskiego. The antibiotic activity of native and European propolis. Post Fitoter. 2013;2:97–107.
5. Veiga RS, De Mendonça S, Mendes PB, Paulino N, Mimica MJ, Lagareiro Netto AA, Marcucci MC. Artepillin C and phenolic compounds responsible for antimicrobial and antioxidant activity of green propolis and *Baccharis dracunculifolia* DC. J Appl Microbiol. 2017;122:911–20. https://doi.org/10.1111/jam.13400.
6. Yoshimasu Y, Ikeda T, Sakai N, Yagi A, Hirayama S, Morinaga Y, Furukawa S, Nakao R. Rapid bactericidal action of propolis against *Porphyromonas gingivalis*. J Dent Res. 2018;97:928–36. https://doi.org/10.1177/0022034518758034.
7. Paulino N, Abreu SRL, Uto Y, Koyama D, Nagasawa H, Hori H, Dirsch VM, Vollmar AM, Scremin A, Bretz WA. Anti-inflammatory effects of a bioavailable compound, artepillin C, in Brazilian propolis. Eur J Pharmacol. 2008;587:296–301. https://doi.org/10.1016/j.ejphar.2008.02.067.
8. Wagh VD. Propolis: a wonder bees product and its pharmacological potentials. Adv Pharmacol Sci. 2013;2013:308249. https://doi.org/10.1155/2013/308249. Epub 2013 Dec 9. PMID: 24382957; PMCID: PMC3872021
9. Kujumgiev A, Tsvetkova I, Serkedjieva Y, Bankova V, Christov R, Popov S. Antibacterial, antifungal and antiviral activity of propolis of different geographic origin. J Ethnopharmacol. 1999;64(3):235–40.
10. Kumar N, Ahmad MKK, Dang R, Husain A. Antioxidant and antimicrobial activity of propolis from Tamil Nadu zone. J Med Plants Res. 2008;2(12):361–4.

11. Cowan MM. Plant products as antimicrobial agents. Clin Microbiol Rev. 1999;12(4):564–82.
12. Laskar RA, Sk I, Roy N, Begum NA. Antioxidant activity of Indian propolis and its chemical constituents. Food Chem. 2010;122(1):233–7.
13. Roy N, Mondal S, Laskar RA, Basu S, Mandal D, Begum NA. Biogenic synthesis of Au and Ag nanoparticles by Indian propolis and its constituents. Colloids Surf B. 2010;76(1):317–25.
14. Ugur A, Arslan T. An *in vitro* study on antimicrobial activity of propolis from Mugla province of Turkey. J Med Food. 2004;7(1):90–4.
15. Yaghoubi MJ, Ghorbani G, Soleimanian Zad S, Satari R. Antimicrobial activity of Iranian propolis and its chemical composition. Daru. 2007;15(1):45–8.
16. Hendi NKK, Naher HS, Al-Charrakh AH. *In vitro* antibacterial and antifungal activity of Iraqi propolis. J Med Plant Res. 2011;5(20):5058–66.
17. Castaldo S, Capasso F. Propolis, an old remedy used in modern medicine. Fitoterapia. 2002;73(1):S1–6.
18. Krol W, Scheller S, Shani J, Pietsz G, Czuba Z. Synergistic effect of ethanolic extract of propolis and antibiotics on the growth of *Staphylococcus aureus*. Arzneimittel-Forschung/Drug Res. 1993;43(5):607–9.
19. Burdock GA. Review of the biological properties and toxicity of bee propolis (propolis). Food Chem Toxicol. 1998;36(4):347–63.
20. Fernandes A, Balestrin ECD, Cunha MLRS. Anti-Staphylococcus aureus activity of bee propolis extracts prepared with different ethanol concentrations. Farm Sci Rev. 2003;24:147–52.
21. Popova M, Bankova V, Tsvetkova I, Kujumgiev A. Comparative study of the biological activity of propolis from different geographic origin: a statistical approach. Macedonian Pharmaceut Bull. 2004;50:9–14.
22. Bosio K, Avanzini C, D'Avolio A, Ozino O, Savoia D. *In vitro* activity of propolis against *streptococcus pyogenes*. Lett Appl Microbiol. 2000;31(2):174–7.
23. Drago L, Mombelli B, De Vecchi E, Fassina MC, Tocalli L, Gismondo MR. In vitro antimicrobial activity of propolis dry extract. J Chemother. 2000;12(5):390–5.
24. Selvan A, Singh R, Prabhu D. Research article: anti-bacteria activity of bee propolis against clinical strains of streptococcus mutants and synergism with chlorhexidine. Int J Pharmaceut Stud Res. 2011;2:85–90.
25. Santos FA, Bastos EMA, Uzeda M, et al. Antibacterial activity of Brazilian propolis and fractions against oral anaerobic bacteria. J Ethnopharmacol. 2002;80(1):1–7.
26. Orsi RO, Sforcin JM, Rall VLM, Funari SRC, Barbosa L, Fernandes A. Susceptibility profile of salmonella against the antibacterial activity of propolis produced in two regions of Brazil. J Venomous Anim Toxins Includ Trop Dis. 2005;11:109–16.
27. Benkovic V, Horvat Knezevic A, Dikic D, et al. Radioprotective effects of propolis and quercetin in γ-irradiated mice evaluated by the alkaline comet assay. Phytomedicine. 2008;15(10):851–8.
28. Grange JM, Davey RW. Antibacterial properties of propolis (bee glue). J R Soc Med. 1990;83(3):159–60.
29. Viuda-Martos M, Ruiz-Navajas Y, Fernández-López J, Pérez-Álvarez JA. Functional properties of honey, propolis, and royal jelly. J Food Sci. 2008;73:R117–24. https://doi.org/10.1111/j.1750-3841.2008.00966.x.
30. Guz NR, Stermitz FR, Johnson JB, Beeson TD, Willen S, Hsiang JF, Lewis K. Flavonolignan and flavone inhibitors of a *Staphylococcus aureus* multidrug resistance pump: structure-activity relationships. J Med Chem. 2001;44:261–8. https://doi.org/10.1021/jm0004190.
31. Seibert JB, Bautista-Silva JP, Amparo TR, Petit A, Pervier P, Dos Santos Almeida JC, Azevedo MC, Silveira BM, Brandão GC, de Souza GHB, et al. Development of propolis nanoemulsion with antioxidant and antimicrobial activity for use as a potential natural preservative. Food Chem. 2019;287:61–7. https://doi.org/10.1016/j.foodchem.2019.02.078.
32. Veloz JJ, Alvear M, Salazar LA. Antimicrobial and antibiofilm activity against *Streptococcus mutans* of individual and mixtures of the main polyphenolic compounds found in Chilean propolis. Biomed Res Int. 2019;2019:7602343. https://doi.org/10.1155/2019/7602343.

33. Soromou LW, Zhang Y, Cui Y, Wei M, Chen N, Yang X, Huo M, Baldé A, Guan S, Deng X, et al. Subinhibitory concentrations of pinocembrin exert anti-*Staphylococcus aureus* activity by reducing α-toxin expression. J Appl Microbiol. 2013;115:41–9. https://doi.org/10.1111/jam.12221.
34. Joray MB, Trucco LD, González ML, Napal GN, Palacios SM, Bocco JL, Carpinella MC. Antibacterial and cytotoxic activity of compounds isolated from *Flourensia oolepis*. Evid Based Complement Alternat Med. 2015;2015:912484. https://doi.org/10.1155/2015/912484.
35. Hernández Tasco AJ, Ramírez Rueda RY, Alvarez CJ, Sartori FT, Sacilotto ACBC, Ito IY, Vichnewski W, Salvador MJ. Antibacterial and antifungal properties of crude extracts and isolated compounds from *Lychnophora markgravii*. Nat Prod Res. 2018:1–5. https://doi.org/10.1080/14786419.2018.1503263.
36. Kharsany K, Viljoen A, Leonard C, van Vuuren S. The new buzz: investigating the antimicrobial interactions between bioactive compounds found in south African propolis. J Ethnopharmacol. 2019;238:111867. https://doi.org/10.1016/j.jep.2019.111867.
37. Nayaka HB, Londonkar RL, Umesh MK, Tukappa A. Antibacterial attributes of apigenin, isolated from *Portulaca oleracea* L. Int J Bacteriol. 2014;2014:175851. https://doi.org/10.1155/2014/175851.
38. Akilandeswari K, Ruckmani K. Synergistic antibacterial effect of apigenin with β-lactam antibiotics and modulation of bacterial resistance by a possible membrane effect against methicillin resistant *Staphylococcus aureus*. Cell Mol Biol. 2016;62:74–82. https://doi.org/10.14715/cmb/2016.62.14.13.
39. Eumkeb G, Chukrathok S. Synergistic activity and mechanism of action of ceftazidime and apigenin combination against ceftazidime-resistant *Enterobacter cloacae*. Phytomedicine. 2013;20:262–9. https://doi.org/10.1016/j.phymed.2012.10.008.
40. Heleno SA, Ferreira IC, Esteves AP, Ćirić A, Glamočlija J, Martins A, Soković M, Queiroz MJ. Antimicrobial and demelanizing activity of *Ganoderma lucidum* extract, p-hydroxybenzoic and cinnamic acids and their synthetic acetylated glucuronide methyl esters. Food Chem Toxicol. 2013;58:95–100. https://doi.org/10.1016/j.fct.2013.04.025.
41. Guzman JD. Natural cinnamic acids, synthetic derivatives and hybrids with antimicrobial activity. Molecules. 2014;19:19292–349. https://doi.org/10.3390/molecules191219292.
42. Yilmaz S, Sova M, Ergün S. Antimicrobial activity of trans-cinnamic acid and commonly used antibiotics against important fish pathogens and nonpathogenic isolates. J Appl Microbiol. 2018;125:1714–27. https://doi.org/10.1111/jam.14097.
43. Vasconcelos NG, Croda J, Simionatto S. Antibacterial mechanisms of cinnamon and its constituents: a review. Microb Pathog. 2018;120:198–203. https://doi.org/10.1016/j.micpath.2018.04.036.
44. Pasupuleti VR, Sammugam L, Ramesh N, Gan SH. Honey, propolis and royal jelly: a comprehensive review of their biological actions and health benefits. Oxidative Med Cell Longev. 2017;2017:1259510. https://doi.org/10.1155/2017/1259510.
45. Park H, Bae SH, Choi H, Suh HJ. Lipase-mediated lipid removal from propolis extract and its antiradiacal and antimicrobial activity. J Sci Food Agric. 2015;95:1697–705. https://doi.org/10.1002/jsfa.6874.
46. Kubiliene L, Laugaliene V, Pavilonis A, Maruska A, Majiene D, Barcauskaite K, Kunilus R, Kasparaviciene G, Savickas A. Alternative preparation of propolis extracts: comparison of their composition and biological activities. Compl Altern Med. 2015;15:156. https://doi.org/10.1186/s12906-015-0677-5.
47. Bridi R, Montenegro G, Nuñez-Quijada G, Giordano A, Morán-Romero FM, Jara-Pezoa I, Speisky H, Atala E, López-Alarcón C. International regulations of propolis quality: required assays do not necessarily reflect their polyphenolic-related in vitro activities. J Food Sci. 2015a;80:C1188–95. https://doi.org/10.1111/1750-3841.12881.
48. Al-Waili N, Al-Ghamdi A, Ansari MJ, Al-Attal Y, Salom K. Synergistic effects of honey and propolis toward drug multi-resistant *Staphylococcus aureus*, *Escherichia coli* and *Candida albicans* isolates in single and polymicrobial cultures. Int J Med Sci. 2012a;9:793–800. https://doi.org/10.7150/ijms.4722.

49. Boyanova L, Kolarov R, Gergova G, Mitov I. In vitro activity of Bulgarian propolis against 94 clinical isolates of anaerobic bacteria. Anaerobe. 2006;12:173–7. https://doi.org/10.1016/j.anaerobe.2006.06.001.
50. Ferreira FB, Torres SA, Rosa OP, Ferreira CM, Garcia RB, Marcucci MC, Gomes BP. Antimicrobial effect of propolis and other substances against selected endodontic pathogens. Oral Surg Oral Med Oral Pathol Oral Radiol Endod. 2007;104:709–16. https://doi.org/10.1016/j.tripleo.2007.05.019.
51. Koru O, Toksoy F, Acikel CH, Tunca YM, Baysallar M, Uskudar GA, Akca E, Ozkok TA, Sorkun K, Tanyuksel M, et al. In vitro antimicrobial activity of propolis samples from different geographical origins against certain oral pathogens. Anaerobe. 2007;13:140–5. https://doi.org/10.1016/j.anaerobe.2007.02.001.
52. Shabbir A, Rashid M, Tipu HN. Propolis, a hope for the future in treating resistant periodontal pathogens. Cureus. 2016;8:e682. https://doi.org/10.7759/cureus.682.
53. Kędzia A. Działanie wyciągu etanolowego z propolisu na bakterie beztlenowe. Herba Pol. 1986;32:53–7.
54. Kędzia A, Kałowski M. Ocena skuteczności działania wyciągu etanolowego z propolisu na bakterie bezwzględnie beztlenowe jamy ustnej. Czas Stomat. 1988;41:757–62.
55. Kędzia A. Wrażliwość bakterii bezwzględnie beztlenowych na wyciąg etanolowy z propolisu. Herba Pol. 1988;34:267–72.
56. Zulhendri F, Chandrasekaran K, Kowacz M, Ravalia M, Kripal K, Fearnley J, Perera CO. Antiviral, antibacterial, antifungal, and Antiparasitic properties of Propolis: a review. Food Secur. 2021;10(6):1360. https://doi.org/10.3390/foods10061360.
57. Przybyłek I, Karpiński TM. Antibacterial properties of propolis. Molecules. 2019b;24:2047.
58. Almuhayawi MS. Propolis as a novel antibacterial agent. Saudi J Biol Sci. 2020;27:3079–86.
59. Silva-Carvalho R, Baltazar F, Almeida-Aguiar C. Propolis: a complex natural product with a plethora of biological activities that can be explored for drug development. Evid Based Complement Alternat Med. 2015;2015:1.
60. Sforcin JM, Bankova V. Propolis: is there a potential for the development of new drugs? J Ethnopharmacol. 2011b;133:253–60.
61. Bogdan Kędzia EH-K. Aktywność antybiotyczna propolisu krajowego i europejskiego. The antibiotic activity of native and European propolis. Postępy Fitoter. 2013;2:97–107.
62. Bridi R, Montenegro G, Nuñez-Quijada G, Giordano A, Fernanda Morán-Romero M, Jara-Pezoa I, Speisky H, Atala E, López-Alarcón C. International regulations of propolis quality: required assays do not necessarily reflect their polyphenolic-related in vitro activities. J Food Sci. 2015b;80:C1188–95.
63. Pamplona-Zomenhan LC, Pamplona BC, da Silva CB, Marcucci MC, Mimica LMJ. Evaluation of the in vitro antimicrobial activity of an ethanol extract of Brazilian classified propolis on strains of Staphylococcus aureus. Braz J Microbiol. 2011;42:1259–64.
64. Ivana Tlak G, Iva P, Mirza B, Ivan K, Siniša S, Toni V, Josipa V. Components responsible for antimicrobial activity of propolis from continental and Mediterranean regions in Croatian. Czech J Food Sci. 2017;35:376–85.
65. Šuran J, Cepanec I, Mašek T, Radić B, Radić S, Tlak Gajger I, Vlainić J. Propolis extract and its bioactive compounds—from traditional to modern extraction technologies. Molecules. 2021;26:2930.
66. Oksuz H, Duran N, Tamer C, Cetin M, Silici S. Effect of propolis in the treatment of experimental Staphylococcus aureus keratitis in rabbits. Ophthalmic Res. 2005;37:328–34.
67. Orsi RO, Fernandes A, Bankova V, Sforcin JM. The effects of Brazilian and Bulgarian propolis in vitro against salmonella Typhi and their synergism with antibiotics acting on the ribosome. Nat Prod Res. 2012;26:430–7.
68. Al-Waili N, Al-Ghamdi A, Ansari MJ, Al-Attal Y, Salom K. Synergistic effects of honey and propolis toward drug multi-resistant staphylococcus aureus, Escherichia coli and Candida Albicans isolates in single and polymicrobial cultures. Int J Med Sci. 2012b;9:793–800.
69. Kowacz M, Pollack GH. Propolis-induced exclusion of colloids: possible new mechanism of biological action. Colloids Interface. Sci Commun. 2020a;38:38.

70. Kowacz M, Pollack GH. Cells in new light: ion concentration, voltage, and pressure gradients across a hydrogel membrane. ACS Omega. 2020b;5:21024–31.
71. Sharaf S, Higazy A, Hebeish A. Propolis induced antibacterial activity and other technical properties of cotton textiles. Int J Biol Macromol. 2013;59:408–16.
72. Abramiuc D, Ciobanu L, Muresan R, Chiosac M, Muresan A. Antibacterial finishing of cotton fabrics using biologically active natural compounds. Fibers Polym. 2013;14:1826–33.
73. Arıkan HK, Solak HH. Propolis extract-PVA nanocomposites of textile design: antimicrobial effect on gram positive and negative bacterias. Int J Second Metab. 2017:218–24.
74. Cheng Y, Moraru CI. Long-range interactions keep bacterial cells from liquid-solid interfaces: evidence of a bacteria exclusion zone near Nafion surfaces and possible implications for bacterial attachment. Colloids Surf B: Biointerfaces. 2018;162:16–24.
75. Dias LG, Pereira AP, Estevinho LM. Comparative study of different Portuguese samples of propolis: Pollinic, sensorial, physicochemical, microbiological characterization and antibacterial activity. Food Chem Toxicol. 2012;50:4246–53.
76. Halder S, Yadav KK, Sarkar R, Mukherjee S, Saha P, Haldar S, Karmakar S, Sen T. Alteration of zeta potential and membrane permeability in bacteria: a study with cationic agents. Springerplus. 2015;4:1–14.

9 Propolis as an Antiviral

9.1 Introduction

Traditional medicine and nutritional supplements have long used propolis, a honeybee resin. However, recent preclinical studies have shown that propolis may have a wide range of therapeutic bioactivities, such as protecting neurons from damage, reducing inflammation, fighting cancer, and preventing the spread of viruses. There is encouraging preclinical evidence that propolis and its constituents can inhibit the growth of several viruses, including adenoviruses, influenza, respiratory tract viruses, herpes simplex virus types 1 and 2, HIV, and SARS-CoV-2. Terpenes, flavonoids, and phenolic acids are only a few of the more than 300 chemical components found in propolis; however, the exact composition varies greatly depending on the place of origin and the flora found there. Through influencing many pathogenic and antiviral pathways, propolis and its components have shown promise as a treatment for SARS-CoV-2 [1].

9.2 Propolis

Honeybee saliva, wax, pollen, and other plant components come together to form propolis, a natural resin that resembles wax made by *Apis mellifera* L. Bees use propolis, a type of cement, to plug holes in their hives. This keeps out parasites and helps keep the beehive at a comfortable temperature and humidity level [2, 3]. The Greek roots of the English words "polis" (meaning "city") and "pro" (meaning "in defense") indicate the significance of propolis in warding off parasites and illnesses as well as halting the progression of bacterial, fungal, and putrefaction [4]. The ancient Egyptians, Greeks, and Romans all attested to propolis's medicinal value, known for thousands of years [5]. London pharmacopeias included propolis as an official medication in the seventeenth century [6], adding to the widespread use of

A. E. Tanuğur Samanci et al., *Propolis: Prevention and Healing Effects in Otorhinolaryngology*, Comprehensive ENT,
https://doi.org/10.1007/978-3-031-68546-0_9

propolis as a remedy for illness over the years. Traditional medicine practitioners often turn to propolis to deal with bacterial and viral infections of the skin and respiratory tract [7]. Health drinks with propolis are still made in particular European, South American, and Asian nations [8]. Also, it is a component of mouthwashes and toothpastes designed to alleviate stomatitis, gingivitis, and cheilitis [9, 10].

Scientific studies have shown that it has several biological actions, including being antibacterial, antifungal, antiulcer, anticancer, wound-healing, immunomodulatory, antimycotic, and anti-inflammatory [11, 12]. In vitro and animal studies have demonstrated that propolis has antiviral properties against various DNA and RNA viruses. These viruses include herpes simplex virus type 1 (HSV-1), an acyclovir-resistant HSV-1 mutant, herpes simplex virus type 2 (HSV-2), adenovirus type 2, vesicular stomatitis virus (VSV), poliovirus type 2 (PV-2) [13, 14], avian influenza virus (H7N7) [15], human rhinoviruses (HRVs) [16], influenza viruses A/HlNl and A/NH3N2 [17], classic coronaviruses [18], and severe acute respiratory syndrome coronavirus 2 (SARS-CoV-2) [19–21]. Propolis comprises various nutrients (intermediate metabolites), bioactive polyphenols (mostly flavonoids and phenolic acids), and wax and essential oils. It also contains 5% pollen and 2% mineral salts. The composition of propolis is as follows: 50% resin, 30% wax, 10% essential oils, 5% pollen, and 2% mineral salts [22, 23]. Some of these chemicals have been extensively studied for their potential antiviral and immunomodulatory effects, and these include kaempferol, p-coumaric acid, apigenin, artepillin C, caffeic acid, and caffeic acid phenyl ester [16, 24, 25].

9.3 Chemical Composition of Propolis

Polyphenolic chemicals, including flavonoids, cinnamic acids, and esters, are abundant in propolis. Extracts from propolis have yielded over 300 distinct compounds, including benzaldehyde derivatives, nicotinic acid, pantothenic acid, chalcones, dihydrochalcones, amino acids, esters, enzymes, ketones, waxy acids, alcohols, fatty acids, and aliphatic hydrocarbons [26]. The active ingredients in propolis differ from one plant species to another and from one region to another [23]. As an example, propolis from the southern Urals (Bashkiria) contained six different flavonoids: pinostrobin, sakuranetin, (2S)-5,4′-dihydroxy-7-methoxyflavanone, pinobanksin-3-acetate, chrysin, 5,7-dihydroxyflavone, and apigenin-7,4′-dimethyl ether [27].

9.4 Antiviral Properties of Propolis

Recent studies have shown that propolis may be effective against SARS-CoV-2, the virus responsible for COVID-19, adding to its long history of usage in treating viral infections [29]. Most viruses that cause illness do not react to the antiviral medications on the market today, and they can develop further strains that are resistant to both treatments and vaccines. Therefore, finding new antiviral candidates is of the utmost importance, especially those derived from natural sources, as these molecules often have low toxicity [28].

The most common viruses that may infect humans are thought to be kinds 1 and 2 of herpes simplex virus (HSV). While herpes simplex virus type 2 is more commonly transmitted sexually and affects the vaginal mucosa, herpes simplex virus type 1 is more common in the mouth and causes blisters that are moist on the skin or mucosa. Resistant virus variants are frequent despite acyclovir's status as a significant antiviral therapy [30]. There was a synergistic effect between acyclovir (the positive control) and propolis from South Turkey (Hatay) at concentrations of 25, 50, and 100 μg/mL, which suppressed the reproduction of both HSV-1 and HSV-2 without harming infected cells [31]. In vitro, antiviral efficacy against acyclovir-resistant HSV was also shown by an ethanolic extract of Brazilian green propolis, which inhibited replication at an early stage of infection [32]. Also, female BALB/c mice were shown to have less epidermal and dermal irritation caused by HSV-2, and a Brazilian hydroalcoholic brown propolis extract (HPE) protected against vaginal lesions [33].

Both water- and alcohol-based propolis extracts demonstrated encouraging antiviral activity in a plaque formation experiment against HSV-1 infection of RC-37 cells. A possible mechanism by which these medicinal effects occur is the masking of viral proteins essential for adsorption or entrance into host cells [34]. When administered at various points throughout the viral infection cycle, both water and alcohol extracts of propolis inhibited HSV-2 growth to an extent similar to that of acyclovir, most likely by obfuscating the viral components that are responsible for entry or adsorption into host cells [35].

Further research on Canadian propolis found that it inhibited the entrance of HSV-2 into Madin-Darby bovine kidney (MDBK) cells and had strong virucidal effects against HSV-1 and -2 [36]. In addition, several strains of PV-2, VSV, and adenovirus type 2 (adeno-2), together with HSV-1, HSV-1-R, and HSV-2, were well inhibited by French propolis. The most effective dosage was 30 μg/mL [28, 37].

The antiviral activities of propolis are effective against several viruses [38]. Chrysin, kaempferol, acacetin, galangin, and quercetin are flavonoids produced from propolis. Debiaggi et al. [18] conducted one of the first investigations on their antiviral properties, testing them against several strains of herpesvirus, adenovirus, rotavirus, and coronavirus [18]. Above all else, research has demonstrated that propolis can inhibit the SARS-CoV-2 virus. When tested against SARS-CoV-2 in vitro, Refaat et al. [39] found that liposomal encapsulated propolis was as effective as remdesivir [39]. Several computational and molecular docking experiments have shown that propolis and its phenolic components effectively interfere with numerous essential SARS-CoV-2 proteins, including proteases and the spike protein [40–43].

Also, propolis does wonders against the illness. The phenolics found in propolis, particularly isopentyl ferulate, showed potent antiviral action against the H3N2 influenza A virus, according to Serkedjieva et al. [17]. Thirteen different ethanolic Brazilian propolis extracts were tested for their antiviral activity against the A/PR/8/34 (H1N1) influenza virus by Shimizu et al. [44]. Each extract exhibited antiviral characteristics, albeit with varying degrees of effectiveness. For instance, one extract (AF-08) mitigated the effects of weight loss and increased the lifespan of sick mice. In lowering the viral load in the bronchoalveolar lavage fluids of the lungs of infected mice, AF-08 extract at a dose of 10 $mg \cdot kg^{-1}$ was nearly as effective as 1 $mg \cdot kg^{-1}$ oseltamivir, an antiviral medication [44].

Influenza A/PR/8/34(H1N1) and influenza A/Toyama/26/2011 (H1N1) viruses, as well as strains of these viruses that are susceptible to or resistant to oseltamivir and peramivir, were all successfully inhibited by the phenolics apigenin, kaempferol, and coumaric acid that were isolated from propolis by Kai et al. [45]. Also, kaempferol increased the infected mice's survival time and decreased the viral load in the bronchoalveolar lavage fluids [45]. In addition, Kuwata et al.'s [46] research showed that propolis water extract might inhibit the growth of influenza A/WSN/33 (H1N1) viruses. Caffeoylquinic acids seemed to be the primary ingredient responsible for the antiviral effects [46]. In a separate study, the same group found that a propolis extract included the anti-influenza molecule 3,4-caffeoylquinic acid [38, 47].

Evidence suggests that propolis may have anti-HIV properties. Triterpenoid moronic acid, derived from Brazilian propolis, suppressed HIV activity in H9 cells [48]. Furthermore, it was shown by Gekker et al. [49] that propolis extracts from several countries and sources, including Brazil, China, and Minnesota (USA), reduced the growth of CD4+ lymphocytes and microglial cell cultures infected with HIV-1 [49]. Above all else, antiretroviral medications like zidovudine and indinavir were not inhibited by propolis [49]. The anti-HIV effect of an ethyl acetate extract of propolis from the northeastern Brazilian state of Ceará was also reported by Silva et al. [50]. The chemicals associated with propolis's antiviral action were phenolics naringenin, quercetin, and diprenylcinnamic acid [50].

If we had to pick one area where propolis's antiviral capabilities have been studied extensively, it would be herpesviruses [38]. Galangin, kaempferol, and quercetin were shown to have anti-herpetic effects by Amoros et al. [13]. Part of propolis's greater effectiveness compared to its separate components was its synergistic interactions between the phenolics generated from it [13]. Also, the chemicals generated from propolis have a synergistic effect, as Schnitzler et al. [51] showed. The anti-herpetic efficacy of propolis aqueous and ethanolic extracts was shown to be superior to that of the individual components, including caffeic acid, p-coumaric acid, benzoic acid, galangin, pinocembrin, and chrysin [51]. Poplar propolis, according to Bankova et al. [52], contains a variety of phenolics that have antiviral properties against herpes simplex virus types 1 and 2 (HSV-1 and -2), including benzoic acid, p-coumaric acid, benzyl p-coumarate, benzyl ferulate, pinocembrin, and pinocembrin chalcone [52].

Stingless bee propolis also has anti-herpetic properties [38]. Coelho et al. [53] demonstrated the antiviral activity against HSV-1 in a hydromethanolic extract of the stingless bee *Scaptotrigona trigona*, which contains C-glycosyl flavones and pyrrolizidine alkaloids [53]. The anti-HSV-1 effects of *Melipona quadrifasciata* propolis were also demonstrated. The mixture of dichloromethane, butanol, and ethyl acetate was particularly effective against herpes [54].

Animal studies have also demonstrated the anti-herpetic efficacy of propolis extract. The herpesvirus may infect mice at different stages. However, Kurokawa et al. [55] found that different propolis extracts inhibited the virus at various stages [55]. Several ethanolic propolis preparations considerably decreased the viral load in the brains and skins of HSV-1-infected mice [55]. Researchers Sartori et al. [56] found that mice infected with HSV-2 had less severe extravaginal lesions and histological damage in the vaginal tissue when given a hydroalcoholic extract (70% ethanol) of propolis [56]. Several viruses, including measles, rhinovirus, dengue, polio, rubella, and picornavirus, are susceptible to propolis's antiviral effects [16, 57, 58].

9.5 How Propolis's Antiviral Properties Work

The possible action mechanisms used by propolis and its components in inactivating SARS-CoV-2 were revealed by molecular docking and in silico research. The 3CL-protease and S1 spike protein of SARS-CoV-2 were both suppressed by rutin and caffeic acid phenethyl ester, as shown by Refaat et al. [59]. The highly conserved residues (substrate-binding pocket) of the Mpro protein of SARS-CoV-2 were likewise demonstrated to be interfered with by caffeic acid phenethyl ester [60]. Molecular docking studies conducted by Sahlan et al. [43] and Dewi et al. [42] showed that compounds derived from propolis, such as Sulabiroins A, (2S)-5,7-dihydroxy-4′-methoxy-8-prenylflavanone acid, glyasperin A, and broussoflavonol F (propolis-derived compounds), can bind to specific residues on the Mpro catalytic sites and so inhibit the activity of the SARS-CoV-2 Mpro protein [42, 43].

Kaempferol and p-coumaric acid were shown by Kwon et al. [16] to suppress viral replication in HeLa cells and to block human rhinovirus entrance [16]. Furthermore, it was shown that ferulic acid, extracted from propolis, inhibits the activity of swine parvovirus [61]. The expression of pro-apoptotic genes Bid, Bad, Bim, and Bak was suppressed and reversed by ferulic acid in response to parvovirus infection. Host cell death and mitochondrial dysfunction have been linked to the expression of these genes [61]. Another finding is that propolis increases the expression of the MX1 gene, which is responsible for myxovirus resistance [62]. The host cell's Mx proteins act as "gatekeepers" against RNA viruses and other groups of viruses that reproduce within the host nucleus [63]. Zinc cation transport across the plasma membrane can be aided by polyphenols even without zinc transport proteins in the plasma membrane [64]. The viral RNA-dependent RNA polymerase can be inhibited by Zn cations [65].

In addition, the viral infection models demonstrated that propolis has immunomodulatory qualities that impact host immunological activities. The 3,4-dicaffeoylquinic acid (3,4-diCQA) component of propolis accelerated viral clearance by increasing the production of tumor necrosis factor-related apoptosis-inducing ligand (TRAIL) [47]. Propolis decreased oxidative stress in the infected host cells by lowering reactive species expression, tyrosine nitration, and myeloperoxidase activity. Infected cells were also shown to have their production of the cellular antioxidant enzyme catalase preserved by propolis [56]. The production of interferon-γ (IFN-γ) was also stimulated by propolis in models of herpes simplex virus infection. The symptoms of viral infections, such as HSV infections, can be alleviated by IFN-γ since it is a significant activator of lymphocyte migration into the skin [55].

Additionally, propolis has shown promise as an in vitro antiviral agent against HIV, the etiological agent of acquired immune deficiency syndrome (AIDS). With over two-thirds of the world's new HIV diagnoses occurring in Africa, the continent is the worst hit, says the World Health Organization (WHO). 4.1% of adult Africans are HIV positive at this time. Several antiretroviral medications can help manage HIV, but they come with significant side effects such as lipodystrophy [66], so new, safer options need to be found. Extracts of propolis from various parts of China and Brazil inhibited viral entry and reverse transcriptase activity, resulting in an 85% reduction in HIV-1 infectivity in CD4+ cell cultures and a 98% reduction in microglial cell cultures [49]. In addition, eight chemicals from Brazilian propolis demonstrated anti-HIV-1 action in H9 lymphocytes. These compounds included four triterpenoids (melliferone, moronic acid, anwuweizonic acid, and betulonic acid) and four aromatic compounds (4-hydroxy-3-methoxypropiophenone, 4-hydroxy-3-methoxybenzaldehyde, 3-(3,4-dimethoxyphenyl)-2-propenal, and 12-acetoxytremetone) [48].

Plaque reduction test results showed that the ethanolic extract of GH 2002 propolis had a substantial antiviral effect against varicella zoster virus (VZV), with an IC50 of 64 μg/mL. Adding propolis extract at various points in the viral infection cycle allowed researchers to identify this antiviral activity. Additionally, during VZV replication, the extract amplified acyclovir's inhibitory effect on viral DNA polymerase. These results prove that propolis's bioactive components can inhibit viral replication and disguise viral proteins, making it harder for the virus to enter host cells [67].

The extraction process determines the antiviral effectiveness, as previously stated. While both ultrasonic extracts showed more activity against bacteriophages MS2 and Av-08 than the maceration extract, a study comparing the antiviral properties of green and red Brazilian propolis extracts using two different methods and maceration found that the maceration extract of red propolis was more active than the corresponding green extract in terms of damaging the viral cell membrane and inhibiting polymerase activity [68]. A recent study indicated that taking an extract from Euro-Asian poplar trees for 4 days might prevent the H1N1 influenza virus from infecting MDCK cells. The therapy reduced viral proliferation and neuraminidase (NA) activity [69]. Using three different human rhinoviruses—HRV-2, HRV-3, and HRV-4—two bioactive components derived from Brazilian propolis, kaempferol and p-coumaric acid, were examined for their ability to prevent HeLa cell infection. Compared to ribavirin (the positive control), kaempferol is the most bioactive molecule, with IC50 values of 7.3, 11.9, and 12.9 μM against HRV-2, HRV-3, and HRV-4, respectively. In contrast, p-coumaric acid demonstrates the least antiviral activity, with IC50 values of 371.2, 454.5, and 604.3 μM. Preliminary research suggests that kaempferol and p-coumaric acid may inhibit virus entrance into host cells, protecting cells against viral reproduction [16].

Researchers in Mexico discovered that when they used propolis to treat MDBK cell monolayers infected with pseudorabies virus (PRV), the treated cells formed an electron-dense layer on their membranes, which blocked the virus's ability to enter [70]. Oral administration to infected mice three times daily for 7 days resulted in antiviral efficacy in vivo; the most effective dose was 10 mg kg^{-1}, and 4 of the 13 ethanolic extracts from South Brazilian propolis showed significant anti-influenza virus activity in vitro [44].

In other studies, the goal was to evaluate the impact of three different materials on poliovirus type 1 (PV1): propolis, *Baccharis dracunculifolia* (essential oil and extract), and two isolated components (caffeic and cinnamic acids). The effects on the virus were evaluated using three protocols: pre-treatment, simultaneous treatment, and post-treatment. Contemporary and post-treatment studies have seen a substantial inhibitory percentage for propolis. As a result of its effects on RNA degradation before viral cell entrance or cell multiplication, propolis partially impacts both phases of the viral life cycle [57].

References

1. Yosri N, Abd El-Wahed AA, Ghonaim R, Khattab OM, Sabry A, Ibrahim MAA, Moustafa MF, Guo Z, Zou X, Algethami AFM, Masry SHD, AlAjmi MF, Afifi HS, Khalifa SAM, El-Seedi HR. Anti-viral and immunomodulatory properties of propolis: chemical diversity, pharmacological properties, preclinical and clinical applications, and in silico potential against SARS-CoV-2. Food Secur. 2021;10(8):1776. https://doi.org/10.3390/foods10081776. PMID: 34441553; PMCID: PMC8391193.
2. Pavlovic R, Borgonovo G, Leoni V, Giupponi L, Ceciliani G, Sala S, Bassoli A, Giorgi A. Effectiveness of different analytical methods for the characterization of propolis: a case of study in northern Italy. Molecules. 2020;25:504. https://doi.org/10.3390/molecules25030504. [PMC free article].
3. Costa AG Jr, Yoshida NC, Garcez WS, Perdomo RT, Matos M.d.F.C., Garcez F.R. Metabolomics approach expands the classification of propolis samples from Midwest Brazil. J Nat Prod. 2020;83:333–43. https://doi.org/10.1021/acs.jnatprod.9b00783.
4. Soroy L, Bagus S, Yongkie IP, Djoko W. The effect of a unique propolis compound (PropoelixTM) on clinical outcomes in patients with dengue hemorrhagic fever. Infect Drug Resist. 2014;7:323–9.
5. Jasprica I, Mornar A, Debeljak Ž, Smolčić-Bubalo A, Medić-Šarić M, Mayer L, Romić Ž, Bućan K, Balog T, Sobočanec S. In vivo study of propolis supplementation effects on antioxidative status and red blood cells. J Ethnopharmacol. 2007;110:548–54. https://doi.org/10.1016/j.jep.2006.10.023.
6. Sforcin JM, Bankova V. Propolis: is there a potential for the development of new drugs? J Ethnopharmacol. 2011;133:253–60. https://doi.org/10.1016/j.jep.2010.10.032.
7. Paulino N, Dantas AP, Bankova V, Longhi DT, Scremin A, de Castro SL, Calixto JB. Bulgarian propolis induces analgesic and anti-inflammatory effects in mice and inhibits in vitro contraction of airway smooth muscle. J Pharmacol Sci. 2003;93:307–13. https://doi.org/10.1254/jphs.93.307.
8. Yuan J, Liu J, Hu Y, Fan Y, Wang D, Guo L, Nguyen TL, Zhao X, Liu X, Liu C. The immunological activity of propolis flavonoids liposome on the immune response against ND vaccine. Int J Biol Macromol. 2012;51:400–5. https://doi.org/10.1016/j.ijbiomac.2012.06.002.
9. Burdock GA. Review of the biological properties and toxicity of bee propolis (propolis). Food Chem Toxicol. 1998;36:347–63. https://doi.org/10.1016/S0278-6915(97)00145-2.

10. Skaba D, Morawiec T, Tanasiewicz M, Mertas A, Bobela E, Szliszka E, Skucha-Nowak M, Dawiec M, Yamamoto R, Ishiai S, et al. Influence of the toothpaste with Brazilian ethanol extract propolis on the oral cavity health. Evid Based Complement Alternat Med. 2013;2013:215391. https://doi.org/10.1155/2013/215391.
11. Sforcin JM. Biological properties and therapeutic applications of propolis. Phyther Res. 2016;30:894–905. https://doi.org/10.1002/ptr.5605.
12. Pasupuleti VR, Sammugam L, Ramesh N, Gan SH Honey, propolis, and royal jelly: a comprehensive review of their biological actions and health benefits. Oxidative Med Cell Longev. 2017;2017. https://doi.org/10.1155/2017/1259510.
13. Amoros M, Sauvager F, Girre L, Cormier M. In vitro antiviral activity of propolis. Apidologie. 1992;23:231–40. https://doi.org/10.1051/apido:19920306.
14. Schnitzler P, Neuner A, Nolkemper S, Zundel C, Nowack H, Sensch KH, Reichling J. Antiviral activity and mode of action of propolis extracts and selected compounds. Phyther Res. 2010;24:S20–8. https://doi.org/10.1002/ptr.2868.
15. Kujumgiev A, Tsvetkova I, Serkedjieva Y, Bankova V, Christov R, Popov S. Antibacterial, antifungal and antiviral activity of propolis of different geographic origin. J Ethnopharmacol. 1999;64:235–40. https://doi.org/10.1016/S0378-8741(98)00131-7.
16. Kwon MJ, Shin HM, Perumalsamy H, Wang X, Ahn Y-J. Antiviral effects and possible mechanisms of action of constituents from Brazilian propolis and related compounds. J Apic Res. 2020;59:413–25. https://doi.org/10.1080/00218839.2019.1695715.
17. Serkedjieva J, Manolova N, Bankova V. Anti-influenza virus effect of some propolis constituents and their analogues (esters of substituted cinnamic acids). J Nat Prod. 1992;55:294–7. https://doi.org/10.1021/np50081a003.
18. Debiaggi M, Tateo F, Pagani L, Luini M, Romero E. Effects of propolis flavonoids on virus infectivity and replication. Microbiologica. 1990;13:207–13.
19. Refaat H, Mady FM, Sarhan HA, Rateb HS, Alaaeldin E. Optimization and evaluation of propolis liposomes as a promising therapeutic approach for COVID-19. Int J Pharm. 2020;592:120028. https://doi.org/10.1016/j.ijpharm.2020.120028.
20. Sahlan M, Irdiani R, Flamandita D, Aditama R, Alfarraj S, Javed Ansari M, Cahya Khayrani A, Kartika Pratami D, Lischer K. Molecular interaction analysis of Sulawesi propolis compounds with SARS-CoV-2 main protease as preliminary study for COVID-19 drug discovery. J King Saud Univ Sci. 2020;33:101234. https://doi.org/10.1016/j.jksus.2020.101234. [PMC free article].
21. Hashem H. In silico approach of some selected honey constituents as SARS-CoV-2 main protease (COVID-19) inhibitors. ChemRxiv. 2020. https://doi.org/10.14744/ejmo.2020.36102.
22. Zabaiou N, Fouache A, Trousson A, Baron S, Zellagui A, Lahouel M, Lobaccaro J-MA. Biological properties of propolis extracts: something new from an ancient product. Chem Phys Lipids. 2017;207:214–22. https://doi.org/10.1016/j.chemphyslip.2017.04.005.
23. Zaccaria V, Garzarella EU, Di Giovanni C, Galeotti F, Gisone L, Campoccia D, Volpi N, Arciola CR, Daglia M. Multi dynamic extraction: an innovative method to obtain a standardized chemically and biologically reproducible polyphenol extract from poplar-type propolis to be used for its anti-infective properties. Materials (Basel). 2019;12:3746. https://doi.org/10.3390/ma12223746.
24. Popova M, Trusheva B, Bankova V. Propolis of stingless bees: a phytochemist's guide through the jungle of tropical biodiversity. Phytomedicine. 2019;86:153098. https://doi.org/10.1016/j.phymed.2019.153098.
25. Tolba MF, Azab SS, Khalifa AE, Abdel-Rahman SZ, Abdel-Naim AB. Caffeic acid phenethyl ester, a promising component of propolis with a plethora of biological activities: a review on its anti-inflammatory, neuroprotective, hepatoprotective, and cardioprotective effects. IUBMB Life. 2013;65:699–709. https://doi.org/10.1002/iub.1189.
26. Anjum SI, Ullah A, Khan KA, Attaullah M, Khan H, Ali H, Bashir MA, Tahir M, Ansari MJ, Ghramh HA. Composition and functional properties of propolis (bee glue): a review. Saudi J Biol Sci. 2019;26:1695–703. https://doi.org/10.1016/j.sjbs.2018.08.013.

27. Zainullin RA, Kunakova RV, Gareev VF, Galyautdinov IV, Sadretdinova ZR, Muslimov ZS, Odinokov VN. Flavanones and flavones from Bashkir propolis. Chem Nat Compd. 2018;54:975–7. https://doi.org/10.1007/s10600-018-2526-5.
28. Przybyłek I, Karpiński TM. Antibacterial properties of propolis. Molecules. 2019;24(11):2047. https://doi.org/10.3390/molecules24112047. PMID: 31146392; PMCID: PMC6600457.
29. Veloz JJ, Alvear M, Salazar LA. Antimicrobial and antibiofilm activity against *Streptococcus mutans* of individual and mixtures of the main polyphenolic compounds found in Chilean propolis. Biomed Res Int. 2019;2019:7602343. https://doi.org/10.1155/2019/7602343.
30. Soromou LW, Zhang Y, Cui Y, Wei M, Chen N, Yang X, Huo M, Baldé A, Guan S, Deng X, et al. Subinhibitory concentrations of pinocembrin exert anti-*Staphylococcus aureus* activity by reducing α-toxin expression. J Appl Microbiol. 2013;115:41–9. https://doi.org/10.1111/jam.12221.
31. Joray MB, Trucco LD, González ML, Napal GN, Palacios SM, Bocco JL, Carpinella MC. Antibacterial and cytotoxic activity of compounds isolated from *Flourensia oolepis*. Evid Based Complement Alternat Med. 2015;2015:912484. https://doi.org/10.1155/2015/912484.
32. Hernández Tasco AJ, Ramírez Rueda RY, Alvarez CJ, Sartori FT, Sacilotto ACBC, Ito IY, Vichnewski W, Salvador MJ. Antibacterial and antifungal properties of crude extracts and isolated compounds from *Lychnophora markgravii*. Nat Prod Res. 2018;34:863. https://doi.org/10.1080/14786419.2018.1503263.
33. Kharsany K, Viljoen A, Leonard C, van Vuuren S. The new buzz: investigating the antimicrobial interactions between bioactive compounds found in South African propolis. J Ethnopharmacol. 2019;238:111867. https://doi.org/10.1016/j.jep.2019.111867.
34. Szeleszczuk Ł, Zielińska-Pisklak M, Goś P. Propolis—panaceum prosto z ula. Lek W Polsce. 2013;23:32–9.
35. Nayaka HB, Londonkar RL, Umesh MK, Tukappa A. Antibacterial attributes of apigenin, isolated from *Portulaca oleracea* L. Int J Bacteriol. 2014;2014:175851. https://doi.org/10.1155/2014/175851.
36. Akilandeswari K, Ruckmani K. Synergistic antibacterial effect of apigenin with β-lactam antibiotics and modulation of bacterial resistance by a possible membrane effect against methicillin resistant *Staphylococcus aureus*. Cell Mol Biol. 2016;62:74–82. https://doi.org/10.14715/cmb/2016.62.14.13.
37. Jabłoński B, Kołtowski Z. Nectar secretion and honey potential of honey plants growing under Poland's conditions. J Api Sci. 2005;49:59.
38. Zulhendri F, Chandrasekaran K, Kowacz M, Ravalia M, Kripal K, Fearnley J, Perera CO. Antiviral, antibacterial, antifungal, and antiparasitic properties of propolis: a review. Food Secur. 2021;10(6):1360. https://doi.org/10.3390/foods10061360.
39. Forouzanfar MH, Afshin A, Alexander LT, Biryukov S, Brauer M, Cercy K, Charlson FJ, Cohen AJ, Dandona L, Estep K, et al. Global, regional, and national comparative risk assessment of 79 behavioural, environmental and occupational, and metabolic risks or clusters of risks, 1990–2015: a systematic analysis for the Global Burden of Disease Study 2015. Lancet. 2016;388:1659–724.
40. Harisna AH, Nurdiansyah R, Syaifie PH, Nugroho DW, Saputro KE, Firdayani, Prakoso CD, Rochman NT, Maulana NN, Noviyanto A, et al. In silico investigation of potential inhibitors to main protease and spike protein of SARS-CoV-2 in propolis. Biochem Biophys Reports. 2021;26:100969.
41. Khayrani AC, Irdiani R, Aditama R, Pratami DK, Lischer K, Ansari MJ, Chinnathambi A, Alharbi SA, Almoallim HS, Sahlan M. Evaluating the potency of Sulawesi propolis compounds as ACE-2 inhibitors through molecular docking for COVID-19 drug discovery preliminary study. J King Saud Univ Sci. 2021;33:101297.
42. Dewi LK, Sahlan M, Pratami DK, Agus A, Agussalim, Sabir A. Identifying propolis compounds potential to be covid-19 therapies by targeting sars-cov-2 main protease. Int J Appl Pharm. 2021;13:103–10.
43. Sahlan M, Irdiani R, Flamandita D, Aditama R, Alfarraj S, Ansari MJ, Khayrani AC, Pratami DK, Lischer K. Molecular interaction analysis of Sulawesi propolis compounds with SARS-

CoV-2 main protease as preliminary study for COVID-19 drug discovery. J King Saud Univ Sci. 2021;33:101234.
44. Shimizu T, Hino A, Tsutsumi A, Yong KP, Watanabe W, Kurokawa M. Anti-influenza virus activity of propolis in vitro and its efficacy against influenza infection in mice. Antivir Chem Chemother. 2008;19:7–13.
45. Kai H, Obuchi M, Yoshida H, Watanabe W, Tsutsumi S, Park YK, Matsuno K, Yasukawa K, Kurokawa M. In vitro and in vivo anti-influenza virus activities of flavonoids and related compounds as components of Brazilian propolis (AF-08). J Funct Foods. 2014;8:214–23.
46. Kuwata K, Urushisaki T, Takemura T, Tazawa S, Fukuoka M, Hosokawa-Muto J, Araki Y. Caffeoylquinic acids are major constituents with potent anti-influenza effects in brazilian green propolis water extract. Evid Based Complement Alternat Med. 2011;2011:254914.
47. Kuwata K, Takemura T, Urushisaki T, Fukuoka M, Hosokawa-Muto J, Hata T, Okuda Y, Hori S, Tazawa S, Araki Y. 3,4-dicaffeoylquinic acid, a major constituent of Brazilian propolis, increases TRAIL expression and extends the lifetimes of mice infected with the influenza a virus. Evid. Based Complement. Altern. Med. 2012;2012:946867.
48. Ito J, Chang FR, Wang HK, Park YK, Ikegaki M, Kilgore N, Lee KH. Anti-AIDS agents. 48. Anti-HIV activity of moronic acid derivatives and the new melliferone-related triterpenoid isolated from Brazilian propolis. J Nat Prod. 2001;64:1278–81.
49. Gekker G, Hu S, Spivak M, Lokensgard JR, Peterson PK. Anti-HIV-1 activity of propolis in CD4+ lymphocyte and microglial cell cultures. J Ethnopharmacol. 2005;102:158–63.
50. da Silva CCF, Salatino A, da Motta LB, Negri G, Salatino MLF. Chemical characterization, antioxidant and anti-HIV activities of a Brazilian propolis from Ceará state. Rev Bras. 2019;29:309–18.
51. Schnitzler P, Neuner A, Nolkemper S, Zundel C, Nowack H, Sensch KH, Reichling J. Antiviral activity and mode of action of propolis extracts and selected compounds. Phyther Res. 2010;24:632.
52. Bankova V, Galabov AS, Antonova D, Vilhelmova N, Di Perri B. Chemical composition of propolis extract ACF® and activity against herpes simplex virus. Phytomedicine. 2014;21:1432–8.
53. Coelho GR, Mendonça RZ, De SennaVilar K, Figueiredo CA, Badari JC, Taniwaki N, Namiyama G, De Oliveira MI, Curti SP, Evelyn Silva P, et al. Antiviral action of hydromethanolic extract of geopropolis from Scaptotrigona postica against antiherpes simplex virus (HSV-1). Evid. Based Complement Alternat Med. 2015;2015:296086.
54. Hochheim S, Guedes A, Faccin-Galhardi L, Rechenchoski DZ, Nozawa C, Linhares RE, da Filho HHS, Rau M, Siebert DA, Micke G, et al. Determination of phenolic profile by HPLC–ESI-MS/MS, antioxidant activity, in vitro cytotoxicity and anti-herpetic activity of propolis from the Brazilian native bee Melipona quadrifasciata. Rev Bras. 2019;29:339–50.
55. Kurokawa M, Shimizu T, Takeshita Y, Takamori Y, Kai H, Sawamura R, Yoshida H, Watanabe W, Tsutsumi A, Park YK, et al. Efficacy of Brazilian propolis against herpes simplex virus type 1 infection in mice and their modes of antiherpetic efficacies. Evid Based Complement Alternat Med. 2011;2011:976196.
56. Sartori G, Pesarico AP, Pinton S, Dobrachinski F, Roman SS, Pauletto F, Rodrigues LC, Prigol M. Protective effect of brown Brazilian propolis against acute vaginal lesions caused by herpes simplex virus type 2 in mice: involvement of antioxidant and anti-inflammatory mechanisms. Cell Biochem Funct. 2012;30:1–10.
57. Búfalo MC, Figueiredo AS, De Sousa JPB, Candeias JMG, Bastos JK, Sforcin JM. Anti-poliovirus activity of Baccharis dracunculifolia and propolis by cell viability determination and real-time PCR. J Appl Microbiol. 2009;107:1669–80.
58. Coelho GR, De Senna Villar K, Figueiredo CA, Badari JC, Mendonca RMZ, Oliveira MI, Curti SP, Silva PES, Do Nascimento RM, Mendonca RZ. Antiviral effects of Scaptotrigona postica propolis and their fractions. BMC Proc. 2014;8:63.
59. Refaat H, Mady FM, Sarhan HA, Rateb HS, Alaaeldin E. Optimization and evaluation of propolis liposomes as a promising therapeutic approach for COVID-19. Int J Pharm. 2021;592:120028.

60. Kumar V, Dhanjal JK, Kaul SC, Wadhwa R, Sundar D. Withanone and caffeic acid phenethyl ester are predicted to interact with main protease (Mpro) of SARS-CoV-2 and inhibit its activity. J Biomol Struct Dyn. 2021;39:3842.
61. Ma X, Guo Z, Zhang Z, Li X, Wang X, Liu Y, Wang X. Ferulic acid isolated from propolis inhibits porcine parvovirus replication potentially through bid-mediate apoptosis. Int Immunopharmacol. 2020;83:106379.
62. Hayakari R, Matsumiya T, Xing F, Tayone JC, Dempoya J, Tatsuta T, Aizawa-Yashiro T, Imaizumi T, Yoshida H, Satoh K. Effects of Brazilian green propolis on double-stranded RNA-mediated induction of interferon-inducible gene and inhibition of recruitment of polymorphonuclear cells. J Sci Food Agric. 2013;93:646–51.
63. Verhelst J, Hulpiau P, Saelens X. Mx proteins: antiviral gatekeepers that restrain the uninvited. Microbiol Mol Biol Rev. 2013;77:551–66.
64. Dabbagh-Bazarbachi H, Clergeaud G, Quesada IM, Ortiz M, O'Sullivan CK, Fernández-Larrea JB. Zinc ionophore activity of quercetin and epigallocatechin-gallate: from hepa 1-6 cells to a liposome model. J Agric Food Chem. 2014;62:8085–93.
65. Kaushik N, Subramani C, Anang S, Muthumohan R, Shalimar, Nayak B, Ranjith-Kumar CT, Surjit M. Zinc salts block hepatitis E virus replication by inhibiting the activity of viral RNA-dependent RNA polymerase. J Virol. 2017;91:e00754–17.
66. Laila U, Akram M, Shariati MA, Hashmi AM, Akhtar N, Tahir IM, Ghauri AO, Munir N, Riaz M, Akhter N, et al. Role of medicinal plants in HIV/AIDS therapy. Clin Exp Pharmacol Physiol. 2019;46:1063–73. https://doi.org/10.1111/1440-1681.13151.
67. Labská K, Plodková H, Pumannová M, Sensch KH. Antiviral activity of propolis special extract GH 2002 against Varicella zoster virus in vitro. Die Pharm Int J Pharm Sci. 2018;73:733–6.
68. Silva-Beltrán NP, Balderrama-Carmona AP, Umsza-Guez MA, Souza Machado BA. Antiviral effects of Brazilian green and red propolis extracts on enterovirus surrogates. Environ Sci Pollut Res. 2020;27:28510–7. https://doi.org/10.1007/s11356-019-07458-z.
69. Governa P, Cusi MG, Borgonetti V, Sforcin JM, Terrosi C, Baini G, Miraldi E, Biagi M. Beyond the biological effect of a chemically characterized poplar propolis: antibacterial and antiviral activity and comparison with flurbiprofen in cytokines release by lps-stimulated human mononuclear cells. Biomedicines. 2019;7:73. https://doi.org/10.3390/biomedicines7040073.
70. Búrquez MdJG, Mosqueda MdLJ, Mendoza HR, Zárate CIS, Miranda LC, Sánchez TAC. Protective effect of a Mexican propolis on MDBK cells exposed to aujeszky's disease virus (pseudorabies virus). African J Tradit Complement Altern Med. 2015;12:106–11. https://doi.org/10.4314/ajtcam.v12i4.16.

Propolis as an Antimycotic 10

10.1 Introduction

According to the scientific literature, a substantial amount of evidence suggests that propolis exhibits antifungal characteristics. The changes in the chemical composition of propolis have been shown to have the potential to affect it [1, 2]. This difference in antifungal action has been seen in many studies that have investigated the effectiveness of propolis originating from various geographical locations against a wide range of fungal species, particularly those that are particularly significant in clinical settings [3–7]. Propolis has been shown to possess antifungal characteristics, and these abilities have been proven against various fungal species, including *Candida albicans*, *Candida parapsilosis*, *Candida tropicalis*, and *Candida glabrata* [8, 9]. The aflatoxigenic impact of this drug has been established against fungi such as *Aspergillus flavus*, where it has been discovered to inhibit the conidial growth of the fungi [1, 10]. This chemical appears to have a positive influence on aflatoxin production.

10.2 Propolis: Overview

The name "propolis" refers to a natural resinous mixture that is formed by honeybees (*Apis mellifera*) using secretions collected from trees and herbaceous plants or resins, mucilage, and gums from the flowers, fruits, branches, stems, and leaves of various plants [11–15]. Honeybees are responsible for the production of propolis. Other common names for propolis include "hive dross" and "bee glue." In addition, and more specifically, propolis is composed of the following sources: (1) resins from plants that *Apis mellifera* collects, (2) wax from the metabolism of bees, (3) chemicals that are added by *Apis mellifera* during the manufacturing process of propolis [12], and (4) other components such as essential oils and pollen [13]. The

A. E. Tanuğur Samanci et al., *Propolis: Prevention and Healing Effects in Otorhinolaryngology*, Comprehensive ENT,
https://doi.org/10.1007/978-3-031-68546-0_10

main composition of raw propolis was described in greater detail by Nainu et al. [16], who included the following percentage range of components: resins and balms (ranging from 50% to 60%), waxes and fatty acids (ranging from 30% to 40%), essential oils (ranging from 5% to 10%), and other chemical compounds other chemical compounds (to 5%), primarily enzymes (such as glucose-6-phosphatase, adenosine triphosphatase, and acid phosphatase), vitamins, and minerals.

Propolis has been recognized and exploited as a form of medicine since the time of the ancient Greeks, Romans, and Egyptians, and this practice has continued until the present day [17]. As a result of its intricate composition, the natural chemical known as propolis can produce a wide range of pharmacological effects. The origin of propolis, as well as the influence of geographical and environmental factors on its chemical makeup [12, 14, 18] and pharmacological activity [19–21], is one of the scientific problems that have received much attention in recent years. This is one of the issues that have been the subject of a significant amount of research.

In addition to honey, royal jelly, and bee venom, propolis is a significant source of natural chemical compounds [22, 23]. Propolis is also a source of other bee products. Bee products come in a variety of forms, one of which is royal jelly. A substantial amount of research has been carried out on propolis in various fields. The increase in the number of discoveries made regarding propolis can be attributed to the advancement of research procedures as well as the ever-increasing curiosity of the scientific community. The continuation of this trend is following the demand to utilize products produced from natural sources, not only for the treatment of a variety of diseases but also for the prevention of those disorders [11].

10.3 Antifungal Properties of Propolis

The fungi that are responsible for the spoilage of juice, such as *Candida famata*, *Candida glabrata*, *Candida kefyr*, *Candida pelliculosa*, *Candida parapsilosis*, and *Pichia ohmeri*, are susceptible to the beneficial effects of propolis, which have been proved to have fungicidal properties [15, 24]. To be more specific, it was demonstrated that the presence of flavonoids was associated with the fungicidal action [25]. Propolis has antifungal activity as tested with 40 yeast strains, including *Candida albicans*, *Candida glabrata*, *Candida krusei*, and *Trichosporon* species. Propolis was shown to have the highest antifungal activity of any bee product tested, according to the findings of our investigation [26]. The growth of *Candida albicans* (MIC 0.2–3.75 μg/mL), *Candida glabrata* (MIC 0.03–7.5 μg/mL), and *Trichosporon* spp. can be inhibited by the inclusion of propolis in the environment (minimum inhibitory concentration 0.1–0.4 μg/mL) and Rhodotorula species (MIC is less than 0.01 μg/mL) and the most sensitive strain was Rhodotorula species, especially. It consists of the strain most vulnerable to the effects of propolis. The C. albicans strain, among all strains, was the most resistant. Indian propolis was shown to be more effective than the anticaries agents typically used in conventional dentistry, according to a study carried out in Bangalore but that was not published [27]. *Streptococcus mutans* is a common cause of dental caries, and it was found that

Indian propolis was able to suppress the growth of this bacteria. Oliveira et al. [28] researched the 67 yeast samples that were isolated and identified from onychomycosis samples. These yeast samples included the following species: *Candida albicans*, *Candida parapsilosis*, *Candida tropicalis*, *Candida kefyr*, *Candida guilliermondii*, *Candida lusitaniae*, *Candida glabrata*, *Candida stellatoidea*, and *Trichosporon* sp. in addition to *T. asahii*, *T. ovoides*, as well as *T. cutaneum*, one *Geotrichum candidum*, and three *Saccharomyces cerevisiae* that were collected from the soil. In the species known as *Trichosporon* sp. [1], with a minimum inhibitory concentration (MIC50) and a minimum inhibitory concentration (MIC90) of 1.25×10^{-2} mg/mL of flavonoids, the flavonoids exhibited the highest level of sensitivity. The *Candida tropicalis* strain, on the other hand, demonstrated the highest level of resistance, as seen by its CFM50 value of 5×10^{-2} mg/mL of flavonoids and its MFC90 value of 10×10^{-2} mg/mL [28]. The disc diffusion method demonstrated an increase in the activity of the ethanolic extraction of propolis when the concentration was increased to 20% and 30%, respectively. The effectiveness of EEP in treating *Candida albicans* was not demonstrated [15, 29].

In vitro investigations carried out against yeasts identified as agents of onychomycosis have demonstrated that propolis extract has demonstrated exceptional efficiency. Within the scope of these experiments, it was shown that propolis has both fungicidal and fungistatic characteristics when present at low levels. According to empirical research carried out by Ota et al. in 2001 [3], Brazilian propolis was examined to determine whether it could inhibit the growth of 80 distinct strains of *Candida* yeast. These strains included 20 *Candida albicans* strains, 20 *Candida tropicalis* strains, 20 *Candida krusei*, and 15 strains of *Candida guilliermondii*. A definitive antifungal action of propolis was reported in the following order of sensitivity: *Candida albicans* > *Candida tropicalis* > *Candida krusei* > *Candida guilliermondii*, with *Candida albicans* being the most sensitive and *Candida guilliermondii* being the most resistant. Propolis was found to be effective against all of the *Candida* species investigated. It was shown that the minimum inhibitory concentrations (MICs) were influential within the 8–12 mg/mL range. Additionally, it was found that patients with complete dentures who utilized a hydroalcoholic extract of propolis saw a reduction in the amount of *Candida* species that were present in their saliva [1, 3].

Several fungal species belonging to the genus *Trichophyton*, which are the agents responsible for dermatophytosis, are susceptible to the antifungal activity of Brazilian propolis. On the other hand, red Brazilian propolis is more effective than green Brazilian propolis [5]. According to research, the n-hexane extract of Brazilian red propolis is effective against *Candida* species that are resistant to antifungal medicines such as fluconazole [30]. Under the supervision of Oliveira et al. [28], an alcoholic extract of Brazilian propolis was put to the test against fungal isolates of *Candida parapsilosis*, *Candida tropicalis*, and *Candida albicans*, in addition to additional yeast species isolated from onychomycosis lesions. The propolis extract was effective against all of these yeast species. The finding was that the propolis flavonoids that could inhibit all yeasts had a concentration of 50 μg/mL. On the contrary, the flavonoids fostered the death of yeast cells when they were present at a concentration of 20 μg/mL. Upon investigation, it was found that *Trichosporon* sp. [28] was the species that exhibited the highest level of sensitivity.

Quiroga and colleagues [31] analyzed the antifungal characteristics of propolis sourced from the northwest of Argentina [31]. The inquiry was part of a more extensive study conducted in 2006. When it came to yeasts, xylophagous fungi, and phytopathogenic fungi, their research primarily focused on the antimycotic and cytotoxic characteristics of propolis extract that had been partially purified. Additionally, propolis's activity was assessed compared to other compounds, such as pinocembrin and galangin, which were extracted from the same propolis. In addition, the effectiveness of propolis was evaluated in comparison to that of synthetic drugs like ketoconazole and clotrimazole. An extract of propolis that had been partially purified was found to be capable of inhibiting the growth of fungi, as demonstrated by the researchers' findings. It was established that propolis was a reliable source of antifungal agents by comparing its relative biocide potency and cytotoxicity with the separated components and the medicines manufactured [31]. Argentinian propolis extract was utilized by Agüero et al. [32] in their inquiry, which was conducted in a different piece of research material. It was tested against a wide range of yeasts and fungi to determine how efficient the antifungal activity was. According to the findings, the *Microsporum gypseum*, *Trichophyton mentagrophytes*, and *Trichophyton rubrum* were reportedly the most susceptible species to the disease. Propolis extracts were shown to have a considerable inhibitory effect on the other dermatophytes and yeasts that were investigated. These extracts' minimum inhibitory concentration (MIC) values ranged from 16 to 125 μg/mL [32].

A study was carried out by Falcao and colleagues in 2014 to examine the antifungal characteristics of Portuguese propolis and its probable floral sources against three distinct types of fungi. These fungi were *Candida albicans*, *Trichoderma rubrum*, and *Aspergillus fumigatus*. The *T. rubrum* strain was the one that proved to be the most significant, while the *A. fumigatus* strain [33] demonstrated the least significant essential effect. Szweda et al. [34] investigated the antifungal properties of an ethanolic extract of propolis (Poland), essential oils, and silver nanoparticles dropped on TiO_2. To establish the efficacy of these chemicals using fluconazole-resistant *Candida albicans*, *Candida glabrata*, and *Candida krusei*, the researchers examined the antifungal activities of these substances against these three types of *Candida*. In their investigation, they discovered that every drug possessed adequate fungicidal action against *C. albicans* and *C. glabrata* isolates that have been successfully isolated indicating to control and prevent candidiasis [34]. Boisard et al. [35] investigated the antifungal properties of organic extracts of French propolis by testing them against a set of different types of fungi. The researchers discovered that the extracts were effective against *Candida albicans* and *Candida glabrata*. However, they only demonstrated a relatively low level of action against *A. fumigatus* [35].

It is possible that the delivery methods and vehicles that serve to make propolis accessible could affect the antifungal activity of the substance. In a study that was conducted by Bruschi and colleagues [6], the antifungal activity of propolis ethanolic extract (PEE) and propolis microparticles (PMs) derived from a Brazilian propolis sample was evaluated in vitro against clinical isolates of yeast that are responsible for vulvovaginal candidiasis. The results of this study were published in the journal *Scientific Reports*. Their experiment showed that PEE and PMs efficiently blocked *C. albicans* and non-*C. albicans* [6]. An investigation into the fungicidal effectiveness of propolis extracts, propolis material microparticles, and propolis soluble dry extract was carried out by Berretta et al. [36] utilizing an in vivo experimental animal model [36]. The impact of the treatment was evaluated against three distinct morphotypes of *Candida albicans*, namely yeast, pseudohyphae, and hyphae, after a period ranging from 6 to 8 h following the administration of the medication. PEE was the most potent among all the extracts, followed by PSDE, PM, and PWE in sequential order. The PWE extract had the lowest potency of all the extracts. An investigation was conducted by Bonfim et al. [37] to examine the efficacy of a novel mucoadhesive thermoresponsive platform for propolis delivery (MTS-PRPe) in the treatment of vulvovaginal candidiasis that was generated by *C. elegans*. The examination was conducted both in vitro and in vivo—albicans in a mouse model used for preclinical research [37]. The researchers performed many different types of analyses, including a chemical analysis, an evaluation of the rheological and mucoadhesive features of propolis formulations, an antifungal assessment in vitro and in vivo, histological assessments, and electron microscopy of the vaginal mucosa. Researchers established that propolis extract and MTS-PRPe possess antifungal properties by using them against a clinical *C. albicans* isolate resistant to fluconazole, in addition to the strain of the typically used fungus. It was shown that this activity occurred in rats and in vitro. The researchers indicate that the MTS-PRPe did not negatively affect propolis's efficacy [1, 37]. The findings of the study demonstrated this.

10.3.1 Vaginal Use

Additionally, they evaluated the effectiveness of the propolis extract (PE) against clinical yeast *C. albicans* while they were in the process of synthesizing the propolis microparticles (PMs) from Brazilian propolis [38, 39] as well as 31 non-*C. albicans* organisms' isolates that are significant in the context of vulvovaginal candidiasis (VVC). *C. glabrata*, *C. tropicalis*, *C. guilliermondii*, as well as *C. parapsilosis* isolates were examined in this study. In addition, the principal antifungal drugs utilized in the treatment of VVC were also investigated. Isolates of *Candida albicans* either resisted the azolic drugs and amphotericin B or exhibited a dose-dependent susceptibility to these treatments. As opposed to the letter, *C. albicans*, which is not C. isolates of albicans, showed a higher level of resistance to the azolic medicines of interest and a dose-dependent sensitivity to those medications.

On the other hand, each of them was either sensitive to amphotericin B or dose-dependently susceptible to its present effects. With only a little difference, PE and PMs could inhibit the growth of all yeasts. This was the case independent of the species of yeast that was considered. Individually, the findings provided helpful information that might be exploited for the potential application of PMs in the treatment of VVC and the possible prevention of the start of future symptomatic episodes [15, 38]. This information could be utilized for the prospective application of PMs.

10.4 Antifungal Mechanisms of Action of Propolis

Wagh [15] carried out an exhaustive evaluation of the research that has been undertaken on propolis and the pharmacological properties it possesses. In conclusion, he concluded that the fungicidal effect against *Candida* was believed to be caused by the presence of phenolic chemicals in propolis. It is *C. pelliculosa*, *C. parapsilosis*, often known as *C. famata*, *C. glabrata* [15], and *Pichia ohmeri* [15]. In a study conducted by Banskota et al. [40], it was discovered that the elements of propolis, such as 3-acetylpinobanksin, pinobanksin-3-acetate, pinocembrin, p-coumaric acid, and caffeic acid, had antifungal properties. Of the 26 or more ingredients discovered in propolis, these chemicals were among them. Aguero et al. [32] concluded that the principal bioactive components responsible for the antifungal activity that was found in the propolis extract were 2′,4′-dihydroxy-3-methoxychalcone and 2′,4′-dihydroxychalcone. This conclusion was reached as a result of their observations. There were two clinical isolates of T. in addition to T. The minimum inhibitory concentrations (MICs) and minimum fungicidal concentrations (MFCs) of mentagrophytes ranged from 1.9 to 2.9 μg/mL, indicating that they exhibited a high activity level. In addition, galangin, pinocembrin, and 7-hydroxy-8-methoxyflavanone were successfully extracted from propolis samples and *Zuccagnia punctata* exudates, and each of these compounds showed a moderate amount of antifungal activity [32]. In vitro, tests were conducted on human pathogenic fungi, two yeasts (*C. albicans* and *C. glabrata*), and one filamentous opportunistic mold (*A. fumigatus*) to determine the antifungal and antibacterial activity of a mixture of French propolis samples. The extracts were aqueous and organic. It was Boisard et al. [35] that were responsible for carrying out the in vitro evaluation. As a result of the obtained findings, they concluded that the high flavonoid content of the material was responsible for the antifungal activity of propolis against *Candida albicans* and *Candida glabrata* [35].

According to the notion detailed in Ref. [41], the fundamental explanation for the antifungal activity of propolis is believed to be the potential of propolis to produce apoptosis through the action of metacaspase and Ras signaling. Furthermore, propolis can make changes to the expression of several genes that are involved in the process of pathogenicity, cell adhesion, biofilm formation, filamentous development, and phenotypic flipping. HST7, GIN4, VPS34, HOG1, ISW2, SUV3, MDS3, HDA2, KAR3, YHB1, NUP85, CDC10, MNN9, ACE2, FKH2, and SNF5 are some of the genes that are included in this compilation. Furthermore, propolis can block the shift from yeast-like development to hyphal growth [41]. Propolis, specifically its phenolic component pinocembrin, disrupts various critical cellular activities in a dose-dependent manner. Among these activities are the maintenance of energy balance and the formation of mycelia. As previously established, the number of phosphorylated adenosine nucleotides found in the hyphae of *Penicillium italicum* is reduced by the presence of pinocembrin. It is also responsible for the ionic leakage and the soluble protein in *P. italicum* [1, 42]. Pinocembrin is accountable for the damage it causes to the structure of the hyphae and the cell membrane.

References

1. Zulhendri F, Chandrasekaran K, Kowacz M, Ravalia M, Kripal K, Fearnley J, Perera CO. Antiviral, antibacterial, antifungal, and antiparasitic properties of propolis: a review. Food Secur. 2021;10(6):1360. https://doi.org/10.3390/foods10061360.
2. Kujumgiev A, Tsvetkova I, Serkedjieva Y, Bankova V, Christov R, Popov S. Antibacterial, antifungal and antiviral activity of propolis of different geographic origin. J Ethnopharmacol. 1999;64:235–40.
3. Ota C, Unterkircher C, Fantinato V, Shimizu MT. Antifungal activity of propolis on different species of Candida. Mycoses. 2001;44:375–8.
4. Murad JM, Calvi SA, Soares AMVC, Bankova V, Sforcin JM. Effects of propolis from Brazil and Bulgaria on fungicidal activity of macrophages against Paracoccidioides brasiliensis. J Ethnopharmacol. 2002;79:331–4.
5. Siqueira ABS, Gomes BS, Cambuim I, Maia R, Abreu S, Souza-Motta CM, De Queiroz LA, Porto ALF. Trichophyton species susceptibility to green and red propolis from Brazil. Lett Appl Microbiol. 2009;48:90–6.
6. Bruschi ML, Dota KFD, Consolaro MEL, Svidzinski TIE. Antifungal activity of Brazilian propolis microparticles against yeasts isolated from vulvovaginal candidiasis. Evid Based Complement Alternat Med. 2011;2011:201953.
7. Bonvehí JS, Gutiérrez AL. The antimicrobial effects of propolis collected in different regions in the Basque Country (Northern Spain). World J Microbiol Biotechnol. 2012;28:1351–8.
8. Al-Waili N, Al-Ghamdi A, Ansari MJ, Al-Attal Y, Salom K. Synergistic effects of honey and propolis toward drug multi-resistant Staphylococcus Aureus, Escherichia coli and Candida Albicans isolates in single and polymicrobial cultures. Int J Med Sci. 2012;9:793–800.
9. Mutlu Sariguzel F, Berk E, Koc AN, Sav H, Demir G. Antifungal activity of propolis against yeasts isolated from blood culture: in vitro evaluation. J Clin Lab Anal. 2016;30:513–6.
10. Ghaly MF, Ezzat SM, Sarhan MM. Use of propolis and ultragriseofulvin to inhibit aflatoxigenic fungi. Folia Microbiol. 1998;43:156–60.
11. Ożarowski M, Karpiński TM, Alam R, Łochyńska M. Antifungal Properties of chemically defined propolis from various geographical regions. Microorganisms. 2022;10(2):364. https://doi.org/10.3390/microorganisms10020364. PMID: 35208818; PMCID: PMC8880174.
12. Dezmirean DS, Paşca C, Moise AR, Bobiş O. Plant sources responsible for the chemical composition and main bioactive properties of poplar-type propolis. Plants. 2020;10:22. https://doi.org/10.3390/plants10010022.
13. Tran TD, Ogbourne SM, Brooks PR, Sánchez-Cruz N, Medina-Franco JL, Quinn RJ. Lessons from exploring chemical space and chemical diversity of propolis components. Int J Mol Sci. 2020;21:4988. https://doi.org/10.3390/ijms21144988.
14. Anjum SI, Ullah A, Khan KA, Attaullah M, Khan H, Ali H, Bashir MA, Tahir M, Ansari MJ, Ghramh HA, et al. Composition and functional properties of propolis (bee glue): a review. Saudi J Biol Sci. 2019;26:1695–703. https://doi.org/10.1016/j.sjbs.2018.08.013.
15. Wagh VD. Propolis: a wonder bees product and its pharmacological potentials. Adv Pharmacol Sci. 2013;2013:308249. https://doi.org/10.1155/2013/308249.
16. Nainu F, Masyita A, Bahar MA, Raihan M, Prova SR, Mitra S, Emran TB, Simal-Gandara J. Pharmaceutical prospects of bee products: special focus on anticancer, antibacterial, antiviral, and antiparasitic properties. Antibiotics. 2021;10:822. https://doi.org/10.3390/antibiotics10070822.

17. Kuropatnicki AK, Szliszka E, Krol W. Historical aspects of propolis research in modern times. Evid Based Complement Alternat Med. 2013;2013:964149. https://doi.org/10.1155/2013/964149.
18. Maldonado L, Marcinkevicius K, Borelli R, Gennari G, Salomón V, Isla MI, Vera N, Borelli V. Differentiation of Argentine propolis from different species of bees and geographical origins by UV spectroscopy and chemometric analysis. J Saudi Soc Agric Sci. 2020;19:185–91. https://doi.org/10.1016/j.jssas.2018.09.003.
19. Dudoit A, Mertz C, Chillet M, Cardinault N, Brat P. Antifungal activity of Brazilian red propolis extract and isolation of bioactive fractions by thin-layer chromatography-bioautography. Food Chem. 2020;327:127060. https://doi.org/10.1016/j.foodchem.2020.127060.
20. Woźniak M, Mrówczyńska L, Kwaśniewska-Sip P, Waśkiewicz A, Nowak P, Ratajczak I. Effect of the solvent on propolis phenolic profile and its antifungal, antioxidant, and in vitro cytoprotective activity in human erythrocytes under oxidative stress. Molecules. 2020;25:4266. https://doi.org/10.3390/molecules25184266.
21. Przybyłek I, Karpiński TM. Antibacterial properties of propolis. Molecules. 2019;24:2047. https://doi.org/10.3390/molecules24112047.
22. Ratajczak M, Kaminska D, Matuszewska E, Hołderna-Kedzia E, Rogacki J, Matysiak J. Promising antimicrobial properties of bioactive compounds from different honeybee products. Molecules. 2021;26:4007. https://doi.org/10.3390/molecules26134007.
23. Kędzia B. The origin of propolis in the theories and scientific research. Herba Pol. 2008;54:179–86.
24. Koc AN, Silici S, Multu-Sariguzel F, Sagdic O. Antifungal activity of propolis in four different fruit juices. Food Technol Biotechnol. 2007;45:57–61.
25. Farnesi AP, Aquino-Ferreira R, De Jong D, Bastos JK, Soares AEE. Effects of stingless bee and honey bee propolis on four species of bacteria. Genet Mol Res. 2009;8(2):635–40.
26. Koç AN, Silici S, Kasap F, Hörmet-Öz HT, Mavus-Buldu H, Ercal BD. Antifungal activity of the honeybee products against Candida spp. and Trichosporon spp. J Med Food. 2011;14(1–2):128–34.
27. Selvan A, Singh R, Prabhu D. Research article: anti-bacteria activity of bee propolis against clinical strains of Streptococcus mutants and synergism with chlorhexidine. Int J Pharm Stud Res. 2011;2:85–90.
28. Oliveira ACP, Shinobu CS, Longhini R, Franco SL, Svidzinski TIE. Antifungal activity of propolis extract against yeasts isolated from onychomycosis lesions. Mem Inst Oswaldo Cruz. 2006;101(5):493–7.
29. Hendi NKK, Naher HS, Al-Charrakh AH. In vitro antibacterial and antifungal activity of Iraqi propolis. J Med Plant Res. 2011;5(20):5058–66.
30. Pippi B, Lana AJD, Moraes RC, Güez CM, Machado M, de Oliveira LFS, Lino von Poser G, Fuentefria AM. In vitro evaluation of the acquisition of resistance, antifungal activity and synergism of Brazilian red propolis with antifungal drugs on Candida spp. J Appl Microbiol. 2015;118:839–50.
31. Quiroga EN, Sampietro DA, Soberón JR, Sgariglia MA, Vattuone MA. Propolis from the northwest of Argentina as a source of antifungal principles. J Appl Microbiol. 2006;101:103–10.
32. Agüero MB, Gonzalez M, Lima B, Svetaz L, Sánchez M, Zacchino S, Feresin GE, Schmeda-Hirschmann G, Palermo J, Daniel Wunderlin AND, et al. Argentinean propolis from Zuccagnia punctata cav. (Caesalpinieae) exudates: phytochemical characterization and antifungal activity. J Agric Food Chem. 2010;58:194–201.
33. Falcão SI, Vale N, Cos P, Gomes P, Freire C, Maes L, Vilas-Boas M. In vitro evaluation of portuguese propolis and floral sources for antiprotozoal, antibacterial and antifungal activity. Phyther Res. 2014;28:437–43.
34. Szweda P, Gucwa K, Kurzyk E, Romanowska E, Dzierżanowska-Fangrat K, Zielińska Jurek A, Kuś PM, Milewski S. Essential oils, silver nanoparticles and propolis as alternative agents against fluconazole resistant candida albicans, candida glabrata and candida krusei clinical isolates. Indian J Microbiol. 2015;55:175–83.

35. Boisard S, Le Ray AM, Landreau A, Kempf M, Cassisa V, Flurin C, Richomme P. Antifungal and antibacterial metabolites from a French poplar type propolis. Evid Based Complement Alternat Med. 2015;2015:319240.
36. Berretta AA, De Castro PA, Cavalheiro AH, Fortes VS, Bom VP, Nascimento AP, Marquele-Oliveira F, Pedrazzi V, Ramalho LNZ, Goldman GH. Evaluation of mucoadhesive gels with propolis (EPP-AF) in preclinical treatment of candidiasis vulvovaginal infection. Evid. Based Complement Alternat Med. 2013;2013:641480.
37. Bonfim AP, Sakita KM, Faria DR, Arita GS, Vendramini FAVR, Capoci IRG, Braga AG, dos Santos RS, Bruschi ML, Becker TCA, et al. Preclinical approaches in vulvovaginal candidiasis treatment with mucoadhesive thermoresponsive systems containing propolis. PLoS One. 2020;15:e0243197.
38. Dota KFD, Consolaro MEL, Svidzinski TIE, Bruschi ML. Antifungal activity of brazilian propolis microparticles against yeasts isolated from vulvovaginal candidiasis. Evid Based Complement Alternat Med. 2011;2011:8 pages. 201953.
39. Park YK, Koo MH, Abreu JAS, Ikegaki M, Cury JA, Rosalen PL. Antimicrobial activity of propolis on oral microorganisms. Curr Microbiol. 1998;36(1):24–8.
40. Banskota AH, Tezuka Y, Kadota S. Recent progress in pharmacological research of propolis. Phyther Res. 2001;15:561–71.
41. De Castro PA, Bom VLP, Brown NA, de Almeida RSC, Ramalho LNZ, Savoldi M, Goldman MHS, Berretta AA, Goldman GH. Identification of the cell targets important for propolis-induced cell death in Candida albicans. Fungal Genet Biol. 2013;60:74–86.
42. Peng L, Yang S, Cheng YJ, Chen F, Pan S, Fan G. Antifungal activity and action mode of pinocembrin from propolis against Penicillium italicum. Food Sci Biotechnol. 2012;21:1533–9.

Diseases of the Honeybees

11

11.1 Introduction

Honeybee colonies are vulnerable to various conditions, including illnesses and parasites. Varroa destructor and *Tropilaelaps clareae* are two examples of non-native parasites that have caused significant damage to European and North American colonies. Both of these parasites are considered to be highly destructive. Colony collapse disorder (CCD), first identified in the United States in 2006, was responsible for the death of many colonies and posed considerable difficulties for agricultural pollination, a vital service provided by the beekeeping sector in North America. In addition, the discovery of CCD heightened worries previously expressed over possible decreases in honeybee populations in the United States and other countries [1].

Honeybees are susceptible to a wide variety of illnesses when they are alive. The Varroa mite poses a significant danger to European honeybees. When honeybees are in the larval and pupal stages, they are susceptible to illnesses that harm their brood, such as American foulbrood (AFB) and European foulbrood (EFB). Nosema is a sickness brought on by a microorganism that only possesses one cell. There is a high probability that bee colonies have dormant forms of viral illnesses such as chronic bee paralysis virus (CBPV) and deformed wing virus (DWV). There are a wide variety of insects that, in some way or another, benefit from honeybees. These insects include wax moths and pollen mites.

11.2 Varroa Destructor

The disease known as varroatosis is caused by the ectoparasite Varroa destructor caused by the Varroa mite. This foreign parasite poses a significant risk to the honeybees native to Europe. Although there is widespread agreement about the many

A. E. Tanuğur Samanci et al., *Propolis: Prevention and Healing Effects in Otorhinolaryngology*, Comprehensive ENT,
https://doi.org/10.1007/978-3-031-68546-0_11

factors that contribute to bee mortality, the fact that this mite is present in every single bee colony places a significant amount of strain on the colonies' health [2].

In many instances, honeybees' winter mortality can be linked to the Varroa mite in conjunction with secondary viral illnesses that the mite carries [2].

11.3 The Small Beetle of the Hive

In the Calabria region, located in Southern Italy, the small hive beetle, also known as *Aethina tumida*, was recently imported. The bee colonies infected by this species, new to Europe, are subject to detrimental consequences [2].

11.3.1 Biology of Beetles

Sub-Saharan Africa is the place of origin for the little hive beetle, also known as *Aethina tumida*. As a result of the fact that the majority of honeybee colonies can tolerate its presence, it is not seriously considered a plague within its native area. The beetle is only capable of causing damage to colonies that are already weak and infected with illness. In addition, this is true to a certain extent in regions not within its native range, such as the United States and Australia. The larvae, which feed on combs and everything else that may be found in them, are the ones who do the most damage. It is also possible for frames that have been kept to become contaminated. While eating their way through the combs, the larvae will defecate, leaving the honey itself for yeast to consume. The intake of honey that has been contaminated is not recommended [2].

11.4 Brood Diseases: *American Foulbrood (AFB), European Foulbrood (EFB), and Chalkbrood*

When honeybees are in the larval and pupal stages, they are susceptible to infections that damage their brood. Although these illnesses do not typically result in the death of a colony, they might hinder the colony's development anyway. Swarming and actively leaving the brood are two methods that bees might use to defend themselves against brood sickness. Brood illnesses can threaten the colony's existence if the beekeeper manages to suppress or disrupt these processes [2].

11.5 Viruses: *Deformed Wing Virus (DWV) and Chronic Bee Paralysis Virus (CBPV)*

Most viral infections are dormant in bee colonies and often do not cause any problems. Bees, on the other hand, are susceptible to experiencing severe repercussions as a result of viral infections that are made worse by stressful settings. Several viruses have begun to play a more significant role in the health of bee colonies [2] ever since the introduction of Varroa destructor in 1983.

Twenty-three viruses have been identified as being connected with the genus *Apis*. Most of the time, viruses remain dormant in honeybee populations and cause very little to no harm to bee colonies. Nevertheless, the replication of the virus can be encouraged or activated (often under stressful settings), which might lead to the manifestation of symptoms of the disease of interest. Consequently, this may result in accidental harm or even the death of the colony [2].

11.5.1 Deformed Wing Virus (DWV) Infection

In this case, the deformed wing virus (DWV) represents an exception to the norm. As a result of the introduction of Varroa destructor, this virus has developed into a significant danger and is now a structural concern for the health of honeybees. This condition is mainly brought on by the Varroa mite, responsible for the successful transmission of DWV. Additionally, the virus replicates in Varroa mites. In addition, when they feed on bees, Varroa mites can trigger an immunological response. The replication of virus particles in bee tissue is an immunological response activated by this immune response. Deformed wings are one of the physical signs that can be caused by DWV, which in turn can impact the lifetime of bees [2].

11.5.2 Chronic Bee Paralysis Virus (CBPV)

The chronic bee paralysis virus (CBPV) can become an issue during the growth season when there are extended periods of cold weather. The virus is responsible for paralysis. Bees afflicted with this virus may be recognized by their dark coloration and the absence of hair on their bodies [2].

11.5.3 Additional Viruses

The tools used to identify viruses have improved, resulting in a greater understanding of viruses' function in the health of bees. As a result, viruses are receiving an increasing amount of attention. Concerning the mortality rate of bees, the additional viruses that are being researched into [2] are as follows:

Potential Viruses (Adopted from Reference 2)

Virus	Distributed in the EU
Acute bee paralysis virus (ABPV)	+
Kashmir bee virus (KBV)	+
Israeli acute paralysis virus (IAPV)	+
Black queen cell virus (BQCV)	+

Virus	Distributed in the EU
Deformed wing virus (DWV)	+
Varroa destructor virus 1 (VDV-1)	+
Sacbrood virus (SBV)	+
Slow bee paralysis virus (SBPV)	+
Chronic bee paralysis virus (CBPV)	+
Cloudy wing virus (CWV)	+
Bee virus X (BVX)	+
Bee virus Y (BVY)	+
Arkansas bee virus (ABV)	?
Berkeley bee virus (BBPV)	?
Macula-like virus (MLV)	+
Filamentous virus (AmFv)	+
Apis iridescent virus (AIV)	?
Aphid lethal paralysis virus (ALPV)	?
Big Sioux River virus (BSRV)	?
Lake Sinaï virus 1 (LSV1)	?
Lake Sinaï virus 2 (LSV2)	?
Invertebrate iridescence virus (IIV)	?
Kakugo virus	?

11.6 *Nosema apis* and *Nosema ceranae*

A condition that affects adult honeybees called nosema is brought on by a parasite that only has one cell on the tissue located in the midgut, where the parasite dwells. Nosema is rather common all around the world. There is also a high incidence of the illness in Belgium and the Netherlands. *Nosema apis* has the potential to inflict significant harm.

The *Nosema ceranae* species has also been found in the Netherlands since 2008. It is uncertain how and whether this species, which is most likely an invasive species, causes illness or death in bee colonies in the Netherlands [2]. However, it is found in practically all bee colonies.

11.6.1 Microsporidia

Microsporidia, which are parasites called *Nosema apis* and *Nosema ceranae*, are only found in the host cell. This indicates that they cannot exist and multiply outside of the host cell. The cells of insects and other invertebrates are the sites of microsporidia's residence. Recently, parasites belonging to the genus Microsporidia were also found in humans [2].

11.6.2 *Nosema apis*

It is common for *Nosema apis* to attack in the spring when the weather is often chilly and wet. When there is a prolonged period of cold and rain, it might lead to an insufficient amount of pollen being produced. As a consequence, bees make themselves more susceptible to this intestinal parasite. This can result in death as well as vomiting and diarrhea. There are also dead and squished bees within and in front of the hive, another indicator of a *Nosema* infestation [2]. These bees represent one of the characteristics of the infestation.

11.6.3 Living Outside of the Confines of the Cell

The spore stage is a fundamental component of microsporidia's life cycle. During this stage, the parasite can persist for extended periods outside of a cell. The disease is transmitted from one organism to another and from one cell to another during this stage [2].

11.7 *Tropilaelaps* Mite

Four species make up the genus *Tropilaelaps*. These species are *T. clareae*, *T. koenigerum*, and the two species only recently described, *T. mercedesae* and *T. thaii*. *Tropilaelaps* was initially found in the colonies of the giant honeybee, also known as *Apis dorsata*. However, they have also been found in colonies of other species of bees. It has been found that both *T. clareae* and *T. mercedesae* are present in Europe, and both species are capable of reproducing in honeybees of the species *Apis mellifera*. It has yet to be reported that *Tropilaelaps* has been seen in the Netherlands [2].

There is a similarity between the life cycle of Varroa destructor and *Tropilaelaps* spp. in colonies of *Apis mellifera*. Under typical circumstances, one to four adult mites will join the brood, and each of these mites will generate one to two offspring. The ratio of drone brood to worker brood is 3:1, which indicates that the mites favor employee brood. The number of boys and girls that are generated is equal. At the same time as a juvenile bee emerges from the brood cell, the adult female mites also depart the cell. The adult men and immature children are left behind and eventually perish. There is a maximum of 2 days that the mites are allowed to remain on the adult bees before they return to the brood cell to replicate themselves [2].

11.8 *Acarapis* Mite

Adult honeybees are susceptible to *Acarapis* mites, also known as *Acarapis woodi*, parasites that attach themselves to the first pair of trachea, the breathing tubes. The drones, workers, and the queen can potentially get infected [2].

The mite is tiny, measuring between 85 and 116 micrometers in length and 57 and 85 micrometers in width. It is yellow-white and has eight legs. There is a mechanism that allows for piercing and sucking, and the mouthparts are well developed. To facilitate piercing, the mite most likely creates a chemical that undermines the strength of chitin. Within the first pair of legs are the organs responsible for touch [2].

11.9 Amoebic Diseases

The amoeba *Malpighamoeba mellificae* Prell is classified as a member of the protozoa, which are unicellular creatures that resemble animals. Using pseudopodia, often known as fake feet, these protozoa move about and eat through phagocytosis [2].

These cysts can be caused by *Malpighamoeba mellificae*. The cell walls of these cysts are extremely tough, and they have a spherical shape with a cross section that measures around 7.5 micrometers. The amoebae are freed and discharged into the environment when the cysts, which are digested by the bees along with their food, reach the rectum of the bee. They go back through the small intestine and into the Malpighian tubules, where they multiply and eventually form cysts once more. After that, feces finally eliminate these cysts [2].

The Malpighian tubules are harmed and clogged as a result of the amoebae. Consequently, waste products from the bee's metabolism accumulate, and the bee becomes poisonous. There is also a disruption in the water balance of the bee, which results in dysentery [2].

11.10 Wax Moths

Experienced beekeepers follow a general rule of thumb when it comes to keeping honeycombs and other hive materials: use caution. Moreover, there is a rationale behind this! It is possible for wax moths to consume honeycombs in their entirety. In addition, they can ruin the wooden frame! Wax moths do not threaten honeybees on their own; nevertheless, when they are in weak colonies, they can consume their way through the honeycombs [2].

11.11 "Bee Louse": *Braula coeca*

The organism known as *Braula coeca* is also referred to as the bee louse. It is a fly that does not have wings and wholly relies on honeybees for its continued existence. There is no longer any evidence of the bee louse in the Netherlands. Introducing the Varroa mite into the environment most likely led to the extinction of this species. Products used to manage the Varroa mite are toxic to this commensal organism [2]. These products are used to control the mite.

References

1. Bee. Britannica. Last Updated: Dec 1, 2023. https://www.britannica.com/animal/honeybee. Accessed online at 08 Dec 2023.
2. Bee diseases. Wageningen University & Research. https://www.wur.nl/en/research-results/research-institutes/plant-research/biointeractions-plant-health/bees-1/bee-diseases.htm#:~:text=The%20honeybee%20is%20susceptible%20to,caused%20by%20a%20unicellular%20parasite

Propolis and Benefits

12

12.1 Introduction

Bees generate a substance that resembles resin called propolis by combining the sap of needle-leaved trees with their saliva and beeswax. Propolis is a resinlike substance. Propolis is a sealant that bees use to construct their hives, but there is some evidence that it may also have health benefits for people. Bee glue, bee propolis, and Baume de Propolis are other names for this substance [1, 2].

Researchers are investigating the anti-inflammatory effects of propolis, which they believe may improve wound healing and protect the body from germs and viruses. However, not much research has been conducted on this topic. Propolis may also help alleviate burns and swelling. Therefore, researchers partly attribute these possible advantages to the trials being conducted with small sample numbers and the methodology used [1].

According to research [1], propolis has been shown to potentially benefit various health issues, including tooth decay, inflammation, and allergies.

The term "propolis" refers to a combination of compounds bees use to protect their hive. As part of this defense, cavities in the hive's walls are filled, the entry is reduced on days when the temperature is low, and the invaders who are needed are mummified, preventing their deterioration [3, 4]. The reason that propolis is frequently referred to as bee glue is because of this [1]. "At the entrance to the city" is what the Greek term "propolis" means, and it comes from the word "propolis" [6, 7]. Since ancient times, people have continued discussing where the propolis came from. Questions have been raised regarding whether or not it originates from plants or bees. At this point, thanks to the advancement of analytical methods, the approximate composition of propolis and the elements that influence it are known [4].

Bees produce propolis by collecting resins from buds, exudates, and other sections of plants and then combining these resins with their salivary enzymes and beeswax to make the substance [8, 9]. Different continents, areas, and plant species

A. E. Tanuğur Samanci et al., *Propolis: Prevention and Healing Effects in Otorhinolaryngology*, Comprehensive ENT,
https://doi.org/10.1007/978-3-031-68546-0_12

are utilized to manufacture propolis, resulting in the composition of propolis being distinct from one another. While having a particular chemical makeup, propolis possesses actions comparable to those of other substances, including antibacterial, antifungal, antiviral, antiparasitic, anti-inflammatory, antiproliferative, and antioxidant properties [10–13].

12.2 The Chemical Compounds of Propolis

It is possible to draw a direct connection between the resins and balsams of plant sources used to manufacture propolis and the chemical composition of propolis. During the study, more than 300 chemical components of propolis were discovered. Except for resins, the primary categories of chemical substances that are present in propolis include waxes, polyphenols (phenolic acids, flavonoids), and terpenoids [3].

In addition, polyphenols and terpenoids are regarded as being among the most active compounds [14]. Chrysin, pinocembrin, apigenin, galangin, kaempferol, quercetin, tectochrysin, pinostrobin, and other flavonoids are all members of the flavonoid group. The aromatic acids found in propolis are another important category of substances. The aromatic acids that are found in propolis most frequently include ferulic, cinnamic, caffeic, benzoic, salicylic, and p-coumaric acids 15–17. On average, flavonoid components made up between 6.2% and 18.8% of the total composition of Polish propolis. Pinocembrin (mean 4.7%), pinobenchin (mean 3.1%), galangin (mean 2.2%), and chrysin (mean 2.1%) were the flavonoids that were found in the greatest concentrations [15]. Moreover, propolis contains several additional phenolic compounds, such as tefillin C, as well as terpenes, such as terpineol, camphor, geraniol, nerol, and farnesol, which are responsible for the distinctive aroma that it exudes. The micro and macro elements manganese, iron, silicon, magnesium, zinc, selenium, calcium, sodium, and copper, as well as vitamins B1, B2, B6, C, and E, may be found in propolis [4, 5, 16–20]. As an antibacterial agent, propolis possesses an extra benefit as a result of the variety of its chemical makeup. The establishment of bacterial resistance is prevented by the combination of many active components and the presence of these compounds in various proportions [21].

12.3 The Antibacterial Activity of Propolis

It is essential to consider the antibacterial activity of propolis on two different levels. First, it is associated with a direct effect on the microorganism. In the second place, it is related to stimulating the immune system, ultimately activating the organism's protective mechanisms [8]. By examining the mechanisms of propolis, it is possible to deduce its impact on the permeability of the cellular membrane of microorganisms, the disruption of membrane potential, the synthesis of adenosine triphosphate (ATP), and the reduction of bacterial motility. In general, it has been discovered that the antibacterial activity of propolis is stronger concerning Gram-positive bacteria than with Gram-negative bacteria. The species-specific structure of the outer membrane of Gram-negative bacteria and the development of hydrolytic enzymes, which are responsible for breaking down the active compounds of propolis [19, 22], explain this phenomenon. Another one of the several phenolic chemicals (prenyl derivatives of p-coumaric acid) that may be found in propolis is tefillin C, also known as 3,5-diprenyl-p-coumaric acid.

Compared to hexane extracts, the content of tefillin C in ethanolic propolis extracts was found to be much more significant, according to research carried out in Brazil by Veiga and colleagues. These extracts also demonstrated significant antibacterial activity against methicillin-resistant *S. aureus* [23]. Research conducted against the anaerobic bacteria *Porphyromonas gingivalis* showed that artepillin C had bacteriostatic action with membrane blebbing [24]. Artepillin C has additional anti-inflammatory properties, which are mediated through the regulation of NF-kappaB and the suppression of prostaglandin E [2] and nitric oxide [25].

Propolis contains several other prenyl derivatives, including 3-prenyl-cinnamic acid allyl ester and 2-dimethyl-8-prenylchromene, which have an antibacterial activity comparable to that of propolis [26]. There is evidence that kaempferide has an antibacterial impact on skin infection-related microorganisms, such as *S. aureus* [27]. Antioxidant and antibacterial action was demonstrated by the ethanolic extract of propolis against *S. aureus*, *S. saprophyticus*, *Listeria monocytogenes*, and *E. faecalis* [28]. The extract included significant kaempferide, artepillin C, drupanin, and p-coumaric acid.

Propolis contains several flavonoids, including pinocembrin and apigenin, among others. In a study conducted by Veloz et al. on Chilean propolis, it was discovered that the antibacterial activity of both of these compounds against *Streptococcus mutans* is greater than the activity of polyphenol mixture or even chlorhexidine (MICs = 1.6 μg/mL). These compounds' minimum inhibitory concentrations (MICs) were 1.4 μg/mL and 1.3 μg/mL, respectively [29]. Extracted pinocembrin has been shown to possess antibacterial properties against several different bacteria, including *S. mutans*, *S. sobrinus*, *S. aureus*, *E. faecalis*, *L. monocytogenes*, *Pseudomonas aeruginosa*, and *K. pneumoniae*, according to several investigations [30–33]. The Gram-negative bacteria *P. aeruginosa*, *K. pneumoniae*, *Salmonella enterica* serotype Typhimurium, *Proteus mirabilis*, and *Enterobacter aerogenes* are all susceptible to the therapeutic effects of apigenin that have been isolated [34]. It was also reported that apigenin, combined with β-lactam antibiotics, had synergistic antibacterial activity against methicillin-resistant *S. aureus* (MRSA) [35]. Additionally, when combined with ceftazidime, apigenin exhibited a synergistic effect against ceftazidime-resistant *Enterobacter cloacae* [36].

Cinnamic acid and its derivatives are a category of aromatic carboxylic acids frequently discovered in the kingdom of plants worldwide. Both the green sections of plants and the flowers contain them in some form or another. Cinnamic acid and esters may be found in abundance in propolis, a substance formed by a significant number of plant secretions. Many investigations have demonstrated that cinnamic acid has antibacterial properties against a wide variety of microorganisms, including *Aeromonas* species, *Vibrio* species, *Escherichia coli*, *Listeria monocytogenes*, *Mycobacterium* TB, *Bacillus* species, and *Staphylococcus* species. The following bacteria were found to be present: *Streptococcus pyogenes*, *Micrococcus flavus*, *P. aeruginosa*, *S. enterica* serotype Typhimurium, *Enterobacter cloacae*, and *Yersinia ruckeri* [37–39]. Cinnamic acid and its derivatives can impede the growth of bacteria by destroying the cell membrane, inhibiting ATPases, cell division, and biofilm creation. In addition to this, they exhibited anti-quorum sensing activity [40].

12.4 Health Benefits of Propolis

12.4.1 Supports Oral Health

According to the authors of a review published in 2015, propolis has the potential to assist in reducing calcium phosphate production, which is the primary component that produces dental plaque [41].

It is explained in the study that propolis has antibacterial properties since it was able to lower the amount of bacteria that were present in individuals who suffered from periodontitis [41].

According to the Centers for Disease Control and Prevention (CDC), periodontitis is an illness of the gums that occurs when bacteria accumulate in a person's gums and teeth. It can cause gum swelling, foul breath, and tooth sensitivity. People with diabetes, crooked teeth, and poor oral hygiene practices are the most likely to be affected by this condition [1, 42].

12.4.2 Reduces Inflammation

The research looked at the effects of mouthwashes that included propolis and chlorhexidine on people with dental plaque and gingivitis, a gum disease that causes bleeding gums, discomfort, and inflammation [43]. Smoking and not flossing your teeth are two factors that increase the likelihood of developing gingivitis [44].

According to the study's findings, mouthwashes containing propolis have the potential to decrease plaque and inflammation. The number of people who experienced adverse reactions to chlorhexidine products increased, including a burning sensation, discoloration of the teeth, and a shift in the way they perceived the taste [43].

The research is based on a limited sample size and does not specify whether or not the subjects are regular smokers. More studies are necessary to ascertain whether mouthwashes containing propolis are helpful and safe for use in clinical settings [43].

12.4.3 Reduces Acne Breakouts

Because of its anti-inflammatory and antibacterial qualities, propolis has the potential to be an effective alternative option for treating acne. Propolis ethanolic extract was proven to be an effective treatment for acne vulgaris, according to a study that involved 40 people who suffered from acne. The participants in the research also determined it to be safe and well tolerated. The individuals had a positive response to the therapy; however, they experienced some slight discomfort. It is necessary to do more research to identify the application of propolis in various skin disorders [45].

12.4.4 Prevents Cancer Spread

According to one study's findings, propolis may possess anticancer effects. It is possible that it may help prevent cancer cells from growing and that it will impede the routes that cancer cells use to communicate with one another [46].

A further investigation reveals that Chinese propolis possesses anti-tumor properties, and it is possible for individuals who have breast cancer to utilize it as an extra treatment [47].

12.4.5 Speeds Up Wound Healing

Recent research has shown that propolis has the potential to speed up wound healing. A number of medical professionals could suggest it as an alternate treatment for diabetic ulcers or burns on the skin. However, more research is needed to outline the use of propolis for improving wound healing [48].

12.5 How to Use Propolis?

Propolis is available as a mouthwash, a skin cream, and an oral supplement to maintain good dental health [1].

It is highly recommended that you seek the advice of a healthcare expert before purchasing any propolis products. In addition to advising you on how to use them, your physician may verify whether or not they are safe for your health [1].

In addition, they can recommend that you have a patch test to determine whether or not you have an allergy to the component [1].

12.5.1 Dosage

There is evidence that oral propolis at 70 mg per day is safe for human consumption [49, 50]. Propolis has also been administered to adults in dosages ranging from 400 to 500 mg per day for up to 13 months [2].

12.6 Is Propolis Safe?

When used in modest amounts, propolis products are still considered safe [1].

If you are a nurse, your healthcare professional may advise you to take 300 mg of oral propolis daily. Large amounts of propolis can be detrimental [2].

If you are pregnant, you should attempt to avoid using products that include propolis. The use of these methods during pregnancy is not well supported by the available data [2].

If you are allergic to bee products, you should avoid using creams, as they can trigger an allergic response on the skin. Lozenges can also cause inflammation and ulcers in the mouth [2].

The Food and Drug Administration (FDA) strongly advises that individuals should not assume that dietary supplements classified as natural are risk free. If the components are consumed in excessive quantities over an extended period, they may still be hazardous to health. They can also interact with meals or even pharmaceuticals [51].

Furthermore, dietary supplements should not mention that they are capable of treating or curing an illness, as this is something that can only be accomplished by a medicine that has been licensed for use [2].

12.7 Potential Drug Interactions

Interactions may occur if you take propolis in conjunction with other drugs or supplements that you are already taking. Blood clotting can be slowed down by propolis. As a result of the fact that herbal supplements like garlic, ginger, and *Ginkgo biloba* have effects that are comparable to those of propolis, taking them together might raise the risk of bleeding [2].

To treat blood clots and reduce the likelihood of you having a heart attack, your physician may prescribe warfarin. Propolis can lessen the effects of warfarin, which can lead to an increased risk of blood clots [2].

12.7.1 Medications That Are Altered by the Liver Because They Are Substrates of Cytochrome P450 1A2 (CYP1A2)

The liver is responsible for modifying and breaking down some drugs. Propolis may alter the rate at which the liver breaks down certain medicines, which may alter the effects and adverse reactions that these drugs cause [2].

12.7.2 Medications Altered by the Liver That Are Called Ssubstrates of Cytochrome P450 2C19 (CYP2C19)

The liver is responsible for modifying and breaking down some drugs. Propolis may alter the rate at which the liver breaks down certain drugs, which could alter the effects and adverse reactions that these drugs cause [2].

12.7.3 Pharmaceuticals That Are Altered by the Liver (Substrate of Cytochrome P450 2C9, Also Known as CYP2C9)

The liver is responsible for modifying and breaking down some drugs. Propolis may alter the rate at which the liver breaks down certain drugs, which could alter the effects and adverse reactions that these drugs cause [2].

12.7.4 Medications That Are Altered by the Liver Because They Are Substrates of Cytochrome P450 2D6 (CYP2D6)

The liver is responsible for modifying and breaking down some drugs. Propolis may alter the rate at which the liver breaks down certain medicines, which may change the effects and adverse reactions that these drugs cause [2].

12.7.5 Substances That Are Altered by the Liver (Substances That Are Substrates of Cytochrome P450 2E1 (CYP2E1))

The liver is responsible for modifying and breaking down some drugs. Propolis may alter the rate at which the liver breaks down certain medicines, which may change the effects and adverse reactions that these drugs cause [2].

12.7.6 Medications Changed by the Liver (Cytochrome P450 3A4 (CYP3A4) Substrates)

The liver is responsible for the modification and breakdown of some medications. Propolis may alter the rate at which the liver breaks down certain drugs, which could alter the effects and adverse reactions that these drugs cause [2].

12.7.7 Anticoagulant/Antiplatelet Drugs

Blood-clotting medications, often known as anticoagulants and antiplatelet medicines, may cause propolis to slow down the process of blood clotting. It is possible that the risk of bruising and bleeding was increased when propolis was used in conjunction with drugs that also decreased the coagulation of blood [2].

12.7.8 Warfarin (Coumadin)

To prevent blood from clotting, warfarin is administered. Propolis may lessen the effects of warfarin. As a result, the likelihood of clotting might be increased [2].

References

1. Iavarone K. Health benefits of propolis. Health. https://www.health.com/propolis-7106541. Accessed online at 08 Dec 2023.
2. Propolis. Medlineplus. https://medlineplus.gov/druginfo/natural/390.html. Accessed online at 08 Dec 2023.
3. Przybyłek I, Karpiński TM. Antibacterial properties of propolis. Molecules. 2019;24(11):2047. https://doi.org/10.3390/molecules24112047.
4. Kędzia B. Pochodzenie propolisu w świetle teorii i badań naukowych. The origin of propolis in the theories and scientific research. Herba Pol. 2008;54:179–86.
5. Zabaiou N, Fouache A, Trousson A, Baron S, Zellagui A, Lahouel M, Lobaccaro JA. Biological properties of propolis extracts: something new from an ancient product. Chem Phys Lipids. 2017;207:214–22. https://doi.org/10.1016/j.chemphyslip.2017.04.005.
6. Wagh VD. Propolis: a wonder bees product and its pharmacological potentials. Adv Pharmacol Sci. 2013;2013:308249. https://doi.org/10.1155/2013/308249.
7. Toreti VC, Sato HH, Pastore GM, Park YK. Recent progress of propolis for its biological and chemical compositions and its botanical origin. Evid Based Complement Alternat Med. 2013;2013:697390. https://doi.org/10.1155/2013/697390.
8. Sforcin JM, Bankova V. Propolis: is there a potential for the development of new drugs? J Ethnopharmacol. 2011;133:253–60. https://doi.org/10.1016/j.jep.2010.10.032.
9. Silva JC, Rodrigues S, Feás X, Estevinho LM. Antimicrobial activity, phenolic profile and role in the inflammation of propolis. Food Chem Toxicol. 2012;50:1790–5. https://doi.org/10.1016/j.fct.2012.02.097.
10. Schnitzler P, Neuner A, Nolkemper S, Zundel C, Nowack H, Sensch KH, Reichling J. Antiviral activity and mode of action of propolis extracts and selected compounds. Phytother Res. 2010;24(Suppl. 1):S20–8. https://doi.org/10.1002/ptr.2868.

11. Ramanauskiene K, Inkeniene A. Propolis oil extract: quality analysis and evaluation of its antimicrobial activity. Nat Prod Res. 2011;25:1463–8. https://doi.org/10.1080/14786419.2010.529440.
12. Franchin M, Cólon DF, Castanheira FV, da Cunha MG, Bueno-Silva B, Alencar SM, Cunha TM, Rosalen PL. Vestitol isolated from Brazilian red propolis inhibits neutrophils migration in the inflammatory process: elucidation of the mechanism of action. J Nat Prod. 2016;79:954–60. https://doi.org/10.1021/acs.jnatprod.5b00938.
13. De Freitas MCD, de Miranda MB, de Oliveira DT, Vieira-Filho SA, Caligiorne RB, de Figueiredo SM. Biological activities of red propolis: a review. Recent Pat Endocr Metab Immun Drug Discov. 2017;11:3–12. https://doi.org/10.2174/1872214812666180223120316.
14. Pimenta HC, Violante IM, Musis CR, Borges ÁH, Aranha AM. In vitro effectiveness of Brazilian brown propolis against *Enterococcus faecalis*. Braz Oral Res. 2015;29:1–6. https://doi.org/10.1590/1807-3107BOR-2015.vol29.0058.
15. Kędzia B, Hołderna-Kędzia E. Pinocembryna—flawonoidowy składnik krajowego propolisu o działaniu opóźniającym rozwój choroby Alzheimera. Pinocembrin—flavonoid component of domestic propolis with delaying effect of the development of Alzheimer's disease. Post Fitoter. 2017;18:223–8.
16. Bankova VS, Castro DSL, Marcucci MC. Propolis: recent advances in chemistry and plant origin. Apidologie. 2000;31:3–15. https://doi.org/10.1051/apido:2000102.
17. Kędzia B. Skład chemiczny i aktywność biologiczna propolisu pochodzącego z różnych rejonów świata. Post Fitoter. 2006;1:23–35.
18. Wolska K, Górska A, Adamiak A. Właściwości przeciwbakteryjne propolisu. Post Mikrobiol. 2016;55:343–50.
19. Sforcin JM. Biological properties and therapeutic applications of propolis. Phytother Res. 2016;30:894–905. https://doi.org/10.1002/ptr.5605.
20. Pasupuleti VR, Sammugam L, Ramesh N, Gan SH. Honey, propolis and royal jelly: a comprehensive review of their biological actions and health benefits. Oxidative Med Cell Longev. 2017;2017:1259510. https://doi.org/10.1155/2017/1259510.
21. Pamplona-Zomenhan LC, Pamplona BC, da Silva CB, Marcucci MC, Mimica LM. Evaluation of the in vitro antimicrobial activity of an ethanol extract of Brazilian classified propolis on strains of *Staphylococcus aureus*. Braz J Microbiol. 2011;42:1259–64. https://doi.org/10.1590/S1517-83822011000400002.
22. Kędzia B, Hołderna-Kędzia E. Aktywność antybiotyczna propolisu krajowego i europejskiego. The antibiotic activity of native and European propolis. Post Fitoter. 2013;2:97–107.
23. Veiga RS, De Mendonça S, Mendes PB, Paulino N, Mimica MJ, Lagareiro Netto AA, Marcucci MC. Artepillin C and phenolic compounds responsible for antimicrobial and antioxidant activity of green propolis and *Baccharis dracunculifolia* DC. J Appl Microbiol. 2017;122:911–20. https://doi.org/10.1111/jam.13400.
24. Yoshimasu Y, Ikeda T, Sakai N, Yagi A, Hirayama S, Morinaga Y, Furukawa S, Nakao R. Rapid bactericidal action of propolis against *Porphyromonas gingivalis*. J Dent Res. 2018;97:928–36. https://doi.org/10.1177/0022034518758034.
25. Paulino N, Abreu SRL, Uto Y, Koyama D, Nagasawa H, Hori H, Dirsch VM, Vollmar AM, Scremin A, Bretz WA. Anti-inflammatory effects of a bioavailable compound, artepillin C, in Brazilian propolis. Eur J Pharmacol. 2008;587:296–301. https://doi.org/10.1016/j.ejphar.2008.02.067.
26. Viuda-Martos M, Ruiz-Navajas Y, Fernández-López J, Pérez-Álvarez JA. Functional properties of honey, propolis, and royal jelly. J Food Sci. 2008;73:R117–24. https://doi.org/10.1111/j.1750-3841.2008.00966.x.
27. Guz NR, Stermitz FR, Johnson JB, Beeson TD, Willen S, Hsiang JF, Lewis K. Flavonolignan and flavone inhibitors of a *Staphylococcus aureus* multidrug resistance pump: structure-activity relationships. J Med Chem. 2001;44:261–8. https://doi.org/10.1021/jm0004190.
28. Seibert JB, Bautista-Silva JP, Amparo TR, Petit A, Pervier P, Dos Santos Almeida JC, Azevedo MC, Silveira BM, Brandão GC, de Souza GHB, et al. Development of propolis nanoemulsion

with antioxidant and antimicrobial activity for use as a potential natural preservative. Food Chem. 2019;287:61–7. https://doi.org/10.1016/j.foodchem.2019.02.078.
29. Veloz JJ, Alvear M, Salazar LA. Antimicrobial and antibiofilm activity against *Streptococcus mutans* of individual and mixtures of the main polyphenolic compounds found in Chilean propolis. Biomed Res Int. 2019;2019:7602343. https://doi.org/10.1155/2019/7602343.
30. Soromou LW, Zhang Y, Cui Y, Wei M, Chen N, Yang X, Huo M, Baldé A, Guan S, Deng X, et al. Subinhibitory concentrations of pinocembrin exert anti-*Staphylococcus aureus* activity by reducing α-toxin expression. J Appl Microbiol. 2013;115:41–9. https://doi.org/10.1111/jam.12221.
31. Joray MB, Trucco LD, González ML, Napal GN, Palacios SM, Bocco JL, Carpinella MC. Antibacterial and cytotoxic activity of compounds isolated from *Flourensia oolepis*. Evid Based Complement Alternat Med. 2015;2015:912484. https://doi.org/10.1155/2015/912484.
32. Hernández Tasco AJ, Ramírez Rueda RY, Alvarez CJ, Sartori FT, Sacilotto ACBC, Ito IY, Vichnewski W, Salvador MJ. Antibacterial and antifungal properties of crude extracts and isolated compounds from *Lychnophora markgravii*. Nat Prod Res. 2018;34:863–7. https://doi.org/10.1080/14786419.2018.1503263.
33. Kharsany K, Viljoen A, Leonard C, van Vuuren S. The new buzz: investigating the antimicrobial interactions between bioactive compounds found in South African propolis. J Ethnopharmacol. 2019;238:111867. https://doi.org/10.1016/j.jep.2019.111867.
34. Nayaka HB, Londonkar RL, Umesh MK, Tukappa A. Antibacterial attributes of apigenin, isolated from *Portulaca oleracea* L. Int J Bacteriol. 2014;2014:175851. https://doi.org/10.1155/2014/175851.
35. Akilandeswari K, Ruckmani K. Synergistic antibacterial effect of apigenin with β-lactam antibiotics and modulation of bacterial resistance by a possible membrane effect against methicillin resistant *Staphylococcus aureus*. Cell Mol Biol. 2016;62:74–82. https://doi.org/10.14715/cmb/2016.62.14.13.
36. Eumkeb G, Chukrathok S. Synergistic activity and mechanism of action of ceftazidime and apigenin combination against ceftazidime-resistant *Enterobacter cloacae*. Phytomedicine. 2013;20:262–9. https://doi.org/10.1016/j.phymed.2012.10.008.
37. Heleno SA, Ferreira IC, Esteves AP, Ćirić A, Glamočlija J, Martins A, Soković M, Queiroz MJ. Antimicrobial and demelanizing activity of *Ganoderma lucidum* extract, p-hydroxybenzoic and cinnamic acids and their synthetic acetylated glucuronide methyl esters. Food Chem Toxicol. 2013;58:95–100. https://doi.org/10.1016/j.fct.2013.04.025.
38. Guzman JD. Natural cinnamic acids, synthetic derivatives and hybrids with antimicrobial activity. Molecules. 2014;19:19292–349. https://doi.org/10.3390/molecules191219292.
39. Yilmaz S, Sova M, Ergün S. Antimicrobial activity of trans-cinnamic acid and commonly used antibiotics against important fish pathogens and nonpathogenic isolates. J Appl Microbiol. 2018;125:1714–27. https://doi.org/10.1111/jam.14097.
40. Vasconcelos NG, Croda J, Simionatto S. Antibacterial mechanisms of cinnamon and its constituents: a review. Microb Pathog. 2018;120:198–203. https://doi.org/10.1016/j.micpath.2018.04.036.
41. Martinotti S, Ranzato E. Propolis: a new frontier for wound healing? Burns Trauma. 2015;3:9. https://doi.org/10.1186/s41038-015-0010-z.
42. Centers for Disease Control and Prevention. Periodontal disease. https://www.cdc.gov/oralhealth/conditions/periodontal-disease.html. Accessed online at 08 Dec 2023.
43. Halboub E, Al-Maweri SA, Al-Wesabi M, et al. Efficacy of propolis-based mouthwashes on dental plaque and gingival inflammation: a systematic review. BMC Oral Health. 2020;20(1):198. https://doi.org/10.1186/s12903-020-01185-5.
44. National Health Service. Gum disease. https://www.nhs.uk/conditions/gum-disease/. Accessed online at 08 Dec 2023.
45. Mohammad Ali B, Ghoname N, Hodeib A, Elbadawy M. Significance of topical propolis in the treatment of facial acne vulgaris. Egypt J Dermatol Venerol. 2015;35(1):29. https://doi.org/10.4103/1110-6530.162468.

46. Chan GCF, Cheung KW, Sze DMY. The immunomodulatory and anticancer properties of propolis. Clinic Rev Allerg Immunol. 2013;44(3):262–73. https://doi.org/10.1007/s12016-012-8322-2.
47. Xuan H, Li Z, Yan H, et al. Antitumor activity of Chinese propolis in human breast cancer mcf-7 and mda-mb-231 cells. Evid Based Complement Alternat Med. 2014;2014:1–11. https://doi.org/10.1155/2014/280120.
48. da Rosa C, Bueno IL, Quaresma ACM, Longato GB. Healing potential of propolis in skin wounds evidenced by clinical studies. Pharmaceuticals. 2022;15(9):1143. https://doi.org/10.3390/ph15091143.
49. Braakhuis A. Evidence on the health benefits of supplemental propolis. Nutrients. 2019;11(11):2705. https://doi.org/10.3390/nu11112705.
50. Vagish Kumar LS. Propolis in dentistry and oral cancer management. N. Am J Med Sci. 2014;6(6):250–9. https://doi.org/10.4103/1947-2714.134369.
51. U.S. Food & Drug Administration. FDA 101: dietary supplements. https://www.fda.gov/consumers/consumer-updates/fda-101-dietary-supplements

Bee Products in Facial Plastic Surgery Procedures and Otolaryngology

13

13.1 Introduction

Honey is a natural substance produced by bees collected using nectar and honeydew as their primary ingredients. Honey is a supersaturated solution of carbohydrates with a wide range of applications and exhibits various features. Propolis is a resinous material gathered by bees from the buds of trees, shrubs, and green plants. Bee glue is another name for propolis. Honey and propolis were used in ancient times for embalming bodies. Honey was also utilized in folk medicine to mend wounds and provide pain relief [1, 2]. In pollen loads, bees collect pollen from plants and then transfer it to the hive, where they are assembled. The pollen process of moistening with nectar or honey leads to the creation of loads. The pollen used for winter supplies is deposited in the honeycomb cells, where it is subjected to lactic fermentation, which results in the production of bee bread. Both antibacterial and bacteriostatic properties can be attributed to bee bread and pollen [3, 4]. The glands found in the bee's abdomen are responsible for the production of beeswax. A helpful element that is utilized in the fields of cosmetics and medicine is wax, which is derived from honeycombs. The bees generate the venom of honeybees, also known as apitoxin. Because of its medicinal and cosmetic characteristics, it is utilized in various fields [5, 6]. It comprises a complex combination of several peptides and mast cell degranulating peptides.

13.2 Biological Features of the Honey

There are at least 181 components found in honey [7]. Research states that honey is a solution of supersaturated carbohydrates mainly consisting of glucose and fructose [8]. Additionally, honey may contain the following sugars in its composition: sucrose, rhamnose, trehalose, nigerobiose, isomaltose, maltose, maltotetraose,

A. E. Tanuğur Samanci et al., *Propolis: Prevention and Healing Effects in Otorhinolaryngology*, Comprehensive ENT,
https://doi.org/10.1007/978-3-031-68546-0_13

maltotriose, maltulose, melezitose, melibiose, nigerose, palatinose, raffinose, and erlose [9, 10]. Several enzymes are also present in it including glucose oxidase, amylase, catalase, peroxidase, invertase, and lysozyme. The enzyme glucose oxidase is responsible for the production of hydrogen peroxide, which is one of the chemicals that contribute to the bactericidal impact of honey [11]. Gluconic acid, citric acid, malic acid, lactic acid, succinic acid, oxalic acid, tartaric acid, formic acid, acetic acid, benzoic acid, and pyruvic acid are some of the organic acids that may be found in honey. The bee bodies and the enzymatic transformations that take place during the manufacture of honey are the potential sources of the acids.

Honeys that have reached maturity have a higher concentration of these acids. Honey contains phenolic acids and flavonoids, which are responsible for a wide variety of biological activities and can inhibit the production of free radicals. Hydroxycinnamic acid and hydroxybenzoic acid derivatives are included in the phenolic acid category. P-coumaric, caffeic, ferulic, and sinapic acids are all hydroxycinnamic acid derivatives. Others include sinapic acid. P-hydroxybenzoic acid, vanillic acid, syringic acid, salicylic acid, and gallic acid are all hydroxybenzoic acid derivatives. Ellagic acid, a dimer of gallic acid, is also included in this category [10]. Among the flavonoids that may be found in honey are naringenin, hesperetin, pinocembrin, chrysin, galangin, quercetin, and kaempferol. Honey that has been heated, on the other hand, results in a considerable reduction in the concentration of galangin, kaempferol, and myricetin, whereas the process of pasteurization results in a significant decrease in the concentration of myricetin [12].

Honey also contains essential oils, which are made up of terpenes such as thymol, bisabolol, farnesol, and cineol according to their chemical makeup. Other components of honey include water, proteins, and amino acids. Honey also contains proteins. A rise in the proline level, which accounts for 50–80% of all amino acids, indicates honey's maturity [9]. Honey is a source of a small group of compounds, the majority of which are vitamins. These vitamins include thiamine, riboflavin, pyridoxine, p-aminobenzoic acid, folic acid, pantothenic acid, and vitamins A, C, and E. Honey also contains minerals, including phosphorus, potassium, calcium, magnesium, sulfur, iron, copper, manganese, and zinc. The trace elements present in honey are very bioavailable, eventhough they are only present in trace amounts. It has been observed that the bioavailability of copper, calcium, zinc, iron, manganese, and magnesium derived from honey is between 80 and 90% [5, 13].

13.3 Propolis

Regarding its chemical composition, propolis is a product that presents a wide range of possibilities. At the current time, a minimum of 300 active chemicals have been discovered inside it [14]. Several chemicals, including flavonoids, benzoic acid, cinnamic acid, and phenolic acids (including caffeic, ferulic, chlorogenic, and p-coumaric), are considered the most significant physiologically active substances. Several flavonoids may be listed, including chrysin, luteolin, apigenin, galangin, kaempferol, quercetin, pinostrobin, pinocembrin, and terpene compounds with a concentration of 0.5% (bisabolol), as well as alcohols (cetyl, myricyl, mannitol, and inositol) [15–17]. Additionally, propolis is a source of minerals such as calcium, magnesium, manganese, zinc, copper, iron, cobalt, and selenium, as well as vitamins B1, B2, B6, C, and E, and enzymes such as succinate dehydrogenase, glucose-6-phosphatase, adenosine triphosphatase, and acid phosphatase [5, 17, 18].

13.4 Pollen from Bees

Pollen from bees contains at least 200 different compounds that have biological activity. Methionine, lysine, threonine, histidine, leucine, isoleucine, valine, phenylalanine, and tryptophan are among the essential amino acids that make up 10.4% of the content of bee pollen. Proteins make up around 22.7% of the total composition of bee pollen. The proportion of reduced sugars is 25.7%, whereas the percentage of digestible carbs accounts for 30.8%. Bee pollen contains various fatty acids, including gamma-linolenic acid, arachidonic acid, and linoleic acid (0.4%). These acids are among the fatty acids that may be described. In addition, nucleic acids and nucleosides are essential components of bee pollen because of their beneficial properties [19, 20]. Minerals and vitamins are also present in it, including potassium, calcium, phosphorus, iron, zinc, copper, and manganese [21]. Vitamins include B1, B2, B3, B5, B6, C, H, and E.

13.5 Honeybee Venom

Among the several peptides that may be found in bee venom are melittin, apamine, adolapin, sekapin, prokamin, and mast cell degranulating peptide [22]. The primary constituents of bee venom are known as peptides. Regarding peptides, melittin, in particular, plays a significant role in eliciting responses connected with bee stings. In addition to causing membrane permeabilization, melittin also causes cell lysis. Additionally, it has enzymes such as phospholipase A2, hyaluronidase acid, phosphomonoesterase, and lysophospholipase, as well as physiologically active amines such as histamine, adrenaline, dopamine, and norepinephrine. Bee venom contains various additional components in addition to peptides, such as lipids, carbohydrates, and free amino acids [5, 6, 23, 24].

13.6 Bee Products and Their Effects on Skin

13.6.1 Honey

Honey is utilized in the medical field for various reasons, including its antibacterial properties. These properties are attributed to hydrogen peroxide, high osmotic pressure, high acidity, phenolic acids, flavonoids, and lysozyme [25]. Honey reduces the formation of bacteria and fungi on the skin's surface, which in turn restricts the proliferation of these organisms. Honey has been used as a therapy for a variety of skin conditions, including pityriasis, tinea, seborrhea, dandruff, diaper dermatitis, psoriasis, hemorrhoids, and anal fissure [26]. Honey is particularly effective as a covering for wounds and burns. Both lysozyme and pinocembrin are responsible for the antifungal characteristics of the substance. Yeast-like fungi are unable to develop when lysozyme is present [27]. Honey has been shown to have a healing impact on wounds that have been surgically repaired [1]. Five hundred and twenty-two patients had their skin wounds covered with honey dressing. Ratings were given for the cosmetic result after three and 6 months had passed. The scars were narrower than they would have been if they had been treated with standard dressing. Honey dressing was applied to wounds in women who had undergone plastic surgery for 5 days, and the results showed that it had an analgesic effect and speed up the healing process. The entrance of extracellular Ca2+ that is generated by honey leads to the healing of wounds. This is comparable to the function that Ca2+ signaling performs in tissue regeneration [28].

Additionally, honey has a beneficial effect on the healing process of wounds and contributes to the regulation of the epithelial–mesenchymal transition (EMT) process. There is a correlation between the floral and the honey's origin and its effect on EMT [29]. Because honey kills bacteria, can penetrate bacterial biofilms, lowers the pH of wounds, reduces pain and inflammation, promotes fibroblast migration and keratinocyte closure, and promotes collagen deposition, honey can play a role in tissue engineering and regeneration. Honey is an apitherapeutic agent that is used in the treatment of wounds that are applied topically. Consider the possibility of incorporating honey into the biomaterial tissue templates to facilitate tissue regeneration. The electrospun templates, cryogels, and hydrogels created with honey were employed [5, 30].

13.6.2 Propolis

In the field of medicine, propolis is utilized extensively. In dermatology, it is used for treating staphylococcal, streptococcal, and fungal infections due to its antiseptic qualities. In addition to treating purulent skin infections, hidradenitis, intertrigo, cheilosis, and thrush, propolis is also used to treat various other skin conditions. In treating skin burns, it has been found that the propolis preparation known as Propol T is significantly more successful than other treatments [31]. Even though propolis and sulfathiazole both have therapeutic benefits equivalent to one another, bee glue is safer and has fewer unwanted effects. Not only does propolis have antibacterial and anti-inflammatory properties, but it also facilitates the formation of scar tissue and alleviates pain. Chrysin, which is a flavonoid, can relieve both pain and discomfort. Utilizing propolis as a treatment for burn wounds in pigs increased fibroblasts' proliferation, activation, and growth capacity. The buildup of glycosaminoglycan, which is necessary for granulation, tissue development, and wound healing, is stimulated by propolis. It has been demonstrated that propolis is a more effective apitherapeutic agent than silver sulfadiazine. The accumulation of collagen type I in the matrix of an injury is a stimulant for the healing process. This is because collagen type I is essential for the migration and reepithelization of keratinocytes.

Additionally, propolis boosts the formation of collagen type III, which speeds up maintaining a healthy body. As a topical apitherapeutic product for treating burns, propolis ointment can contribute to the reepithelization process [32]. By regulating neutrophil and neutrophil elastase levels, propolis topically reduced the amount of chronic inflammation present in diabetic wounds. The analgesic and anti-inflammatory properties of propolis are attributed to the presence of caffeine [33].

Furthermore, propolis is helpful in the healing process in various animal models, including rats with diabetic wounds and animals with burns [32–34]. Propolis is a highly effective therapy for acne vulgaris with a proven track record. Following the application of an ethanol extract of propolis to the skin, researchers established that the incidence of Cutibacterium acnes, a bacterium that plays a significant role in the development of acne vulgaris, was restricted [35]. The ethanol extract of propolis inhibits both *Staphylococcus epidermidis* and other bacteria. Propolis is utilized in the production of cosmetics for the skin affected by acne and in the production of medications that combat bacterial and fungal infections [36]. In concentrations ranging from 5% to 20%, propolis possesses regenerative and healing capabilities and the ability to defend against external causes. The skin tissue is strengthened and protected from harmful bacteria by this substance, which makes it suitable for use in the production of anti-bedsore products [37]. Due to the inclusion of caffeic acid, coumaric acid, and ferulic acid, propolis can absorb ultraviolet light, which is another way to protect against the harmful effects of ultraviolet radiation. Because of its anti-inflammatory, anti-oxidative, and regenerative characteristics, propolis is an excellent ingredient for sunblock products such as creams, lotions, sticks, and lipsticks [38]. It also can act as a natural filter. Some other researchers demonstrated that applying Romanian propolis to the skin of 30 Swiss mice resulted in photoprotective benefits against ultraviolet B radiation [39].

13.6.3 Royal Jelly

Royal jelly's impact on the skin is determined by a wide range of biological activities, including antibacterial, anti-inflammatory, immunomodulatory, antiallergic, antioxidant, toning, moisturizing, and antiaging properties [40]. Royal jelly possesses a broad spectrum of biological activities. Royal jelly possesses powerful antibacterial action within the skin tissue, which is already noticeable at a concentration of 20%. Royal jelly is a product of bees. As a result of its anti-inflammatory properties, royal jelly is effective in alleviating periodontal disorders and irritation of the oral cavity, tongue, and throat. The capacity of this substance to block the production of pro-inflammatory cytokines (TNF-α, IL-6, and IL-1) is the source of its anti-inflammatory effect and its ability to promote wound healing. Royal jelly protects blood vessels and can alleviate hemorrhoids and varicose veins in the lower extremities. Royal jelly also works to reduce pain. As a treatment for lichen, ulcers, burns, bed sores, shingles, and any other condition in which the regeneration of the epidermis is anticipated, wound epithelialization, nutritional impact, healing, and antibacterial activity are all possible applications of this substance. Research has been conducted to investigate the effect of royal jelly at a concentration of 5% on ulcers that develop on the diabetic foot.

The wound was dressed with sterile royal jelly containing 5% three times a week for the duration of the therapy, which lasted for 3 months. Eight ulcers were treated, seven of which healed, and in one instance, an improvement was noticed [41]. The reepithelization of wounds is facilitated by royal jelly. After being incubated with a water extract of royal jelly, the keratinocytes are responsible for the increased synthesis of MMP-9 (matrix metalloproteinase-9). After administering aqueous extract of royal jelly, there was an increase in the migration of keratinocytes and the pace at which wounds closed. The component of royal jelly known as defensin-1 is the one that is responsible for increasing the creation of MMP-9. In addition, defensin-1 encourages the reepithelization and closure of wounds. In the same way as honey does, defensin-1 is responsible for the closure of cutaneous wounds by increasing the production of keratinocytes and MMP-9 [42].

13.7 Use of Honey Products in Otolaryngology

Honey is recommended as a potential remedy for cough caused by the common cold in children at least 1 year old. Honey can be administered in its purest form, 2.5 to 5 ml (0.5–1 teaspoon), or diluted in liquids such as tea or juice [43]. If honey is unavailable, corn syrup can be used as an alternative. Honey is considered safe for children older than 1 year old and has a moderately favorable effect on nocturnal cough. Honey is not likely to be hazardous to children. Honey is not recommended for consumption by infants and toddlers less than 1 year old due to the possibility of botulism [44].

After doing a comprehensive analysis of 14 randomized studies that compared honey to other treatments in the treatment of upper respiratory tract infections in children and adults, the researchers concluded that honey was superior to the standard treatment, which included placebo, diphenhydramine, and dextromethorphan [45]. Honey was found to lower the frequency of coughing (standard mean difference (SMD) −0.36, 95% confidence interval (CI) −0.50 to −0.21; eight trials, 832 individuals) and the intensity of coughing (SMD −0.44, 95% CI −0.64 to −0.25; five trials, 598 participants) in meta-analyses. Honey was shown to be more effective than diphenhydramine and comparable to dextromethorphan in terms of lowering the frequency and severity of coughing, according to observations made through direct comparisons. Infrequent and moderate adverse effects, such as nausea, were observed.

The World Health Organization (WHO) and the American Academy of Pediatrics (AAP) recommend honey as a viable therapy for upper respiratory infections (URI) in young children older than 1 year old [43, 46]. Honey is relatively safe and inexpensive. The American College of Chest Physicians has suggested that honey is more beneficial than a placebo in treating cough cases caused by the common cold [47].

In the study conducted by Hehlgans and colleagues [48], it was found that propolis activated caspase 3 cleavage and enhanced the rate of apoptosis in HNSCC cell lines. Additionally, propolis was found to produce significant alterations in proteins that have a role in the evolution of tumors, including AKT, ERK1/2, FAK, E-cadherin, and cyclin D. Furthermore, when cancer cells were pre-treated with propolis, they became more sensitive to the effects of ionizing radiation therapy [48]. Similarly, Kuo et al. [49] have confirmed that propolis in HNSCC cells led to the down-regulation of AKT and cyclin D, in addition to FOXO and NF-κB. Furthermore, they demonstrated that the combination of propolis and 5-fluorouracil resulted in an additive impact on the reduction of cell growth. As a result of these findings, it is evident that propolis not only controls many pathways that are connected with the evolution of cancer, but it also appears to promote the processes of radiation and chemotherapy.

Nor et al. [50] found a decrease in endothelial cells' vitality when HDMEC cells were subjected to green, brown, or red propolis extracts. It has been demonstrated that endothelial cells can regulate several aspects of cancer cell activity, such as proliferation, tumor development, invasiveness, and resistance [51, 52]. It was demonstrated by Borovski et al. [53] that administering antiangiogenic treatment to gliomas and eliminating tumor vasculature lead to an increased vulnerability of the CSC to cytotoxic drugs. Bevacizumab, an antibody that neutralizes VEGF, lowered the number of cancer stem cells (CSC) in the body, preventing the formation of tumors. This was accomplished by inhibiting angiogenesis and depleting blood vessels simultaneously. These findings lend credence to angiogenesis' impact on cancer stem cells (CSC) and, subsequently, on the growth of tumors. As a result, the modulation of the perivascular niche by propolis might be a viable treatment method for cancer.

Moon et al. [54] conducted a study to explore the positive benefits of water-soluble ethanol extract propolis on post-tonsillectomy patients. One hundred thirty patients who had undergone tonsillectomy or adenotonsillectomy were randomly divided into the control group and the propolis group, each consisting of 65 patients. An oral application of propolis was administered to the propolis group soon following surgery, and it was also gargled. The pain experienced by patients in the propolis group following post-tonsillectomy was considerably lower than that experienced by patients in the control group on postoperative days 3 and 7–10. Compared to the control group, the propolis group exhibited a reduction in post-tonsillectomy bleeding that was statistically significant ($p < 0.05$). During postoperative days 7–10, the wound healing was substantially better in the group that received propolis than in the group that received the control ($p = 0.002$). The researchers concluded that applying propolis to the wound that was left behind after tonsillectomy positively impacted the patient's recovery by lowering postoperative discomfort, avoiding bleeding, and speeding up the healing process of the tonsillar fossa tissue.

It is well known that propolis can improve the creation of scars and tissue regeneration. The application of propolis to a wound site with open epithelium causes the propolis to penetrate deeply into the tissue, which stimulates cell regeneration, enhances the proliferation of cornification cells, and contributes to wound healing [55]. Propolis was shown to be more effective in wound healing than silver sulfadiazine, a standard treatment for burn wounds [56]. This was the case while investigating burn wounds. These actions would finally allow epithelial regeneration and scar formation [55, 57]. Flavonoid in propolis displays a cicatrization effect by reducing acid secretion, boosting prostaglandin concentration, suppressing lipid peroxidation, and lowering reactive oxygen species. These processes would eventually lead to cicatrization.

Honey has the potential to be a successful (additional) therapy for mucositis, cough in children, chronic cough experienced after an infectious illness, and cough that occurs after tonsillectomy. Propolis might play a part in the treatment of stomatitis, also known as aphthous stomatitis, and in the prevention of acute otitis media. There was evidence that royal jelly prevented mucositis. According to the research, beehive products were shown to be safe, with very few instances of adverse responses [58].

References

1. Goharshenasan P, Amini S, Atria A, Abtahi H, Khorasani G. Topical application of honey on surgical wounds: A randomized clinical trial. Compl Med Res. 2016;23:12–5. https://doi.org/10.1159/000441994.
2. El-Soud A, Helmy N. Honey between traditional uses and recent medicine. Macedon J Med Sci. 2012;5:205–14. https://doi.org/10.3889/mjms.1857-5773.2012.0213.
3. Abouda Z, Zerdani I, Kalalou I, Faid M, Ahami MT. The antibacterial activity of Moroccan bee bread and bee pollen (fresh and dried) against pathogenic bacteria. Res J Microbiol. 2011;6:376–84. https://doi.org/10.3923/jm.2011.376.384.
4. Cornara L, Biagi M, Xiao J, Burlando B. Therapeutic properties of bioactive compounds from different honeybee products. Front Pharmacol. 2017;8:412. https://doi.org/10.3389/fphar.2017.00412.
5. Kurek-Górecka A, Górecki M, Rzepecka-Stojko A, Balwierz R, Stojko J. Bee products in dermatology and skin care. Molecules. 2020;25(3):556. https://doi.org/10.3390/molecules25030556. PMID: 32012913; PMCID: PMC7036894.
6. Han SM, Lee GG, Park KK. Skin sensitization study of bee venom (*Apis mellifera* L.) in Guinea pigs. Toxicol Res. 2012;28:1–4.
7. Viuda-Martos M, Ruiz-Navajas Y, Fernández-López J, Pérez-Álvarez JA. Functional properties of honey, propolis, and royal jelly. J Food Sci. 2008;73:117–24. https://doi.org/10.1111/j.1750-3841.2008.00966.x.
8. Ball DW. The chemical composition of honey. J Chem Educ. 2007;84:1643. https://doi.org/10.1021/ed084p1643.
9. Borawska M, Arciuch L, Puścion-Jakubik A, Lewoc D. Content of sugars (fructose, glucose, sucrose) and proline in different varieties of natural bee honey. Probl Hig Epidemiol. 2015;96:816–20.
10. Da Silva PM, Gauche C, Gonzaga LV, Costa ACO, Fett R. Honey: chemical composition, stability and authenticity. Food Chem. 2016;196:309–23. https://doi.org/10.1016/j.foodchem.2015.09.051.
11. Sak-Bosnar M, Sakač N. Direct potentiometric determination of diastase activity in honey. Food Chem. 2012;135:827–31. https://doi.org/10.1016/j.foodchem.2012.05.006.

12. Truchado P, Ferreres F, Bortolotti L, Sabatini AG, Tomás-Barberán FA. Nectar flavonol rhamnosides are floral markers of acacia (*Robinia pseudacacia*) honey. J Agric Food Chem. 2008;56:8815–24. https://doi.org/10.1021/jf801625t.
13. Stecka H, Gręda K, Pohl P. Total content and the bioavailable fraction of calcium, cooper, iron, magnesium, manganese and zinc in polish commercial bee honeys. Bromatol Chem Toksykol. 2012;45:111–6.
14. De Castro SL. Propolis: biological and pharmacological activities. Therapeutic uses of this bee-product. ARBS Ann Rev Biomed Sci. 2001;3:49–83. https://doi.org/10.5016/1806-8774.2001v3p49.
15. Schnitzler P, Neuner A, Nolkemper S, Zundel C, Nowack H, Sensch KH, Reichling J. Antiviral activity and mode of action of propolis extracts and selected compounds. Phytother Res. 2010;24:20–8. https://doi.org/10.1002/ptr.2868.
16. Kurek-Górecka A, Rzepecka-Stojko A, Górecki M, Stojko J, Sosada M, Świerczek-Zięba G. Structure and antioxidant activity of polyphenols derived from propolis. Molecules. 2013;19:78–101. https://doi.org/10.3390/molecules19010078.
17. Olczyk P, Komosińska-Vassev K, Ramos P, Mencner L, Olczyk K, Pilawa B. Free radical scavenging activity of drops and spray containing propolis—an EPR examination. Molecules. 2017;22:128. https://doi.org/10.3390/molecules22010128.
18. Mărghitaş LA, Dezmirean DS, Bobiş O. Important developments in Romanian propolis research. Evid Based Complement Alternat Med. 2013;2013:1. https://doi.org/10.1155/2013/159392.
19. Komosińska-Vassev K, Olczyk P, Kaźmierczak J, Mencner L, Olczyk K. Bee pollen: chemical composition and therapeutic application. Evid Based Complement Alternat Med. 2015;2015. https://doi.org/10.1155/2015/297425.
20. Feás X, Vázquez-Tato MP, Estevinho L, Seijas JA, Iglesias A. Organic bee pollen: botanical origin, nutritional value, bioactive compounds, antioxidant activity and microbiological quality. Molecules. 2012;17:8359–77. https://doi.org/10.3390/molecules17078359.
21. Campos MG, Bogdanov S, de Almeida-Muradian LB, Szczesna T, Mancebo Y, Frigerio C, Ferreira F. Pollen composition and standardisation of analytical methods. J Apic Res. 2008;47:156–61.
22. Son DJ, Lee JW, Lee YH, Song HS, Lee CK, Hong JT. Therapeutic application of anti-arthritis, pain-releasing, and anti-cancer effects of bee venom and its constituent compounds. Pharmacol Ther. 2007;115:246–70. https://doi.org/10.1016/j.pharmthera.2007.04.004.
23. Pałgan K, Bartuzi Z. Biological properties of bee venom. Alerg Astma Immun. 2009;14:17–9.
24. Kim H, Park S-Y, Lee G. Potential therapeutic applications of bee venom on skin disease and its mechanisms: a literature review. Toxins. 2019;11:374. https://doi.org/10.3390/toxins11070374.
25. Bogdanov S. Nature and origin of the antibacterial substances in honey. LWT-Food Sci Technol. 1997;30:748–53. https://doi.org/10.1006/fstl.1997.0259.
26. Burlando B, Cornara L. Honey in dermatology and skin care: a review. J Cosm Dermatol. 2013;12:306–13. https://doi.org/10.1111/jocd.12058.
27. Kędzia B, Hołderna-Kędzia E. Contemporary opinions on the mechanism of antimicrobial action of honey. Postep Fitoter. 2017;4:290–7. https://doi.org/10.25121/PF.2017.18.4.290.
28. Martinotti S, Laforenza U, Patrone M, Moccia F, Ranzato E. Honey-mediated wound healing: H_2O_2 entry through AQP3 determines extracellular Ca^{2+} influx. Int J Mol Sci. 2019;20:764. https://doi.org/10.3390/ijms20030764.
29. Nordin A, Sainik NQAV, Zulfarina MS, Naina-Mohamed I, Saim A, Idrus RBH. Honey epithelial to mesenchymal transition in wound healing: an evidence-based review. Wound Med. 2017;18:8–20. https://doi.org/10.1016/j.wndm.2017.06.003.
30. Minden-Birkenmaier BA, Bowlin GL. Honey-based templates in wound healing and tissue engineering. Bioengineering. 2018;5:46. https://doi.org/10.3390/bioengineering5020046.
31. Olczyk P, Komosińska-Vassev K, Winsz-Szczotka K, Stojko J, Klimek K, Gajewski K, Olczyk K. The evaluation of chosen extracellular matrix enzymes activity during regeneration of experimental thermal injuries. Leczenie Ran. 2014;11:97–101. https://doi.org/10.15374/LR2014016.

32. Olczyk P, Wisowski G, Komosińska-Vassev K, Stojko J, Klimek K, Olczyk M, Koźma EM. Propolis modifies collagen types I and III accumulation in the matrix of burnt tissue. Evid Based Complement Alternat Med 2013;2013. https://doi.org/10.1155/2013/423809.
33. Al-Waili N, Hozzein WN, Badr G, Al-Ghamdi H, Al-Waili H, Salom K, Al-Waili T. Propolis and bee venom in diabetic wounds; a potential approach that warrants clinical investigation. Afr J Tradit Complement Altern Med. 2015;12:1–11. https://doi.org/10.4314/ajtcam.v12i6.1.
34. Tie L, An Y, Han J, Xiao Y, Xiaokaiti Y, Fan S, Liu S, Chen AF, Li X. Genistein accelerates refractory wound healing by suppressing superoxide and FoxO1/iNOS pathway in type 1 diabetes. J Nutr Biochem. 2013;24:88–96. https://doi.org/10.1016/j.jnutbio.2012.02.011.
35. Ali BMM, Ghoname NF, Hodeib AA, Elbadawy MA. Significance of topical propolis in the treatment of facial acne vulgaris. Egypt J Dermatol Venerol. 2015;35:29–36. https://doi.org/10.4103/1110-6530.162468.
36. Bankova V. Recent trends and important developments in propolis research. Evid Based Complement Alternat Med. 2005;2:29–32. https://doi.org/10.1093/ecam/neh059.
37. Sawicka D, Borawska MH. The use of propolis in skin diseases. Derm Estet. 2013;1:13–7.
38. Nisakorn S. Natural products as photoprotection. J Cosmet Dermatol. 2015;14:47–63. https://doi.org/10.1111/jocd.12123.
39. Bolfa P, Vidrighinescu R, Petruta A, Dezmirean D, Stan L, Vlase L, Damian G, Catoi C, Filip A, Clichici S. Photoprotective effects of Romanian propolis on skin of mice exposed to UVB irradiation. Food Chem Toxicol. 2013;62:329–42. https://doi.org/10.1016/j.fct.2013.08.078.
40. Pavel CI, Mărghitaş LA, Bobiş O, Dezmirean DS, Şapcaliu A, Radoi I, Mădaş MN. Biological activities of royal jelly—review. Sci Pap Anim Sci Biotechnol. 2011;44:108–18.
41. Siavash M, Shokri S, Haghighi S, Mohammadi M, Shahtalebi MA, Farajzadehgan Z. The efficacy of topical royal jelly on diabetic foot ulcers healing: a case series. J Res Med Sci. 2011;16:904–9.
42. Bucekova M, Sojka M, Valachova I, Martinotti S, Ranzato E, Szep Z, Majtan V, Klaudiny J, Majtan J. Bee-derived antibacterial peptide, defensin 1, promotes wound re-epithelialisation in vitro and in vivo. Sci Rep. 2017;7:7340. https://doi.org/10.1038/s41598-017-07494-0.
43. American Academy of Pediatrics. Coughs and colds: medicines or home remedies? http://www.healthychildren.org/English/health-issues/conditions/ear-nose-throat/pages/Coughs-and-Colds-Medicines-or-Home-Remedies.aspx. Accessed 23 Aug 2011.
44. Pappas DE. The common cold in children: management and prevention. In: Edwards MS, Blake D, editors. UpToDate. Last updated: Mar 22, 2023.
45. Abuelgasim H, Albury C, Lee J. Effectiveness of honey for symptomatic relief in upper respiratory tract infections: a systematic review and meta-analysis. BMJ Evid Based Med. 2021;26:57.
46. World Health Organization. Cough and cold remedies for the treatment of acute respiratory infections in young children, 2001. https://apps.who.int/iris/handle/10665/66856. Accessed 18 Oct 2021
47. Malesker MA, Callahan-Lyon P, Ireland B, et al. Pharmacologic and nonpharmacologic treatment for acute cough associated with the common cold: CHEST expert panel report. Chest. 2017;152:1021.
48. Hehlgans S, Lange I, Eke I, Kammerer B, Cordes N. Human head and neck squamous cell carcinoma cell lines are differentially radiosensitised by the honeybee product Propolis. Int J Radiat Biol. 2011;87(3):243–53. https://doi.org/10.3109/09553002.2010.533248.
49. Kuo YY, Jim WT, Su LC, Chung CJ, Lin CY, Huo C, et al. Caffeic Acid phenethyl ester is a potential therapeutic agent for oral cancer. Int J Mol Sci. 2015;16(5):10748–66. https://doi.org/10.3390/ijms160510748.
50. Nör F, Nör C, Bento LW, Zhang Z, Bretz WA, Nör JE. Propolis reduces the stemness of head and neck squamous cell carcinoma. Arch Oral Biol. 2021;125:105087. https://doi.org/10.1016/j.archoralbio.2021.105087. Epub 2021 Feb 19. PMID: 33639480; PMCID: PMC8532192.
51. Song YS, Park EH, Jung KJ, Jin C. Inhibition of angiogenesis by propolis. Arch Pharm Res. 2002;25(4):500–4. https://doi.org/10.1007/bf02976609.

52. de Moura SA, Ferreira MA, Andrade SP, Reis ML, Noviello ML, Cara DC. Brazilian green propolis inhibits inflammatory angiogenesis in a murine sponge model. Evid Based Complement Alternat Med. 2011;2011:182703. https://doi.org/10.1093/ecam/nep197.
53. Borovski T, De Sousa EMF, Vermeulen L, Medema JP. Cancer stem cell niche: the place to be. Cancer Res. 2011;71(3):634–9. https://doi.org/10.1158/0008-5472.CAN-10-3220.
54. Moon JH, Lee MY, Chung YJ, Rhee CK, Lee SJ. Effect of topical propolis on wound healing process after tonsillectomy: randomized controlled study. Clin Exp Otorhinolaryngol. 2018;11(2):146–50. https://doi.org/10.21053/ceo.2017.00647.
55. Viuda-Martos M, Ruiz-Navajas Y, Fernandez-Lopez J, Perez-Alvarez JA. Functional properties of honey, propolis, and royal jelly. J Food Sci. 2008;73(9):R117–24.
56. Akbas Y, Pata YS, Unal M, Gorur K, Micozkadioglu D. The effect of fusafungine on postoperative pain and wound healing after pediatric tonsillectomy. Int J Pediatr Otorhinolaryngol. 2004;68(8):1023–6.
57. Martin MJ, La-Casa C, Alarcon-de-la-Lastra C, Cabeza J, Villegas I, Motilva V. Antioxidant mechanisms involved in gastroprotective effects of quercetin. Z Naturforsch C. 1998;53(1–2):82–8.
58. Henatsch D, Wesseling F, Kross KW, Stokroos RJ. Honey and beehive products in otorhinolaryngology: a narrative review. Clin Otolaryngol. 2016;41(5):519–31. https://doi.org/10.1111/coa.12557.

Nasal Effects of Propolis

14

14.1 Introduction

One of the most common complications that might arise during nasal procedures, such as endoscopic sinus surgery and septoplasty [1], is trauma to the nasal mucosa. Healing the nasal mucosa after it has been injured is very complicated and entails restoring the anatomical and functional integrity of the tissue at the same time [2]. Staffieri and colleagues [3] conducted a study to explore the effects of nasal corticosteroid sprays on the healing of the nasal mucosa following nasal operations.

The resinous substance known as propolis is a product of the beehive made up of plant components that hive workers gather. Afterward, salivary enzymes are added to the wax, and the mixture is combined with wax to make propolis [4]. Bees chew on these components. Flavonoids and caffeic acid esters are propolis fractions with the most significant potential biological activity [5].

Propolis possesses antioxidant properties [7], anti-inflammatory properties [6], antimicrobial properties [8], and most importantly, antibacterial properties [9]. Furthermore, the propolis component known as caffeic acid is powerful in blocking pro-inflammatory proteinase, matrix metalloproteinase-9, which is known to be elevated in ulcers [10].

Propolis topical application has been proven effective in treating ulcers [4]. In light of this, several nations have approved its use in treating ulcers and abrasions [4]. The profile of adverse effects associated with propolis is likewise considered modest [1, 11].

A. E. Tanuğur Samanci et al., *Propolis: Prevention and Healing Effects in Otorhinolaryngology*, Comprehensive ENT,
https://doi.org/10.1007/978-3-031-68546-0_14

14.2 Propolis

The term "propolis" refers to a combination of compounds bees use to protect their hive. As part of this defense, cavities in the hive's walls are filled, the entry is reduced on days when the temperature is low, and the invaders who are needed are mummified, preventing their deterioration [12, 13]. The reason why propolis is often referred to as bee glue is because of this [14]. The Latin term propolis comes from Greek and literally translates to "at the entrance to the city" [4, 15]. Since ancient times, people have continued discussing where the propolis came from. Some questions have been raised regarding whether or not it originates from plants or bees. At this point, thanks to the advancement of analytical methods, the approximate composition of propolis and the elements that influence it are known [13].

Bees produce propolis by collecting resins from buds, exudates, and other sections of plants and then combining these resins with their salivary enzymes and beeswax [16, 17]. Different continents, areas, and plant species are utilized to manufacture propolis, resulting in the composition of propolis being distinct. While having a particular chemical makeup, propolis possesses actions comparable to those of other substances, including antibacterial, antifungal, antiviral, antiparasitic, anti-inflammatory, antiproliferative, and antioxidant properties [18–22].

Throughout Central Europe, including Poland, bees collect secretion from poplar buds (Populus spp.) and alder (Alnus spp.). Various varieties of poplar are also used as a source of resin in other European nations, such as Bulgaria, Hungary, Albania, and England, as well as in countries that are located in the temperate zone, such as the United States of America, Mongolia, West Asia, and North Africa. Birch, also known as Betula species, is a source of propolis in Northern Europe, such as the region of Russia in North Europe. Additionally, propolis is produced by bees from the buds of willow (Salix spp.), oak (Quercus spp.), ash (Fraxinus spp.), chestnut tree (Aesculus spp.), and bark from coniferous trees, such as spruce (Picea spp.), fir (Abies spp.), or pine (Pinus spp.). Bees in tropical regions make use of the secretions of plants such as Xanthorrhoea (in Australia), Acacia (in North Africa), Plumeria (in Hawaii), Clusia (in Central America), and Baccharis, Araucaria, and Eucalyptus (in Brazil) [12–14, 22–24].

Regarding research on goods derived from bees, including propolis, Brazil is the country that leads the pack [25]. Many propolis varieties in Brazil can be identified from one another based on their botanical origin. Because of the climate, bees can collect propolis throughout the year. Within the scope of their research, Bueno-Silva and colleagues analyzed one of the most prevalent varieties of Brazilian propolis, known as red, whose principal plant source is Dalbergia ecastophyllum. An investigation was conducted to determine the impact of the period at which the propolis was collected and its chemical makeup and antibacterial activity. It was noted that the concentrations of vestitol, neovestitol, and isoliquiritigenin varied throughout the year because of seasonal differences. The rainy season, which spans from January to May, was shown to have the highest concentration of these components and the highest antibacterial activity [26].

"Geopropolis" refers to a different propolis produced by stingless bees, such as *Melipona mondury* and *M. scutellaris*. Propolis, generated by bees belonging to the genus Apis, is highly comparable to this substance's chemical makeup and biological activity [27, 28]. In the research conducted by Torres and colleagues, a comparison was made between two ethanolic propolis (EEP) obtained from two different species of stingless bees: *Melipona quadrifasciata* and *Tetragonisca angustula*. For Gram-positive bacteria, such as *Staphylococcus aureus* MSSA and MRSA, and *Enterococcus faecalis*, geopropolis extracts demonstrated much higher levels of activity than Gram-negative bacteria, such as *Klebsiella pneumoniae* and *Escherichia coli*, according to the findings of the study. Compared to the other two geopropolis which were investigated, the Melipona species was shown to be more effective [12, 29].

In its raw form, propolis cannot be utilized directly in an analytical or therapeutic setting. To begin, it is necessary to remove it to dissolve and release the most active components. The following solvents are utilized to extract the substance: ethanol, methanol, water, hexane, acetone, dichloromethane, and chloroform. There is a concentration of propolis in the extracts that is around 70% [30, 31]. The presence of chemicals such as flavonoids and phenolic compounds is significant in their ability to inhibit the growth of bacteria [32–34].

On the other hand, the biological activity discovered varies according to the solvent utilized. Extracts of brown, green, and red propolis obtained by ethanolic extraction were found to have roughly two times greater amounts of phenolic chemicals than extracts obtained using supercritical extraction, according to the findings of Devequi-Nunes and colleagues. On the other hand, compared to the results of supercritical extraction, the amounts of flavonoids were more significant in ethanolic extracts of green and red propolis. At the same time, they were shown to be lower in brown propolis extraction [35]. The research conducted by Wieczyńska and colleagues showed that the antibacterial activity of ethanolic extracts from Polish propolis was much higher than that of hexane extracts [36].

The measurement of the total phenolics content (TP) and flavonoids (FP) of propolis extracts has recently become the basis for the evaluation of the antibacterial activity of these extracts to be conducted. Bridi and colleagues discovered in their research that TP and FP tests of antimicrobial activity in vitro may only sometimes provide an accurate reflection of the activity. The findings of the TP in the samples with the greatest and the lowest content were closely related to the amount of flavonoids and antioxidant characteristics present in the samples from both groups. However, they did not provide a clear and unequivocal answer in the case of antibacterial activity. In the process of establishing international quality standards for propolis, it is recommended that additional tests, such as ORAC (Oxygen Radical Absorbance Capacity) and antimicrobial testing, be taken into consideration [12, 37].

Considering that propolis and other bee products include antibacterial properties, the combination of these two substances ought to amplify the impact. Researchers Al-Waili and colleagues investigated the possibility of relying on the mixture of propolis and honey gathered in Egypt and Saudi Arabia. It has been demonstrated via the findings of this research that the antibacterial properties of propolis and honey are enhanced when combined. This is the case for both *S. aureus* and *E. coli*. An approximately twofold reduction in the MIC value was observed due to this impact, which was substantial for Saudi propolis. The activity level of Egyptian raw materials was significantly lower [38].

Propolis's effect on anaerobic bacteria has only been the subject of a small amount of research. On the other hand, the findings of this study suggest that this bee product possesses a high level of action against a variety of bacterial species, including Clostridium, Bacteroides, Porphyromonas, Prevotella, Fusobacterium, Actinomyces, and Propionibacterium [39–42]. The anaerobic bacteria from the Fusobacterium genus were shown to be the most vulnerable to low concentrations of ethanolic extract from propolis (EEP) in Polish research. These values ranged from 0.01 to 0.06 mg/mL. On the other hand, bacteria belonging to the genera Actinomyces, Bacteroides, Clostridium, Peptococcus, Peptostreptococcus, and Propionibacterium were susceptible to EEP when it was present in high quantities (ranging from 1 to 3 mg/mL) [43–45].

Bees utilize a mixture of chemicals called "propolis" to defend their colony. This defense mechanism includes sealing up openings in the hive's walls, limiting access on cold days, and mummifying necessary intruders to keep them from deteriorating [12, 13]. For this reason, "bee glue" is a common name for propolis [14]. "At the entrance to the city" is the literal translation of the Greek origin of the Latin word "propolis" [4, 15]. The origin of propolis has been a topic of debate since ancient times. Whether it comes from plants or bees is a matter of some debate. The development of analytical tools has allowed us to determine the factors that affect propolis and its approximate makeup [13].

Bees collect resins from various parts of plants, such as buds and exudates, then mix these resins with beeswax and salivary enzymes to make propolis [16, 17]. The composition of propolis is distinct because it is made from various plant species from different continents, places, and countries. Propolis has a unique chemical composition but a wide range of useful qualities, such as antimicrobial, antiviral, antiparasitic, anti-inflammatory, antiproliferative, and antioxidant [18, 21, 22].

In Poland and the rest of Central Europe, bees gather pollen from alder and poplar buds. Other temperate zone countries, including the United States, Mongolia, West Asia, and North Africa, utilize different types of poplar as a resin supply. In contrast, other European nations like Bulgaria, Hungary, Albania, and England do the same. Northern Europe, including the Russian Federation, relies on birch trees—also called Betula species—for its propolis supply. Also, bees make propolis from the other plant parts, including the buds of trees like willow, oak, ash, chestnut, and coniferous trees like spruce, fir, and pine. From Xanthorrhoea in Australia to Acacia in North Africa, Plumeria in Hawaii, Clusia in Central America, and Baccharis, Araucaria, and Eucalyptus in Brazil, bees in tropical climates utilize plant secretions [12–14, 22–24].

Regarding studies on bee products, such as propolis, Brazil is at the forefront of the field [25]. Different types of propolis in Brazil can be distinguished according to their botanical ancestry. The weather allows bees to gather propolis at any time of year. As part of their study, Bueno-Silva and colleagues examined red propolis, a type of Brazilian propolis derived primarily from the Dalbergia ecastophyllum plant. A study was carried out to ascertain the effect of the collection period on the chemical composition and antibacterial activity of the propolis. Vestitol, neovestitol, and isoliquiritigenin concentrations fluctuated throughout the year due to seasonal variations. The antibacterial activity and concentration of these components were found to be maximum during the rainy season, which begins in January and ends in May [26].

The term "geopropolis" describes a distinct kind of propolis made by stingless bees like *Melipona mondury* and *M. scutellaris*. This material's chemical composition and biological activity are quite similar to those of propolis, which is produced by bees of the species Apis [27, 28]. The study by Torres and colleagues compared two types of stingless bees, *Melipona quadrifasciata* and *Tetragonisca angustula*, using ethanolic extract of propolis (EEP). The study found that geopropolis extracts were much more active against Gram-positive bacteria like *Staphylococcus aureus*, MSSA and MRSA, as well as *Enterococcus faecalis*, compared against Gram-negative bacteria like *Klebsiella pneumoniae* and *Escherichia coli*. The results showed that the Melipona species were more effective than the other geopolises [12, 29].

There is no analytical or therapeutic use for propolis in its unprocessed state. To start, you need get rid of it so the active ingredients may dissolve and be released. Hexane, acetone, dichloromethane, chloroform, ethanol, methanol, water, and hexane are the solvents used to extract the chemical. The extracts contain a concentration of propolis of approximately 70% [30, 31]. The capacity of substances like flavonoids and phenolic compounds to suppress bacterial growth is strong [32–34].

Conversely, the biological activity that has been found differs depending on the solvent used. According to the research conducted by Devequi-Nunes and colleagues, the phenolic chemical content of brown, green, and red propolis extracts obtained through ethanolic extraction was about double that of extracts acquired using supercritical extraction. However, the flavonoid concentrations in the ethanolic extracts of the green and red propolis were much higher than in the supercritical extraction results. Simultaneously, brown propolis extraction demonstrated that they were lower [35]. Wieczyńska and colleagues' investigation demonstrated that ethanolic extracts of Polish propolis had much more antibacterial activity than hexane extracts [36].

A new standard for determining whether or not propolis extracts have antibacterial properties is to assess their total phenolics (TP) and flavonoids (FP) content. In their study, Bridi and colleagues found that TP and FP tests for antimicrobial activity in vitro don't always give a true picture of the activity. The levels of flavonoids and antioxidant properties in the two groups of samples were significantly correlated with the TP results for the highest and lowest content samples, respectively. When asked about their antibacterial action, though, they were evasive. Additional tests like ORAC (Oxygen Radical Absorbance Capacity) and antimicrobial testing should be considered when setting international quality standards for propolis [12, 37].

Combining these two chemicals should increase their antibacterial effects, as propolis and other bee products already have them. Scientists Al-Waili and colleagues explored the prospect of using a combination of honey and propolis collected in Saudi Arabia and Egypt. The results of this study show that combining propolis and honey increases their antibacterial effects. The same holds true for *Escherichia coli* and *Staphylococcus aureus*. As a result of this effect, which was significant for Saudi propolis, the MIC value was found to have decreased by around half. There was a considerable decrease in the activity level of Egyptian raw materials [38].

Minimal studies have been conducted on the effects of propolis on anaerobic bacteria. Conversely, this study's results imply that this bee product has a high level of action against several bacterial species, such as Clostridium, Bacteroides, Porphyromonas, Prevotella, Fusobacterium, Actinomyces, and Propionibacterium [39–42, 46]. Polish researchers found that modest amounts of propolis (EEP) ethanolic extract were particularly effective against anaerobic bacteria from the Fusobacterium genus. Between 0.01% and 0.06%, in mg/mL, these readings fell. However, at high concentrations (1–4.6) of EEP, bacteria from the genera Actinomyces, Bacteroides, Clostridium, Peptococcus, Peptostreptococcus, and Propionibacterium were vulnerable to it.

14.3 Effects of Propolis on Nasal Mucosa

The findings of the research conducted by El-Anwar et al. [1] showed that the injection of propolis decreased the intensity of inflammation and retained both ciliated and goblet cells following experimental damage to the nasal mucosa. The fact that the group treated with propolis did not develop ulcerations indicates that the healing process was accelerated due to the administration of this substance. On the other hand, the groups that were not treated and those that had gum tragacanth had significant inflammation and ulceration, along with the loss of ciliated and goblet cells.

Henshaw et al. [45] discovered that weekly topical propolis expedited wound closure in human diabetic foot ulcers and improved the healing process of wounds in this particular context. Their findings demonstrated that propolis has a significant antibacterial activity, which reduces the amount of germs present in diabetic foot ulcers. Furthermore, Kinis et al. [2] discovered that caffeic acid phenethyl ester, one of the active components of propolis, had a positive impact on the healing process of wounds in the nasal mucosa of rats.

Up to this point, more than 300 distinct chemicals have been identified in propolis. These compounds include aliphatic acids, esters, fatty acids, aromatic acids, aldehydes, carbohydrates, amino acids, chalcones, dihydrochalcones, terpenoids, ketones, vitamins, and inorganic elements. When compared to other substances, flavonoids receive more scientific attention [47].

The in vitro antibacterial activity of propolis results from synergistic activities of propolis components, namely pinocembrin and galangin flavonoids. This activity has been effective against various Gram-negative and Gram-positive bacteria.

Several other flavonoids, including chrysin and kaempferol, have demonstrated antiviral action, reducing the intracellular growth of certain viruses, including herpes simplex [48].

Inflammatory mediators are produced due to the tissue alterations brought about by trauma and the possibility of infection. These mediators are responsible for future inflammatory processes. The release of interleukin-1 (IL-1) and tumor necrosis factor-alpha (TNF-α) by macrophages that have been activated leads to vasodilation, which in turn leads to the relaxing of smooth muscle and an increase in the flow of blood in the local area. Microvascular alterations related to increased vascular permeability occur, leading to an increase in plasmatic exudation, an accumulation of phagocytes (including neutrophils, macrophages, and monocytes), and an increase in the amount of endogenous chemical mediators. At the same time, phagocytic cells, mast cells, and endothelial cells all use the lipids found in plasma membranes to create significant inflammatory mediators [49].

In the prospective epidemiological multicenter research that Marti et al. [50] conducted 40 children between the ages of 2 and 12 years old experiencing symptoms of AR and the common cold were included in the study. A therapy consisting of administering propolis nasal spray three times per day for 7 days was carried out, and a comparison of symptomatology, subjective global improvement, and quality of life (QoL) was carried out between the initial visit (on day 1) and the final visit (on day 7). Using Jackson's scoring test, the primary objective was to assess the alterations in the severity of symptoms. After 7 days of therapy, there was a substantial reduction in the number of symptoms, both in terms of the overall score (p less than 0.0001) and each AR symptom (p less than 0.01). About the sample, no symptoms were reported by day 7, and the remission of symptoms occurred approximately around day 4.

Furthermore, there was no requirement for additional therapy. After receiving treatment, patients appeared to have a considerable increase in their quality of life and their subjective perception of worldwide improvement. Not a single adverse event (AE) was discovered worldwide. It is possible to conclude that propolis nasal spray is an excellent solution in the treatment of this condition, as it does not require any adjuvant therapy [50]. This is because it efficiently improves recovery from infectious AR and common cold symptoms in children.

Tanugur Samanci and colleagues [51] investigated the effects of applying propolis topically to the nasal epithelial cells to determine whether or not this had any detrimental impact on the cells. After applying propolis topically, they concluded that it did not have a cytotoxic effect on the cells that comprise the nasal epithelium. It has been shown that topical use in treating sinonasal inflammatory illnesses (such as acute and chronic rhinosinusitis) may have an auxiliary impact on the treatment process. This conclusion was reached after considering the substances' antibacterial and antioxidant actions. Furthermore, there is a minor inducement of proliferation of the primary cells by propolis, which may assist in the healing of wounds that have been subjected to epistaxis and septal operations.

References

1. El-Anwar MW, Abdelmonem S, Abdelsameea AA, AlShawadfy M, El-Kashishy K. The effect of propolis in healing injured nasal mucosa: an experimental study. Int Arch Otorhinolaryngol. 2016;20(3):222–5. https://doi.org/10.1055/s-0036-1579664. Epub 2016 Feb 26. PMID: 27413403; PMCID: PMC4942295.
2. Kınıs V, Ozbay M, Akdag M, et al. Effects of caffeic acid phenethyl ester on wound healing of nasal mucosa in the rat: an experimental study. Am J Otolaryngol. 2014;35(4):482–6.
3. Staffieri A, Marino F, Staffieri C, et al. The effects of sulfurous-arsenical-ferruginous thermal water nasal irrigation in wound healing after functional endoscopic sinus surgery for chronic rhinosinusitis: a prospective randomized study. Am J Otolaryngol. 2008;29(4):223–9.
4. Wagh VD. Propolis: a wonder bees product and its pharmacological potentials. Adv Pharmacol Sci. 2013;2013:308249.
5. Banskota AH, Nagaoka T, Sumioka LY, et al. Antiproliferative activity of The Netherlands propolis and its active principles in cancer cell lines. J Ethnopharmacol. 2002;80(1):67–73.
6. Grunberger D, Banerjee R, Eisinger K, et al. Preferential cytotoxicity on tumor cells by caffeic acid phenethyl ester isolated from propolis. Experientia. 1988;44(3):230–2.
7. Talas ZS, Ozdemir I, Ciftci O, Cakir O, Gulhan MF, Pasaoglu OM. Role of propolis on biochemical parameters in kidney and heart tissues against L-NAME induced oxidative injury in rats. Clin Exp Hypertens. 2014;36(7):492–6.
8. Gekker G, Hu S, Spivak M, Lokensgard JR, Peterson PK. Anti-HIV-1 activity of propolis in CD4(+) lymphocyte and microglial cell cultures. J Ethnopharmacol. 2005;102(2):158–63.
9. Astani A, Zimmermann S, Hassan E, Reichling J, Sensch KH, Schnitzler P. Antimicrobial activity of propolis special extract GH 2002 against multidrug-resistant clinical isolates. Pharmazie. 2013;68(8):695–701.
10. Liu Y, Min D, Bolton T, et al. Increased matrix metalloproteinase-9 predicts poor wound healing in diabetic foot ulcers. Diabetes Care. 2009;32(1):117–9.
11. Gallo E, Lucenteforte E, Firenzuoli F, et al. Herbalists' perception of risks involving commonly sold medicinal plants in Italy. Complement Ther Med. 2014;22(1):81–6.
12. Przybyłek I, Karpiński TM. Antibacterial properties of propolis. Molecules. 2019;24(11):2047. https://doi.org/10.3390/molecules24112047. PMID: 31146392; PMCID: PMC6600457.
13. Kędzia B. Pochodzenie propolisu w świetle teorii i badań naukowych. The origin of propolis in the theories and scientific research. Herba Pol. 2008;54:179–86.
14. Zabaiou N, Fouache A, Trousson A, Baron S, Zellagui A, Lahouel M, Lobaccaro JA. Biological properties of propolis extracts: something new from an ancient product. Chem Phys Lipids. 2017;207:214–22. https://doi.org/10.1016/j.chemphyslip.2017.04.005.
15. Toreti VC, Sato HH, Pastore GM, Park YK. Recent progress of propolis for its biological and chemical compositions and its botanical origin. Evid Based Complement Alternat Med. 2013;2013:697390. https://doi.org/10.1155/2013/697390.
16. Sforcin JM, Bankova V. Propolis: is there a potential for the development of new drugs? J Ethnopharmacol. 2011;133:253–60. https://doi.org/10.1016/j.jep.2010.10.032.
17. Silva JC, Rodrigues S, Feás X, Estevinho LM. Antimicrobial activity, phenolic profile and role in the inflammation of propolis. Food Chem Toxicol. 2012;50:1790–5. https://doi.org/10.1016/j.fct.2012.02.097.
18. Schnitzler P, Neuner A, Nolkemper S, Zundel C, Nowack H, Sensch KH, Reichling J. Antiviral activity and mode of action of propolis extracts and selected compounds. Phytother Res. 2010;24(Suppl. 1):S20–8. https://doi.org/10.1002/ptr.2868.
19. Ramanauskiene K, Inkeniene A. Propolis oil extract: quality analysis and evaluation of its antimicrobial activity. Nat Prod Res. 2011;25:1463–8. https://doi.org/10.1080/14786419.2010.529440.
20. Franchin M, Cólon DF, Castanheira FV, da Cunha MG, Bueno-Silva B, Alencar SM, Cunha TM, Rosalen PL. Vestitol isolated from Brazilian red propolis inhibits neutrophils migration in

the inflammatory process: elucidation of the mechanism of action. J Nat Prod. 2016;79:954–60. https://doi.org/10.1021/acs.jnatprod.5b00938.
21. De Freitas MCD, de Miranda MB, de Oliveira DT, Vieira-Filho SA, Caligiorne RB, de Figueiredo SM. Biological activities of red propolis: a review. Recent Pat Endocr Metab Immun Drug Discov. 2017;11:3–12. https://doi.org/10.2174/1872214812666180223120316.
22. Warakomska Z, Maciejewicz W. Microscopic analysis of propolis from Polish regions. Apidologie. 1992;23:277. https://doi.org/10.1051/apido:19920401.
23. Jabłoński B, Kołtowski Z. Nectar secretion and honey potential of honey plants growing under Poland's conditions. J Api Sci. 2005;49:59.
24. Szeleszczuk Ł, Zielińska-Pisklak M, Goś P. Propolis—panaceum prosto z ula. Lek W Polsce. 2013;23:32–9.
25. Şenel E, Demir E. Bibliometric analysis of apitherapy in complementary medicine literature between 1980 and 2016. Complement Ther Clin Pract. 2018;31:47–52. https://doi.org/10.1016/j.ctcp.2018.02.003.
26. Bueno-Silva B, Marsola A, Ikegaki M, Alencar SM, Rosalen PL. The effect of seasons on Brazilian red propolis and its botanical source: chemical composition and antibacterial activity. Nat Prod Res. 2016;31:1318–24. https://doi.org/10.1080/14786419.2016.1239088.
27. da Cunha MG, Franchin M, de Carvalho Galvão LC, de Ruiz AL, de Carvalho JE, Ikegaki M, de Alencar SM, Koo H, Rosalen PL. Antimicrobial and antiproliferative activities of stingless bee *Melipona scutellaris* geopropolis. BMC Complement Altern Med. 2013;13:23. https://doi.org/10.1186/1472-6882-13-23.
28. Santos TLAD, Queiroz RF, Sawaya ACHF, Lopez BG, Soares MBP, Bezerra DP, Rodrigues ACBC, Paula VF, Waldschmidt AM. *Melipona mondury* produces a geopropolis with antioxidant, antibacterial and antiproliferative activities. An Acad Bras Cienc. 2017;89:2247–59. https://doi.org/10.1590/0001-3765201720160725.
29. Torres AR, Sandjo LP, Friedemann MT, Tomazzoli MM, Maraschin M, Mello CF, Santos ARS. Chemical characterization, antioxidant and antimicrobial activity of propolis obtained from *Melipona quadrifasciata quadrifasciata* and *Tetragonisca angustula* stingless bees. Braz J Med Biol Res. 2018;51:e7118. https://doi.org/10.1590/1414-431x20187118.
30. Gómez-Caravaca AM, Gómez-Romero M, Arráez-Román D, Segura-Carretero A, Fernández-Gutiérrez A. Advances in the analysis of phenolic compounds in products derived from bees. J Pharm Biomed Anal. 2006;41:1220–34. https://doi.org/10.1016/j.jpba.2006.03.002.
31. Miguel MG, Nunes S, Dandlen SA, Cavaco AM, Antunes MD. Phenols and antioxidant activity of hydro-alcoholic extracts of propolis from Algarve, South of Portugal. Food Chem Toxicol. 2010;48:3418–23. https://doi.org/10.1016/j.fct.2010.09.014.
32. Inui S, Hatano A, Yoshino M, Hosoya T, Shimamura Y, Masuda S, Ahn MR, Tazawa S, Araki Y, Kumazawa S. Identification of the phenolic compounds contributing to antibacterial activity in ethanol extracts of Brazilian red propolis. Nat Prod Res. 2014;28:1293–6. https://doi.org/10.1080/14786419.2014.898146.
33. Brodowska KM. Natural flavonoids: classification, potential role, and application of flavonoid analogues. Eur J Biol Res. 2017;7:108–23.
34. Górniak I, Bartoszewski R, Króliczewski J. Comprehensive review of antimicrobial activities of plant flavonoids. Phytochem Rev. 2019;18:241–72. https://doi.org/10.1007/s11101-018-9591-z.
35. Devequi-Nunes D, Machado BAS, Barreto GA, Rebouças SJ, da Silva DF, da Rocha JLC, Brandão HN, Borges VM, Umsza-Guez MA. Chemical characterization and biological activity of six different extracts of propolis through conventional methods and supercritical extraction. PLoS One. 2018;13:e0207676. https://doi.org/10.1371/journal.pone.0207676.
36. Wieczyńska A, Weżgowiec J, Więckiewicz W, Czarny A, Kulbacka J, Nowakowska D, Gancarz R, Wilk KA. Antimicrobial activity, cytotoxicity and total phenolic content of different extracts of propolis from the west Pomeranian region in Poland. Acta Pol Pharm. 2017;74:715–22.
37. Bridi R, Montenegro G, Nuñez-Quijada G, Giordano A, Morán-Romero FM, Jara-Pezoa I, Speisky H, Atala E, López-Alarcón C. International regulations of propolis quality: required

assays do not necessarily reflect their polyphenolic-related in vitro activities. J Food Sci. 2015;80:C1188–95. https://doi.org/10.1111/1750-3841.12881.
38. Al-Waili N, Al-Ghamdi A, Ansari MJ, Al-Attal Y, Salom K. Synergistic effects of honey and propolis toward drug multi-resistant *Staphylococcus aureus*, *Escherichia coli* and *Candida albicans* isolates in single and polymicrobial cultures. Int J Med Sci. 2012;9:793–800. https://doi.org/10.7150/ijms.4722.
39. Boyanova L, Kolarov R, Gergova G, Mitov I. In vitro activity of Bulgarian propolis against 94 clinical isolates of anaerobic bacteria. Anaerobe. 2006;12:173–7. https://doi.org/10.1016/j.anaerobe.2006.06.001.
40. Ferreira FB, Torres SA, Rosa OP, Ferreira CM, Garcia RB, Marcucci MC, Gomes BP. Antimicrobial effect of propolis and other substances against selected endodontic pathogens. Oral Surg Oral Med Oral Pathol Oral Radiol Endod. 2007;104:709–16. https://doi.org/10.1016/j.tripleo.2007.05.019.
41. Koru O, Toksoy F, Acikel CH, Tunca YM, Baysallar M, Uskudar Guclu A, Akca E, Ozkok Tuylu A, Sorkun K, Tanyuksel M, et al. In vitro antimicrobial activity of propolis samples from different geographical origins against certain oral pathogens. Anaerobe. 2007;13:140–5. https://doi.org/10.1016/j.anaerobe.2007.02.001.
42. Shabbir A, Rashid M, Tipu HN. Propolis, a hope for the future in treating resistant periodontal pathogens. Cureus. 2016;8:e682. https://doi.org/10.7759/cureus.682.
43. Kędzia A, Kałowski M. Ocena skuteczności działania wyciągu etanolowego z propolisu na bakterie bezwzględnie beztlenowe jamy ustnej. Czas Stomat. 1988;41:757–62.
44. Kędzia A. Wrażliwość bakterii bezwzględnie beztlenowych na wyciąg etanolowy z propolisu. Herba Pol. 1988;34:267–72.
45. Henshaw FR, Bolton T, Nube V, et al. Topical application of the bee hive protectant propolis is well tolerated and improves human diabetic foot ulcer healing in a prospective feasibility study. J Diabetes Complicat. 2014;28(6):850–7.
46. Kędzia A. Działanie wyciągu etanolowego z propolisu na bakterie beztlenowe. Herba Pol. 1986;32:53–7.
47. Havsteen BH. The biochemistry and medical significance of the flavonoids. Pharmacol Ther. 2002;96(2–3):67–202.
48. Marcucci MC. Propolis: chemical composition, biological properties and therapeutic activity. Apidologie (Celle). 1995;26:83–99.
49. Lopes RE, Chapadeiro E, Raso P, Tafuri LW. Patologia. Rio de Janeiro: Guanabara, 1987, 67–112.
50. Marti J, López F, Gascón I, Julve J. Propolis nasal spray effectively improves recovery from infectious acute rhinitis and common cold symptoms in children: a pilot study. J Biol Regul Homeost Agents. 2017;31(4):943–50.
51. Tanugur Samanci AE, Bayar Muluk N, Vejselova Sezer C, Kutlu HM, Topsakal V, Cingi C. Efficacy and toxicity of Anatolian propolis on healthy nasal epithelial cells. Eur Rev Med Pharmocol Sci. 2022;26(2 Suppl):103–11. https://doi.org/10.26355/eurrev_202212_30493.

15 Pulmonary Effects of Propolis

15.1 Introduction

Propolis, which continues to be a fascinating source of these chemicals, is related to several natural chemical substances that have antibacterial, antifungal, antiviral, antioxidant, and anti-inflammatory properties. These are just some of the natural chemical substances and their effects. The ever-increasing prevalence of respiratory tract infections brought on by a wide range of pathogenic viruses has led to the ongoing search for complementary methods of prevention and treatment that can be employed with medication. The characteristics of propolis could be of substantial value in preventing and treating respiratory tract illnesses caused by viruses. These viruses include severe acute respiratory syndrome coronavirus 2, influenza, parainfluenza, and rhinoviruses. The severe acute respiratory syndrome coronavirus 2 (SARS-CoV-2), the virus that causes COVID-19, has been one of the most significant challenges over the previous few years. In recent years, there has been a rise in research focused on the efficacy of various propolis formulations against SARS-CoV-2 as an adjuvant therapy for this infection. Several primary pathways of anti-SARS-CoV-2 action have been proven to be associated with propolis. These methods include inhibiting the connection between the S1 spike protein and the ACE-2 protein, reducing viral replication via limiting the generation of RNA transcripts in cells, and reducing coronavirus particles [1]. All of these mechanisms are listed in the previous sentence.

According to Yusuf [2], among the many therapeutic options that are accessible to patients who have COVID-19 and diabetes mellitus, propolis, which is a source of phenolic compounds, can be considered to be among the most effective forms of treatment. Even though hyperglycemia may enhance the risk (severity?) of SARS-CoV-2 infections, propolis has been shown to minimize the synergy between SARS-CoV-2- and COVID-19-mediated morbidity. Because hyperglycemia may increase the probability of SARS-CoV-2 infections, this treatment method is appropriate

A. E. Tanuğur Samanci et al., *Propolis: Prevention and Healing Effects in Otorhinolaryngology*, Comprehensive ENT,
https://doi.org/10.1007/978-3-031-68546-0_15

because of this potential danger. In his article, Ghosh [3] highlights the fact that people who have been diagnosed with COVID-19 typically have one or more comorbidities, such as hypertension, cardiovascular illness, and chronic lung disease. According to the outcomes of a review that was carried out by Balica et al. [4], which included 22 preclinical investigations and eight clinical research, the utilization of propolis was revealed to yield beneficial benefits in patients who were suffering from diabetes mellitus, dyslipidemia, and obesity.

Propolis was discovered to have a beneficial effect on chronic obstructive pulmonary disease (COPD) by simultaneously lowering the levels of proinflammatory cytokines and reducing acute lung inflammation, as indicated by several studies [5, 6]. Researchers discovered that propolis possesses antihypertensive, anticoagulant, and antihemostatic activities [7]. This is an additional advantage of using propolis. It is essential to consider that propolis possesses antibacterial characteristics that are effective against many microorganisms [8–10]. Pathogens that may infect a patient during the development of COVID-19, such as co-infections and secondary bacterial infections, are the targets of these actions directed against these pathogens. According to Farrell [11], there is a need to increase the collection of death information about subsequent bacterial illnesses. There is a possibility that the COVID-19 infection will cause damage to the lung parenchyma.

Furthermore, persons infected with the sickness are more likely to face long-term repercussions such as bacterial infections. According to Pourajam [12], 11% of patients had secondary bacterial infections caused by *Klebsiella pneumoniae* and *Acinetobacter baumannii*. The fact that secondary infections caused by *Chlamydia pneumonia*, *Haemophilus influenza*, *Legionella pneumophila*, *Mycoplasma pneumoniae*, *Streptococcus pneumoniae*, and *Staphylococcus aureus* have also been reported has been brought to the notice of other individuals on multiple occasions [13]. Recent research has shown that propolis possesses antibacterial properties not only against *Klebsiella pneumoniae* but also against *Enterococcus faecalis*, *Listeria monocytogenes*, *Pseudomonas aeruginosa*, *Staphylococcus aureus*, *Streptococcus sobrinus*, *Streptococcus mutans* [14, 15], *Bacillus subtilis*, *Clostridium difficile*, *Escherichia coli*, *Proteus mirabilis*, and Salmonella species. These antibacterial properties have been discovered in recent times. Additionally, Streptococcus epidermidis [1, 10] is present.

15.2 Effects of Propolis on the Airways

Several primary pathways of anti-SARS-CoV-2 action have been proven to be associated with propolis. One way is to inhibit the interaction between the S1 spike protein and the ACE-2 protein. Other mechanisms include reducing coronavirus particles and viral replication through decreased cell RNA transcript production. Using extracts and the single physiologically active compounds found in propolis (such as apigenin, caffeic acid, chrysin, kaempferol, and quercetin), the antiviral activity of propolis has been proven. A condition known as hyperglycemia, which is associated with an increased likelihood of contracting SARS-CoV-2 infections [1], can be effectively treated with propolis.

Cohen et al. [16] conducted a randomized double-blind placebo-controlled study to determine whether or not a herbal preparation that contained propolis (50 mg/mL), echinacea (50 mg/mL), and vitamin C (10 mg/mL) was effective in preventing upper respiratory tract infections in children (between the ages of 1 and 5). The purpose of the study was to determine whether or not the herbal preparation was effective in controlling the infection. A total of 12 weeks were spent administering dosages of 5.0 and 7.5 mL to patients on a twice-daily basis. They received this mixture that was brought to them. It was noted that patients who were administered the preparation reported a reduction of 55% in the number of episodes of sickness, a decrease of 62% in the number of days with fever, and an overall reduction in the total number of days with symptomatic disease following the administration of the preparation.

Many individuals have acknowledged the anti-inflammatory properties of propolis, which have been demonstrated to be effective. As shown by animal models, lipopolysaccharide (LPS) causes inflammation and lung harm. It has been shown that propolis and its bioactive components, including CAPE and galangin, can considerably reduce the activity of lung cyclooxygenase (COX) and myeloperoxidase (MPO), in addition to malonaldehyde (MDA), tumor necrosis factor-alpha (TNF-α), and interleukin-6 (IL-6). Nevertheless, it has been demonstrated that propolis can boost the activity of catalase (CAT) and superoxide dismutase (SOD) in the context of lung injury caused by lipopolysaccharide (LPS) [17–21]. Chrysin also lessens the amount of oxidative damage in the lungs of mice that have been made septic by LPS. This is because chrysin inhibits the creation of oxidative damage. Chrysin can decrease the expression of oxidative and inflammatory indicators, including aspartate transaminase (AST), alanine aminotransferase (ALT), interleukin-1β, interleukin-10, tumor necrosis factor-alpha (TNF-α), and malondialdehyde (MDA), while simultaneously elevating the levels of antioxidant parameters, including superoxide dismutase (SOD), catalase (CAT), and glutathione peroxidase (GPx) [22]. In addition, it has been demonstrated that propolis can reduce the expression of toll-like receptor 4 (TLR4) as well as macrophage infiltration, MPO activity, and apoptosis in the lung tissues of mice subjected to septic therapy [23].

15.3 Effects of Propolis on the Pulmonary System

In particular, it has been proven that infectious diseases involving bacterial and viral respiratory pathogenic microorganisms significantly impact life and impose financial costs [17]. Illnesses of the respiratory system, such as infections of the respiratory tract, influenza, and asthma, have been determined to be the ones that impose the most significant social and economic consequences, as stated by Ferkol et al. [24]. This was discovered through research conducted by the researchers above. The severe acute respiratory syndrome coronavirus 2 (SARS-CoV-2) has been recognized as one of the most critical challenges in recent years. This virus is responsible for COVID-19 and has been projected to have a direct medical cost of one hundred sixty-three billion dollars [25]. As a result, there is an urgent requirement to search for techniques that are both more cost-effective and less expensive to treat respiratory problems. Antivirals, anti-inflammatory drugs, antibodies produced from convalescent plasma, anticoagulants, and monoclonal antibodies are some of the treatments utilized in treating persons who have been diagnosed with COVID-19 up until this time [26]. Research conducted in the field of pharmacology indicates that the use of propolis in conjunction with a wide range of other pharmaceutical treatments, such as antibiotics, antifungals, and antiviral medications, has the potential to produce synergistic effects.

Additionally, there is a possibility that propolis will result in a reduction in the dosages of these medications that are required [27]. In addition to propolis, approximately 30 additional medicinal plant species are also used to treat SARS-CoV-2 infection. This is something that has been seen. Forsythia suspensa (Thunb.) Vahl, Glycyrrhiza glabra L., and Platycodon grandiflorum (Jacq.) A. are a few examples of plants that fall under this category. Nigella sativa L., more precisely DC.) ([28–32] respectively).

The antiviral properties of propolis extracts have been demonstrated to be effective against SARS-CoV-2-related infections. These effects are attributed to several mechanisms, including the inhibition of the interaction between the S1 spike protein and the ACE-2 protein, the reduction of the replication of viruses by reducing the synthesis of RNA transcripts in cells, the reduction of the number of virions, the inhibition of the activity of neuraminidase, and the reduction of the viral load (influenza virus A) in the bronchoalveolar lavage fluids of the lungs [1].

Additionally, it was demonstrated that quercetin has an effect against human CoV-229E in vitro [33]. The experiments demonstrated this. Flavonoids found in propolis, such as naringin and rutin, were found to have anti-SARS-CoV-2 activity in vitro, and the extent of this activity depended on the quantity of the flavonoids. This was highlighted by Ali et al. [34] in their study. According to Yosri et al. [35], these antiviral activities were also found to be presented by chrysin, broussoflavonol F, glycerin A, kaempferol, sulabiroins A, caffeic acid, 3-phenylacetic acid, and lumichrome.

Moreover, lumichrome was demonstrated to possess these capabilities. Furthermore, several secondary metabolites, such as phenolic compounds, which inhibit the activity of the SARS-3CLpro enzyme; quercetin, which inhibits the cellular entry of SARS-CoV and the activity of SARS-CoV 3Clpro; kaempferol, which inhibits the 3a ion channel of coronavirus; luteolin, which binds the surface spike protein of SARS-CoV; and apigenin and luteolin, which inhibit the activity of SARS-CoV 3CLpro, are among the secondary metabolites that exhibit antiviral action. The ability of chrysin to inhibit the production of viral capsid proteins and the replication of RNA in enterovirus 71 [36–39] is proof that chrysin also possesses antiviral properties. Among the naturally occurring chemical substances that have been demonstrated to inhibit the spike protein, PLpro, and 3CLpro of SARS-CoV-2, curcumin, kaempferol, licoleafol, myricitrin, and silybin are among the chemicals that have been identified. The findings of Jamshidnia et al. [32], which were recently disclosed, indicate that this information was recently disclosed.

Furthermore, Malekmohammad and Rafieian-Kopaei [31] found that in addition to quercetin, apigenin, kaempferol, and curcumin, baicalin, glycyrrhizin, scutellarin, and ursolic acid, these compounds have the potential to be evaluated as potential candidates for the treatment of symptoms associated with SARS-CoV-2 infection. Their findings suggest that these compounds could be used to treat symptoms related to SARS-CoV-2 infection. Furthermore, chrysin has been proven to block the interaction between the spike protein and the ACE2 receptor [40]. Hesperidin has been shown to interact with the ACE2 protein and the spike protein of SARS-CoV2, as demonstrated by a study that was carried out using molecular docking [41].

In a study conducted not too long ago, Silva-Beltrán and his colleagues [33] showed that extracts produced from green and brown propolis exhibited antiviral activity against human CoV-229E in MRC-5 cells. These extracts had EC50 values of 19.08 μg/mL and 11.24 μg/mL, respectively when measured against the standard. Several studies have demonstrated that propolis extracts can inhibit the activity of SARS-CoV-2 in vitro [42–45]. The researchers Berretta et al. [45] conducted an exhaustive investigation into the potential antiviral mechanisms of propolis and a wide range of natural chemical compounds, focusing on SARS-CoV-2 as the subject of their investigation. Propolis was found to prevent the invasion of SARS-CoV-2 into the host body's cells by interacting with angiotensin-converting enzyme 2 (ACE-2) and transmembrane serine protease 2 (TMPRSS2). The researchers noticed this. These enzymes are crucial targets for developing effective treatment alternatives because SARS-CoV-2 has a significant binding affinity for ACE-2, which promotes pathogenetic pathways. For this reason, these enzymes are essential targets.

On the other hand, only three in vitro studies have been carried out in this industry that are associated with propolis, according to the findings of a survey that was carried out by Guler et al. [44], an ethanolic extract of Anatolian propolis that was 70% ethanolic and contained a more substantial number of polyphenols was found to prevent the interaction between the S1 spike protein (SARS-CoV-2) and the ACE-2 protein. The researchers discovered this. In addition, using an ELISA kit test and in silico methods, the study project demonstrated that hesperetin and pinocembrin had inhibitory activity against the SARS-CoV-2 S1 spike protein and the ACE-2 protein (IC50 = 11.13 mM and IC50 = 14.15 mM, respectively) [44]. This was accomplished by demonstrating the inhibitory action of hesperetin and pinocembrin. Furthermore, Sberna and colleagues [42] observed that the incorporation of an extract of poplar-type propolis at a concentration of 25 μg/mL, which constituted 80% of the total population, into a kidney epithelial cell line and human lung epithelial cells that were infected with SARS-CoV-2 led to a decrease in the replication of the virus and a subsequent reduction in the production of RNA transcripts within the cells. In addition, the application of propolis extract reduced the number of virions and decreased the number of infected cells [42].

To investigate the therapeutic effects of propolis dissolved in isopropanol in conjunction with methanolic extract of *Hyoscyamus niger*, a randomized clinical trial [46] was carried out at the Akhavan and Sepehri Clinics of the Kashan University of Medical Sciences in Iran. This experiment intended to determine whether or not the combination of these two substances would be effective. According to the syrup, which included 1.6 milligrams of the extract of H. niger, the participants ranged from 18 to 65. It was administered three times a day for 6 days. Ten milliliters of niger and four hundred and fifty milligrams of propolis were administered. The findings showed that patients who received the syrup saw a reduction in the intensity of chest discomfort, dry cough, breath score, and sore throat. This was determined by comparing the patients who received the syrup to those who did not. It is possible to attach statistical significance to these observations.

15.4 Respiratory Tract Infections

It has been established that propolis possesses antiviral properties that are effective against various respiratory viruses, including strains of influenza viruses, parainfluenza viruses, rhinoviruses, and respiratory syncytial virus (RSV). According to the research conducted by [47–52], the effective concentration varied between 5 and 300 μg/mL depending on the geographical origins of the extract and the kinds of extract. According to the findings of Shimizu et al. [52], propolis was proven to have antiviral activity comparable to that of oseltamivir when used as a first treatment for mice infected with influenza A (H1N1). This was demonstrated to be accurate at the most significant amount examined 10 mg/kg of body weight. Additionally, Kai et al. [49] revealed that apigenin, coumaric acid, and kaempferol, all of which were derived from propolis, were able to alleviate the symptoms of influenza in mice, with kaempferol being the most effective of the three [49].

There is additional evidence that propolis has antibacterial properties, namely against germs that cause respiratory pathology. Some of the bacteria that fall under this category are as follows: *Staphylococcus aureus* (including strains that are resistant to methicillin), *Pseudomonas aeruginosa*, *Streptococcus pneumoniae*, *Moraxella catarrhalis*, *Haemophilus influenzae*, *Klebsiella pneumoniae*, and *Streptococcus pyogenes*. Both in vitro and animal models have used this activity to illustrate its effectiveness [53–61]. There was a range that extended from 64 to 460 μg/mL. In addition, propolis can kill germs, specifically Mycobacteria, a type of bacteria. Propolis extract has been effective against various mycobacteria species and strains, including *Mycobacterium tuberculosis*, which appear throughout a wide range of concentrations, from 44 to 800 μg/mL. *M. kansasii contains many wild-type* strains, including M. The xenopei, M. with M. intracellulare—the BCG. The following are examples: [61–64] H37Rv, M.H37Ra, and M.223.

To determine whether or not pharmaceuticals, nutritional supplements, or nutraceuticals that contain propolis are effective as a primary treatment for reducing and treating symptoms of respiratory tract infections caused by respiratory bacteria and viruses, several clinical investigations involving human subjects have been conducted throughout the years. One of the oldest randomized placebo-controlled trials (RCT) that the authors uncovered was carried out by Cohen et al. [16]. A Chizukit supplement that contained echinacea, propolis, and vitamin C was administered to 328 youngsters who participated in the randomized controlled trial. According to the researchers' findings, the therapy group had a significant decrease (more than 50%) in the number of cases of upper respiratory tract infections, acute otitis media, pneumonia, and tonsillopharyngitis [16]. Marchisio et al. [65] found that a supplement comprising zinc and propolis extract could dramatically reduce the frequency of recurrent acute otitis media and respiratory-related morbidity in children. This was demonstrated by the fact that the supplement did not contain any other ingredients. For this study, a randomized controlled trial was conducted, with 122 participants in the sample. The substantial reduction in respiratory infections, particularly *S. pneumoniae* and *H. influenzae*, was associated with alleviating symptoms [65]. In addition, Marti et al. [66] discovered that a proprietary propolis nose spray dubbed "Child Free Nose Propolis" significantly decreased the amount of time that signs and symptoms of acute rhinitis and the common cold lasted [66]. This was a significant finding. In a manner comparable to what was previously shown, several randomized controlled studies [67–69] have provided additional evidence that propolis has a beneficial impact on treating respiratory tract infections. The participants reported no notable adverse events or side effects in these clinical studies [17], and these studies were not recorded.

In addition to its antiviral and antibacterial activities, propolis appears to change the hosts' immune responses in relation to respiratory tract infections. This is in addition to propolis, which has antibacterial and antiviral properties. Propolis and one of its bioactive components, 3,4-caffeoylquinic acid, were found to promote the production of tumor necrosis factor-related apoptosis-inducing ligand (TRAIL), which increased viral clearance in mice infected with influenza A [70]. In a study conducted by Takeshita et al. [71], it was discovered that propolis could significantly reduce viral titers and the production of interferon-γ (IFN-γ), tumor necrosis factor-alpha (TNF-α), and interleukin-6 (IL-6) in mice that were infected with RSV. Because of this, the severity of the disease, which was made worse by tetrabromobisphenol-A, was lessened. In a model of viral infection and double-stranded RNA transfection, it has been demonstrated that propolis can boost the expression of myxovirus resistance-1 (MX1) while concurrently lowering the production of interferon-gamma (IFN-β) [72]. In addition, it has been established that propolis can stimulate the proliferation of lymphocytes and the formation of serum antibodies in hens injected with the avian influenza vaccine [73]. This was demonstrated by propolis promoting the development of serum antibodies. After being inoculated, immunosuppressed animals can experience an increase in lymphocyte proliferation, antibody titer, and the concentration of IgG and IgM when exposed to propolis [17, 74].

Propolis has been shown to have a beneficial impact as an adjuvant therapy in this area, and at least two clinical trials, including humans, have revealed that this effect has been demonstrated. An increase in the expression of interferon-gamma (IFN-γ) and the activity of superoxide dismutase (SOD) was observed in patients with multiple-drug resistant tuberculosis (MDR) who were receiving treatment with anti-MDR-TB drugs. The findings of the study by Permatasari and Hasan [75] demonstrated that the presence of propolis led to this increase. Conversely, the control group observed a decline in both parameters during the study [75]. As stated by Mahani et al. [76], the researchers who carried out the study [76], propolis supplementation was found to hasten the effectiveness of anti-TB drugs and to accelerate the recovery of body weight in patients suffering from tuberculosis.

References

1. Ożarowski M, Karpiński TM. The effects of propolis on viral respiratory diseases. Molecules. 2023;28(1):359. https://doi.org/10.3390/molecules28010359. PMID: 36615554; PMCID: PMC9824023.
2. Yusuf AP, Zhang JY, Li JQ, Muhammad A, Abubakar MB. Herbal medications and natural products for patients with COVID-19 and diabetes mellitus: potentials and challenges. Phytomed Plus. 2022;2:100280. https://doi.org/10.1016/j.phyplu.2022.100280.
3. Ghosh S, Al-Sharify ZT, Maleka MF, Onyeaka H, Maleke M, Maolloum A, Godoy L, Meskini M, Rami MR, Ahmadi S, et al. Propolis efficacy on SARS-COV viruses: a review on antimicrobial activities and molecular simulations. Environ Sci Pollut Res Int. 2022;29:58628–47. https://doi.org/10.1007/s11356-022-21652-6.
4. Balica G, Vostinaru O, Stefanescu C, Mogosan C, Iaru I, Cristina A, Pop CE. Potential role of propolis in the prevention and treatment of metabolic diseases. Plants. 2021;10:883. https://doi.org/10.3390/plants10050883.
5. Zullkiflee N, Taha H, Usman A. Propolis: its role and efficacy in human health and diseases. Molecules. 2022;27:6120. https://doi.org/10.3390/molecules27186120.
6. Khayyal MT, El-Ghazaly MA, El-Khatib AS, Hatem AM, de Vries PJ, El-Shafei S, Khattab MM. A clinical pharmacological study of the potential beneficial effects of a propolis food product as an adjuvant in asthmatic patients. Fundam Clin Pharmacol. 2003;17:93–102. https://doi.org/10.1046/j.1472-8206.2003.00117.x.
7. Silva H, Francisco R, Saraiva A, Francisco S, Carrascosa C, Raposo A. The cardiovascular therapeutic potential of propolis—a comprehensive review. Biology. 2021;10:27. https://doi.org/10.3390/biology10010027.
8. Magnavacca A, Sangiovanni E, Racagni G, Dell'Agli M. The antiviral and immunomodulatory activities of propolis: an update and future perspectives for respiratory diseases. Med Res Rev. 2022;42:897–945. https://doi.org/10.1002/med.21866.
9. Ozarowski M, Karpinski TM, Alam R, Łochynska M. Antifungal properties of chemically defined propolis from various geographical regions. Microorganisms. 2022;10:364. https://doi.org/10.3390/microorganisms10020364.
10. Przybyłek I, Karpiński TM. Antibacterial properties of propolis. Molecules. 2019;24:2047. https://doi.org/10.3390/molecules24112047.
11. Farrell JM, Zhao CY, Tarquinio KM, Brown SP. Causes and consequences of COVID-19-associated bacterial infections. Front Microbiol. 2021;12:682571. https://doi.org/10.3389/fmicb.2021.682571.
12. Pourajam S, Kalantari E, Talebzadeh H, Mellali H, Sami R, Soltaninejad F, Amra B, Sajadi M, Alenaseri M, Kalantari F, et al. Secondary bacterial infection and clinical characteristics in patients with COVID-19 admitted to two intensive care units of an academic hospital in Iran during the first wave of the pandemic. Front Cell Infect Microbiol. 2022;12:784130. https://doi.org/10.3389/fcimb.2022.784130.
13. Hoque MN, Akter S, Mishu ID, Islam MR, Rahman MS, Akhter M, Islam I, Hasan MM, Rahaman MM, Sultana M, et al. Microbial co-infections in COVID-19: associated microbiota

and underlying mechanisms of pathogenesis. Microb Pathog. 2021;156:104941. https://doi.org/10.1016/j.micpath.2021.104941.
14. Taufik FF, Natzir R, Patellongi I, Santoso A, Hatta M, Junita AR, Syukri A, Primaguna MR, Dwiyanti R, Febrianti A. In vivo and in vitro inhibition effect of propolis on Klebsiella pneumoniae: a review. Ann Med Surg. 2022;81:104388. https://doi.org/10.1016/j.amsu.2022.104388.
15. Almuhayawi MS. Propolis as a novel antibacterial agent. Saudi J Biol Sci. 2020;27:3079–86. https://doi.org/10.1016/j.sjbs.2020.09.016.
16. Cohen HA, Varsano I, Kahan E, Sarrell EM, Uziel Y. Effectiveness of an herbal preparation containing echinacea, propolis, and vitamin C in preventing respiratory tract infections in children: a randomized, double-blind, placebo-controlled, multicenter study. Arch Pediatr Adolesc Med. 2004;158:217–21. https://doi.org/10.1001/archpedi.158.3.217.
17. Zulhendri F, Perera CO, Tandean S, et al. The potential use of propolis as a primary or an adjunctive therapy in respiratory tract-related diseases and disorders: a systematic scoping review. Biomed Pharmacother. 2022;146:112595. https://doi.org/10.1016/j.biopha.2021.112595.
18. Rossi A, Longo R, Russo A, Borrelli F, Sautebin L. The role of the phenethyl ester of caffeic acid (CAPE) in the inhibition of rat lung cyclooxygenase activity by propolis. Fitoterapia. 2002;73:S30. https://doi.org/10.1016/S0367-326X(02)00188-0.
19. Yangi B, Cengiz Ustuner M, Dincer M, Ozbayer C, Tekin N, Ustuner D, Colak E, Kolac UK, Entok E. Propolis protects endotoxin induced acute lung and liver inflammation through attenuating inflammatory responses and oxidative stress. J Med Food. 2018;21:1096–105. https://doi.org/10.1089/jmf.2017.0151.
20. Machado JL, Assunção AKM, da Silva MCP, Reis ASD, Costa GC, de Sousa Arruda D, Rocha BA, de Oliveira Lima Leite Vaz MM, de Andrade Paes AM, Guerra RNM, Berretta AA, do Nascimento FRF. Brazilian green propolis: anti-inflammatory property by an immunomodulatory activity. Evid. Based Complement Altern Med. 2012;2012:157652. https://doi.org/10.1155/2012/157652.
21. Koksel O, Ozdulger A, Tamer L, Cinel L, Ercil M, Degirmenci U, Unlu S, Kanik A. Effects of caffeic acid phenethyl ester on lipopolysaccharide-induced lung injury in rats. Pulm Pharmacol Ther. 2006;19:90–5. https://doi.org/10.1016/j.pupt.2005.03.006.
22. Koc F, Tekeli MY, Kanbur M, Karayigit MÖ, Liman BC. The effects of chrysin on lipopolysaccharide-induced sepsis in rats. J Food Biochem. 2020;44:e13359. https://doi.org/10.1111/jfbc.13359.
23. Silveira MAD, Capcha JMC, Sanches TR, de Sousa Moreira R, Garnica MS, Shimizu MH, Berretta A, Teles F, Noronha IL, Andrade L. Green propolis extract attenuates acute kidney injury and lung injury in a rat model of sepsis. Sci Rep. 2021;11:5925. https://doi.org/10.1038/s41598-021-85124-6.
24. Ferkol T, Schraufnagel D. The global burden of respiratory disease. Ann Am Thorac Soc. 2014;11:404–6. https://doi.org/10.1513/AnnalsATS.201311-405PS.
25. Richards F, Kodjamanova P, Chen X, Li N, Atanasov P, Bennetts L, Patterson BJ, Yektashenas B, Mesa-Frias M, Tronczynski K, et al. Economic burden of COVID-19: a systematic review. ClinicoEcon Outcomes Res. 2022;14:293–307. https://doi.org/10.2147/CEOR.S338225.
26. Ripari N, Sartori AA, Honorio MS, Conte FL, Tasca KI, Santiago KB, Sforcin JM. Propolis antiviral and immunomodulatory activity: a review and perspectives for COVID-19 treatment. J Pharm Pharmacol. 2021;73:281–99. https://doi.org/10.1093/jpp/rgaa067.
27. Salatino A. Perspectives for uses of propolis in therapy against infectious diseases. Molecules. 2022;27:4594. https://doi.org/10.3390/molecules27144594.
28. Yeh CF, Wang KC, Chiang LC, Shieh DE, Yen MH, San CJ. Water extract of licorice had antiviral activity against human respiratory syncytial virus in human respiratory tract cell lines. J Ethnopharmacol. 2013;148:466–73.
29. Zhou W, Yin A, Shan J, Wang S, Cai B, Di L. Study on the rationality for antiviral activity of Flos Lonicerae Japonicae-Fructus Forsythiae herb couple preparations improved by chito-oligosaccharide via integral pharmacokinetics. Molecules. 2017;22:654. https://doi.org/10.3390/molecules22040654.

30. Khan M, Saddique MAB, Tahir H, Amjad MD, Ahmad A, Masood U, Khan D. A short review on key role of plants and their extracts in boosting up immune response to combat COVID-19. Infect Disord Drug Targets. 2022;22:e270521193625. https://doi.org/10.2174/1871526521666210527091939.
31. Malekmohammad K, Rafieian-Kopaei M. Mechanistic aspects of medicinal plants and secondary metabolites against severe acute respiratory syndrome coronavirus 2 (SARS-CoV-2). Curr Pharm Des. 2021;27:3996–4007. https://doi.org/10.2174/1381612827666210705160130.
32. Jamshidnia M, Sewell RDE, Rafieian-Kopaei M. An update on promising agents against COVID-19: secondary metabolites and mechanistic aspects. Curr Pharm Des. 2022;28:2415–25. https://doi.org/10.2174/1381612828666220722124826.
33. Silva-Beltrán NP, Galvéz-Ruíz JC, Ikner LA, Umsza-Guez MA, de Paula Castro TL, Gerba CP. In vitro antiviral effect of Mexican and Brazilian propolis and phenolic compounds against human coronavirus 229E. Int J Environ Health Res. 2022;33:1591–603. https://doi.org/10.1080/09603123.2022.2110576.
34. Ali AM, Kunugi H. Propolis, bee honey, and their components protect against coronavirus disease 2019 (COVID-19): a review of in silico, in vitro, and clinical studies. Molecules. 2021;26:1232. https://doi.org/10.3390/molecules26051232.
35. Yosri N, Abd El-Wahed AA, Ghonaim R, Khattab OM, Sabry A, Ibrahim MAA, Moustafa MF, Guo Z, Zou X, Algethami AFM, et al. Anti-viral and immunomodulatory properties of propolis: chemical diversity, pharmacological properties, preclinical and clinical applications, and in silico potential against SARS-CoV-2. Food Secur. 2021;10:1776. https://doi.org/10.3390/foods10081776.
36. Schwarz S, Sauter D, Wang K, Zhang R, Sun B, Karioti A, Bilia AR, Efferth T, Schwarz W. Kaempferol derivatives as antiviral drugs against the 3a channel protein of coronavirus. Planta Med. 2014;80:177–82. https://doi.org/10.1055/s-0033-1360277.
37. Chen CJ, Michaelis M, Hsu HK, Tsai CC, Yang KD, Wu YC, Cinatl J Jr, Doerr HW. Toona sinensis Roem tender leaf extract inhibits SARS coronavirus replication. J Ethnopharmacol. 2008;120:108–11. https://doi.org/10.1016/j.jep.2008.07.048.
38. Yi L, Li Z, Yuan K, Qu X, Chen J, Wang G, Zhang H, Luo H, Zhu L, Jiang P, et al. Small molecules blocking the entry of severe acute respiratory syndrome coronavirus into host cells. J Virol. 2004;78:11334. https://doi.org/10.1128/JVI.78.20.11334-11339.2004.
39. Wang J, Ting Z, Jiang D, Sheng C, Fan Y, Qi J. Anti-enterovirus 71 effects of chrysin and its phosphate ester. PLoS One. 2014;9:3. https://doi.org/10.1371/journal.pone.0089668.
40. Basu A, Sarkar A, Maulik U. Molecular docking study of potential phytochemicals and their effects on the complex of SARS-CoV2 spike protein and human ACE2. Sci Rep. 2020;10:17699. https://doi.org/10.1038/s41598-020-74715-4.
41. Silveira MAD, De Jong D, Berretta AA, Galvão EBDS, Ribeiro JC, Cerqueira-Silva T, Amorim TC, da Conceicao LFMR, Gomes MMD, Teixeira MB, et al. Efficacy of Brazilian green propolis (EPP-AF®) as an adjunct treatment for hospitalized COVID-19 patients: a randomized, controlled clinical trial. Biomed Pharmacother. 2021;138:111526. https://doi.org/10.1016/j.biopha.2021.111526.
42. Sberna G, Biagi M, Marafini G, Nardacci R, Biava M, Colavita F, Piselli P, Miraldi E, D'Offizi G, Capobianchi MR, et al. In vitro evaluation of antiviral efficacy of a standardized hydroalcoholic extract of poplar type propolis against SARS-CoV-2. Front Microbiol. 2022;13:799546. https://doi.org/10.3389/fmicb.2022.799546.
43. Bijelic K, Hitl M, Kladar N. Phytochemicals in the prevention and treatment of SARS-CoV-2—clinical evidence. Antibiotics. 2022;11:1614. https://doi.org/10.3390/antibiotics11111614.
44. Güler Hİ, Ay ŞF, Can Z, Kara Y, Yildiz O, Beldüz AO, Canakci S, Kolayli S. Targeting CoV-2 spike RBD and ACE-2 interaction with flavonoids of Anatolian propolis by in silico and in vitro studies in terms of possible COVID-19 therapeutics. Turk J Biol. 2021;45:530–48. https://doi.org/10.3906/biy-2104-5.
45. Berretta AA, Silveira MAD, Cóndor Capcha JM, De Jong D. Propolis and its potential against SARS-CoV-2 infection mechanisms and COVID-19 disease: running title: propolis against

SARS-CoV-2 infection and COVID-19. Biomed Pharmacother. 2020;131:110622. https://doi.org/10.1016/j.biopha.2020.110622.
46. Kosari M, Noureddini M, Khamechi SP, Najafi A, Ghaderi A, Sehat M, Banafshe HR. The effect of propolis plus Hyoscyamus niger L. methanolic extract on clinical symptoms in patients with acute respiratory syndrome suspected to COVID-19: a clinical trial. Phytother Res. 2021;35:4000–6. https://doi.org/10.1002/ptr.7116.
47. Serkedjieva J, Manolova N, Bankova V. Anti-influenza virus effect of some propolis constituents and their analogues (esters of substituted cinnamic acids). J Nat Prod. 1992;55:294–7. https://doi.org/10.1021/np50081a003.
48. Urushisaki T, Takemura T, Tazawa S, Fukuoka M, Hosokawa-Muto J, Araki Y, Kuwata K. Caffeoylquinic acids are major constituents with potent anti-influenza effects in Brazilian green propolis water extract. Evid Based Complement Altern Med. 2011;2011:254914. https://doi.org/10.1155/2011/254914.
49. Kai H, Obuchi M, Yoshida H, Watanabe W, Tsutsumi S, Park YKYK, Matsuno K, Yasukawa K, Kurokawa M. In vitro and in vivo anti-influenza virus activities of flavonoids and related compounds as components of Brazilian propolis (AF-08). J Funct Foods. 2014;8:214–23. https://doi.org/10.1016/j.jff.2014.03.019.
50. Kujumgiev A, Tsvetkova I, Serkedjieva Y, Bankova V, Christov R, Popov S. Antibacterial, antifungal and antiviral activity of propolis of different geographic origin. J Ethnopharmacol. 1999;64:235–40. https://doi.org/10.1016/S0378-8741(98)00131-7.
51. Governa P, Cusi MG, Borgonetti V, Sforcin JM, Terrosi C, Baini G, Miraldi E, Biagi M. Beyond the biological effect of a chemically characterized poplar propolis: antibacterial and antiviral activity and comparison with flurbiprofen in cytokines release by LPS-stimulated human mononuclear cells. Biomedicines. 2019;7:73. https://doi.org/10.3390/biomedicines7040073.
52. Shimizu T, Hino A, Tsutsumi A, Yong KPKP, Watanabe W, Kurokawa M. Anti-influenza virus activity of propolis in vitro and its efficacy against influenza infection in mice. Antivir Chem Chemother. 2008;19:7–13. https://doi.org/10.1177/095632020801900102.
53. Valcic S, Montenegro G, Mujica A-M, Avila G, Franzblau S, Singh MP, Maiese WM, Timmermann BN. Phytochemical, morphological, and biological investigations of propolis from Central Chile. Z Naturforsch Sect C J Biosci. 1999;54:406–16. https://doi.org/10.1515/znc-1999-5-617.
54. Drago L, Mombelli B, De Vecchi E, Fassina MCC, Tocalli L, Gismondo MRR. In vitro antimicrobial activity of propolis dry extract. J Chemother. 2001;13:102. https://doi.org/10.1179/joc.2000.12.5.390.
55. Speciale A, Costanzo R, Puglisi S, Musumeci R, Catania MR, Caccamo F, Iauk L. Antibacterial activity of propolis and its active principles alone and in combination with macrolides, beta-lactams and fluoroquinolones against microorganisms responsible for respiratory infections. J Chemother. 2006;18:164–71. https://doi.org/10.1179/joc.2006.18.2.164.
56. Onlen Y, Duran N, Atik E, Savas L, Altug E, Yakan S, Aslantas O. Antibacterial activity of propolis against MRSA and synergism with topical mupirocin. J Altern Complement Med. 2007;13:713–8. https://doi.org/10.1089/acm.2007.7021.
57. Ophori EA, Wemabu EC. Antimicrobial activity of propolis extract on bacteria isolated from nasopharynx of patients with upper respiratory tract infection admitted to central hospital, Benin City, Nigeria, AFRICAN. J Microbiol Res. 2010;4:1719–23.
58. Popova M, Dimitrova R, Al-Lawati HT, Tsvetkova I, Najdenski H, Bankova V. Omani propolis: chemical profiling, antibacterial activity and new propolis plant sources. Chem Cent J. 2013;7:158. https://doi.org/10.1186/1752-153X-7-158.
59. Orodan M, Vodnar DC, Toiu AM, Pop CE, Vlase L, Viorica I, Arsene AL. Phytochemical analysis, antimicrobial and antioxidant effect of some gemmotherapic remedies used in respiratory diseases. Farmacia. 2016;64:224–30.
60. De Marco S, Piccioni M, Pagiotti R, Pietrella D. Antibiofilm and antioxidant activity of propolis and bud poplar resins versus Pseudomonas aeruginosa. Evid Based Complement Altern Med. 2017;2017:5163575. https://doi.org/10.1155/2017/5163575.

61. Scheller S, Kawalski H, Oklek K, Dworniczak S, Matsuno T, Waldemar-Klimmek K, Rajca M, Shani J. Correlation between virulence of various strains of mycobacteria and their susceptibility to ethanolic extract of propolis (EEP). Z Naturforsch C J Biosci. 1998;53:1040–4.
62. Scheller S, Dworniczak S, Waldemar-Klimmek K, Rajca M, Tomczyk A, Shani J. Synergism between ethanolic extract of propolis (EEP) and anti-tuberculosis drugs on growth of mycobacteria. Z Naturforsch Sec C J Biosci. 1999;54:549–53. https://doi.org/10.1515/znc-1999-7-814.
63. Guzmán-Gutiérrez SL, Nieto-Camacho A, Castillo-Arellano JI, Huerta-Salazar E, Hernández-Pasteur G, Silva-Miranda M, Ello-Nájera OA, Sepúlveda-Robles O, Espitia CI, Reyes-Chilpa R. Mexican propolis: a source of antioxidants and anti-inflammatory compounds, and isolation of a novel chalcone and ε-caprolactone derivative. Molecules. 2018;23:334. https://doi.org/10.3390/molecules23020334.
64. de Lima VHM, Almeida KDCR, Alves CCF, Rodrigues ML, Crotti AEM, de Souza JM, Ribeiro AB, Squarisi IS, Tavares DC, Martins CHG, Miranda MLD. Biological properties of volatile oil from Brazilian brown propolis. Rev Bras Farm J Pharmacogn. 2019;29:807–10. https://doi.org/10.1016/j.bjp.2019.07.004.
65. Marchisio P, Esposito S, Bianchini S, Desantis C, Galeone C, Nazzari E, Pignataro L, Principi N. Effectiveness of a propolis and zinc solution in preventing acute otitis media in children with a history of recurrent acute otitis media. Int J Immunopathol Pharmacol. 2010;23:567–75. https://doi.org/10.1177/039463201002300219.
66. Marti J, López F, Gascón I, Julve J. Propolis nasal spray effectively improves recovery from infectious acute rhinitis and common cold symptoms in children: a pilot study. J Biol Regul Homeost Agents. 2017;31:943–50.
67. Esposito C, Garzarella EU, Bocchino B, D'Avino M, Caruso G, Buonomo AR, Sacchi R, Galeotti F, Tenore GC, Zaccaria V, Daglia M. A standardized polyphenol mixture extracted from poplar-type propolis for remission of symptoms of uncomplicated upper respiratory tract infection (URTI): a monocentric, randomized, double-blind, placebo-controlled clinical trial. Phytomedicine. 2021;80:153368. https://doi.org/10.1016/j.phymed.2020.153368.
68. Seçilmis Y, Silici S. Bee product efficacy in children with upper respiratory tract infections. Turk J Pediatr. 2020;62:634–40. https://doi.org/10.24953/turkjped.2020.04.013.
69. Vekic J, Ivanisevic J, Zeljkovic A, Spasojevic-Kalimanovska V, Bogavac-Stanojevic N, Mihajlovic M, Janac J, Vujcic S, Miljkovic M, Zujovic D, Kotur-Stevuljevic J. Effect of propolis and N-acetylcysteine supplementation on lipoprotein subclasses distribution and paraoxonase 1 activity in subjects with acute respiratory infection. J Med Biochem. 2020;39:467–73. https://doi.org/10.5937/jomb0-24695.
70. Kuwata K, Takemura T, Urushisaki T, Fukuoka M, Hosokawa-Muto J, Hata T, Okuda Y, Hori S, Tazawa S, Araki Y, Kuwata K. 3,4-dicaffeoylquinic acid, a major constituent of Brazilian propolis, increases TRAIL expression and extends the lifetimes of mice infected with the influenza a virus. Evid Based Complement Altern Med. 2012;2012:946867. https://doi.org/10.1155/2012/946867.
71. Takeshita T, Watanabe W, Toyama S, Hayashi Y, Honda S, Sakamoto S, Matsuoka S, Yoshida H, Takeda S, Hidaka M, Park YK, Kurokawa M. Effect of Brazilian propolis on exacerbation of respiratory syncytial virus infection in mice exposed to tetrabromobisphenol A, a brominated flame retardant. Evid Based Complement Altern Med. 2013;2013:698206. https://doi.org/10.1155/2013/698206.
72. Hayakari R, Matsumiya T, Xing F, Tayone JCJC, Dempoya J, Tatsuta T, Aizawa-Yashiro T, Imaizumi T, Yoshida H, Satoh K. Effects of Brazilian green propolis on double-stranded RNA-mediated induction of interferon-inducible gene and inhibition of recruitment of polymorphonuclear cells. J Sci Food Agric. 2013;93:646–51. https://doi.org/10.1002/jsfa.5892.

73. Fan Y, Wang D, Liu J, Hu Y, Zhao X, Han G, Nguyen TL, Chang S. Adjuvanticity of epimedium polysaccharide-propolis flavone on inactivated vaccines against AI and ND virus. Int J Biol Macromol. 2012;51:1028–32. https://doi.org/10.1016/j.ijbiomac.2012.08.025.
74. Fan Y, Ma L, Zhang W, Xu Y, Suolangzhaxi X, Zhi E, Cui X, Song X. Microemulsion can improve the immune-enhancing activity of propolis flavonoid on immunosuppression and immune response. Int J Biol Macromol. 2014;63:126–32. https://doi.org/10.1016/j.ijbiomac.2013.09.039.
75. Permatasari A, Hasan H. The effect of ethanol extract propolis (EEP) on the level of IFN-F and superoxide dismutase (SOD) activities in patients with MDR tuberculosis. In: Respirology conference; 2014. p. 58.
76. Mahani M, Sulaeman A, Anwar A, Hardinsyah A, Damanik MR, Ploeger A. Efficacy of propolis supplementation to accelerate healing process and body weight recovery of pulmonary tuberculosis patients. J GIZI DAN Pangan. 2018;13:1–10. https://doi.org/10.25182/jgp.2018.13.1.1-10.

Effect of Propolis on Rhinosinusitis 16

16.1 Introduction

There is a significant cause for worry within the medical community over the growing resistance of microorganisms to antibiotic treatment [1, 2]. The use of specific probiotic strains to inhibit the growth of pathogens due to the release of bacteriocins [3] and the use of phytochemicals that can inhibit biofilms interfere with bacterial quorum sensing signaling pathways, or act as chelating agents and efflux pump inhibitors [4] are two examples of the innovative strategies that have been proposed as a result of this concern. The "wait and see" strategy is less inventive but pragmatic nonetheless. A wait-and-see approach, in which antibacterial medication is postponed for 48–72 h, has been proposed to treat acute otitis media (AOM) in children. This is primarily due to the growing antibiotic resistance of bacteria that cause respiratory infections [5].

16.2 Rhinosinusitis

The defining characteristic of sinusitis is inflammation of the lining of the paranasal sinuses. Since sinusitis rarely occurs without concurrent rhinitis, the term rhinosinusitis is most commonly used to describe this ailment. This is because the nasal mucosa is implicated simultaneously. This condition is more prevalent in females, and the age range between 45 and 64 has the most significant occurrence [6].

16.2.1 Signs and Symptoms

Clinical findings in acute sinusitis may include the following [6]: Pain over the cheek and radiating to the frontal region or teeth, increasing with straining or

A. E. Tanuğur Samanci et al., *Propolis: Prevention and Healing Effects in Otorhinolaryngology*, Comprehensive ENT,
https://doi.org/10.1007/978-3-031-68546-0_16

bending down; redness of nose, cheeks, or eyelids; tenderness to pressure over the floor of the frontal sinus immediately above the inner canthus; referred pain to the vertex, temple, or occiput; postnasal discharge; a blocked nose; persistent coughing or pharyngeal irritation; facial pain; and hyposmia.

Symptoms of acute bacterial rhinosinusitis include the following [6]: facial pain or pressure (especially unilateral); hyposmia/anosmia; nasal congestion/drainage; postnasal drip; fever; cough; fatigue; molar dental pain; and/or ear fullness/pressure.

When one of the following conditions [6] is present, the possibility of a diagnosis of acute bacterial sinusitis should be carefully considered.

- Symptoms or indications of acute rhinosinusitis that have been present for 10 days or more after the beginning of upper respiratory symptoms
- An increase in the severity of symptoms or indicators of acute rhinosinusitis within 10 days following an initial recovery in the condition

16.2.2 Brief History

It is the inflammation of the lining of the paranasal sinuses which is the defining characteristic of sinusitis. As a result of the simultaneous involvement of the nasal mucosa and the relative rarity of sinusitis occurring in the absence of contemporaneous rhinitis, the name rhinosinusitis has emerged as the most appropriate designation for this ailment [7].

It is possible to further categorize rhinosinusitis based on the anatomic site (maxillary, ethmoidal, frontal, or sphenoidal), the pathogenic organism (viral, bacterial, or fungal), the existence of a complication (orbital or intracranial), and the related variables (nasal polyposis, immunosuppression, or anatomic variations).

Because acute sinusitis is a clinical diagnosis, it is essential to thoroughly grasp its manifestations to differentiate this condition from allergy or vasomotor rhinitis and other upper respiratory infections. Because no clinical symptom or sign is sensitive or specific for acute sinusitis, the overall clinical impression should guide therapy throughout the treatment process.

The key objectives of the care of acute sinusitis are the elimination of the infection, the reduction in the severity and duration of symptoms, and prevention of consequences. In the primary care context, the majority of patients who are diagnosed with acute sinusitis are treated. If any of the following conditions are present, it is suggested that you get further assessment from an otolaryngologist [7]:

- If the patient continues to deteriorate despite receiving optimal antibiotic treatment
- If sinusitis attacks come back
- In cases when symptoms continue to be present after two sessions of antibiotic treatment
- If concurrent medical conditions such as immunodeficiency, nosocomial infection, or consequences of sinusitis are present

16.2.3 Pathophysiology

When physiologic circumstances are present, the sinuses are generally clear of pathogens. The ciliary activity in the sinuses causes the secretions generated there to flow down the ostia and then drain into the nasal cavity. Whenever a person is in good health, the flow of sinus secretions is always unidirectional (that is, toward the ostia), which prevents the sinuses from becoming contaminated in the other direction. In most people, the maxillary sinus comprises a single ostium that is the sole outflow channel for drainage. This ostium measures 2.5 mm in diameter and 5 mm squared in a cross-sectional area. In a position independent of the sinus cavity, this thin conduit is positioned high on the medial wall of the sinus cavity. The edema of the mucosa at these apertures, which range from 1 to 3 mm in diameter, most likely becomes congested as a result of some factor (such as an allergy, viruses, or chemical irritation), which results in the blockage of the outflow tract stasis of secretions with negative pressure, which ultimately leads to infection by bacteria.

When mucus is retained, sinusitis can develop as a result of infection. Another explanation proposes that colonized bacteria in the nasopharynx may infect the sinuses, which are ordinarily sterile due to their continuous relationship with the nasal cavity. These bacteria are typically eliminated by mucociliary clearance; thus, if mucociliary clearance is disrupted, bacteria may be inoculated, and infection may occur, resulting in sinusitis [8, 9].

The currently available data support the existence of colonization in healthy sinuses. In a study conducted on 12 people who had undergone corrective surgery for septal deviation [10], the bacterial flora of sinuses that were not inflamed was examined for both aerobic and anaerobic microorganisms. An average of four organisms were recovered from each sinus aspirate, and all of the aspirates included organisms. The species of Prevotella, Porphyromonas, Fusobacterium, and Peptostreptococcus were the most commonly isolated from anaerobic environments. *S. pyogenes*, *S. aureus*, *S. pneumonia*, and *H. influenzae* were the oxygen-consuming bacteria found most often. In a different investigation, materials were analyzed just for aerobic bacteria, and the results showed that alpha-hemolytic streptococci and Staphylococcus species were isolated [11]. Sixty percent of the maxillary sinuses of individuals who had undergone surgical repositioning of the maxilla were found to have retrieved organisms [6].

16.2.4 Obstruction of Sinus Drainage

Regular mucus outflow will be restricted if the natural sinus ostia are blocked. The ostia can become obstructed due to mucosal edema or local reasons (such as trauma or rhinitis), as well as by certain systemic illnesses and immunological disorders that are often linked with inflammation. Systemic disorders that cause a reduction in mucociliary clearance, such as cystic fibrosis, respiratory allergies, and primary ciliary dyskinesia (Kartagener syndrome), can predispose factors for acute sinusitis in sporadic instances. Patients with immunodeficiencies (e.g., agammaglobulinemia, mixed variable immunodeficiency, and immunodeficiency with diminished immunoglobulin G [IgG]– and immunoglobulin A [IgA]–bearing cells) are also at greater risk of developing acute sinusitis [6].

Occlusion can also be caused by mechanical problems, which nasal polyps, foreign substances, deviated septa, or tumors can cause. In particular, the septal deviation, paradoxical middle turbinates, and Haller cells are anatomical anomalies limiting the ostiomeatal complex. These changes render this region more susceptible to blockage caused by mucosal inflammation. For the most part, the edges of the edematous mucosa have a scalloped look. However, in extreme cases, mucus may fully cover a sinus, making it difficult to differentiate between an allergic process and infectious sinusitis. All paranasal sinuses are afflicted, and the nasal turbinates next to them are enlarged, which is characteristic of this condition. Air-fluid levels and bone erosion are not characteristics of uncomplicated allergic sinusitis. On the other hand, swollen mucosa in a sinus that drains poorly is more likely to be affected by subsequent bacterial infection.

Hypoxia within the blocked sinus is believed to produce ciliary dysfunction and changes in mucus production, which would further compromise the typical mechanism for mucus clearance [6].

16.2.5 Impaired Ciliary Function

The drainage patterns of the paranasal sinuses are not dependent on gravity, as was previously believed, but rather on the mucociliary transport process. This diverges from traditional conceptions of sinus physiology. The natural sinus ostia are the destination of the sinus contents, which are propelled toward them by the metachronous coordination of the ciliated columnar epithelial cells. Whenever there is a disturbance in the function of the cilia, there is a buildup of fluid within the sinus. Poor ciliary activity can be caused by several factors, including the loss of ciliated epithelial cells, high airflow, ciliotoxins from viruses, bacteria, or the environment, inflammatory mediators, contact between two mucosal surfaces, scars, and Kartagener syndrome [12].

Genetic variables, such as Kartagener syndrome, can influence the activity of the ciliary system. There is a correlation between Kartagener syndrome and immobile cilia, which results in the retention of secretions and a tendency to sinus infection. A low pH, anoxia, cigarette smoke, chemical pollutants, dehydration, and pharmaceuticals (such as anticholinergic medications and antihistamines) are all factors that can lead to a reduction in ciliary function [6].

Toxins produced by bacteria can also diminish ciliary activity. It is estimated that around 10% of cases of acute sinusitis are caused by the direct injection of the sinus with a significant quantity of germs. Sinusitis can also be caused by dental abscesses or treatments that result in a connection between the oral cavity and the sinuses. In addition, the activity of the cilia might be altered with certain viral infections [6].

Based on the physical examination, the following symptoms may be seen [6]:

- Purulent nasal secretions
- Secretions from the posterior pharynx that are purulent
- Erythema of the mucosa
- Edema of the periorbital region
- Pain that is localized over the sinuses
- To evaluate maxillary sinus disease, the air-fluid levels on the sinuses' transillumination have a 60% repeatability rate.
- The erythema of the face

16.3 Propolis and Rhinosinusitis

Exudates from buds, plants, poplars, conifers, birch, pine, alder, willow, palm, Baccharis dracunculifolia, and Dalbergia ecastaphyllum are used by honeybees to form propolis, which is a well-known natural resinous combination [13]. Honeybees generate propolis. Raw propolis comprises around 50% resins, 30% waxes, 10% essential oils, 5% pollen, and 5% diverse organic compounds [14]. These organic compounds include flavonoids, phenylpropanoids, terpenes, stilbenes, lignans, and coumarins, as well as their prenylated derivatives, along with more than 300 distinct chemicals [15]. It depends on the geographical region, the botanical origin, and the bee species engaged [16–19] to determine the specific chemical composition of propolis. Pinocembrin, pinobanksin, caffeic acid phenyl ester, artepillin C, cinnamic acid, p-coumaric acid, caffeic acid, ferulic acid, isoferulic acid, chrysin, galangin, kaempferol, and quercetin are the primary chemical components found in propolis [20]. These components have been researched primarily in terms of their pharmacological action. Flavonoids, the primary ingredients of propolis, contribute significantly to the pharmacological effects of the substance. Even though they possess antibacterial, antiviral, antifungal, and anti-inflammatory effects [21–25], flavonoids derived from propolis, which are virtually entirely aglycones, are characterized by low solubility and poor bioavailability [26, 27]. It has been observed that using phytochrome forms and grinding technology can boost the oral bioavailability of flavonoids, as well as their solubility [28–30].

In acute otitis media (AOM), using a product containing propolis reduces the intensity of symptoms. In cases of nonstreptococcal pharyngitis, it minimizes the length and severity of symptoms (at least in some instances). It also decreases the rate at which symptoms progress to tracheitis, bronchitis, and rhinosinusitis. The use of this medication in treating acute obstructive pharyngitis and pharyngitis considerably lowers the amount of antipyretics and anti-inflammatory medications that are administered to children, hence lowering the likelihood of adverse effects occurring in the liver and the stomach mucosa. The impact of propolis in decreasing recurrent upper respiratory tract viral infections and episodes of acute obstructive pulmonary disease (AOM) in children was established by other authors in studies that were quite comparable to these [31, 32].

In this study, a proprietary product based on propolis that was created to address the well-known issues of low oral bioavailability and poor solubility was subjected to a retrospective analysis. Because of their chemical and physical features, propolis polyphenols, likely the most essential component of propolis, are inadequately water soluble. As a result, they cannot dissolve and disseminate throughout the throat mucosa, which would prevent them from having the potential to exert a local impact. Furthermore, the same percentage exhibits low gastrointestinal absorption, which results in a minimum amount of systemic availability. The propolis formulation employed in this retrospective investigation blended two different fractions. This was done to address these two primary issues. Cogrinding, or mechanical/chemical activation, was the initial procedure applied to propolis. This process was carried out in off-axis mills with L-lysine as the carrier. During grinding with L-lysine, propolis loses its crystalline structure and transitions toward an amorphous form with the airline. A product with improved water-dissolution kinetics is produced as a consequence of grinding, which causes a remarkable change in the properties of the substance. After that, propolis was connected to a phospholipid carrier, which increased its lipophilicity and made it possible for it to be emulsified by bile salts, after which it could be absorbed and dispersed throughout the body. We know that some writers have attempted to tackle the solubility and bioavailability issues associated with propolis [33, 34] by concentrating primarily on using liposomes and microemulsions. However, to our knowledge, these authors have yet to conduct clinical tests to determine the potential impact of these novel formulations [1].

NAC and propolis have been investigated in fixed combination for their possible synergistic effects on oxidative stress and inflammatory or biochemical parameters in acute and chronic respiratory infections [35–37].

The antibacterial activity of propolis has already been investigated, and the results show that propolis is more effective against Gram-positive bacteria than it is against Gram-negative bacteria [38–41]. In our research, the minimum inhibitory concentration (MIC) for dry propolis extract was between 0.25 and 8 mg/mL, and the Gram-positive bacteria were shown to have the most potent antibacterial activity. Furthermore, our findings demonstrated that the dry propolis extract was similarly effective against Gram-negative bacteria but with a somewhat higher minimum inhibitory concentration (MIC) than Gram-positive bacteria. Although the absolute values cannot be directly correlated, the MIC values are comparable to those reported by other authors [38–41]. We used a standardized dry propolis extract to contain 12% of total polyphenols. In contrast, other authors have primarily used a liquid ethanolic propolis extract of different geographical origins prepared by the official standards for extract production. Our research indicates that the combination of NAC and dry propolis extract synergistically impacted more than 50% of the strains. This was demonstrated by the fact that each component's minimum inhibitory concentration (MIC) in its fixed combination was lowered by two to four times when compared with the MIC of each compound. The additive effect was detected in roughly 40% of the strains, and just 10% were indifferent to this combination. This is yet another favorable pharmacological interaction discovered. It was observed that the inhibitory effect of NAC against Gram-positive and Gram-negative bacteria that were isolated from infections of the upper respiratory tract ranged from 2.5 to more than 40 mg/mL [42–46]. Compared to the above data, our findings indicate that the minimum inhibitory concentration (MIC) for NAC has decreased due to synergistic interactions. In contrast, propolis' minimum inhibitory concentration (MIC) values change depending on the solvent. For both Gram-positive and Gram-negative bacteria, the antimicrobial activity of ethanolic and methanolic extracts is significantly higher than that of non-alcoholic extracts, which include water, DMSO, and hexane. Przybyłek and Karpinski conducted a comprehensive evaluation to examine the antibacterial activity of several propolis extracts. The minimum inhibitory concentration (MIC) values were reported as follows: S. aureus up to 3.1 mg/mL, S. epidermidis up to 1.1 mg/mL, S. pneumoniae up to 1.5 mg/mL, P. aeruginosa 7.9 mg/mL, and H. influenzae 2.5 mg/mL [47]. Our research lowered propolis' minimum inhibitory concentration (MIC) in fixed combination to 0.125–2 mg/mL. This reduction can be due to synergistic effects comparable to those of NAC, and it substantiates the positive impact of this particular combination of NAC and propolis. This observation is particularly significant because the fixed combination of NAC and propolis may be administered through the oral route and as a local mucosal treatment. Furthermore, lower quantities of both compounds are less irritating to mucous membranes and are well tolerated. The processes that underlie the synergistic impact of NAC and propolis may differ from one microbe species to another or from one health condition to another, depending on the respective targets. To achieve a more efficient antibacterial clearance, the combination of propolis and NAC can potentially increase the antimicrobial activities of both substances individually. Both compounds possess immunomodulatory properties [48], and they may have synergistic effects in promoting a balanced immune response and enhancing immune defense mechanisms. Additionally, both compounds possess antioxidative properties [49, 50], providing synergistic antioxidant effects and improved protection against oxidative damage. In vivo, all of the mechanisms that have been highlighted have favorable effects since they can minimize mucosal inflammation and damage and speed up the process of tissue regeneration [35].

References

1. Di Pierro F, Zanvit A, Colombo M. Role of a proprietary propolis-based product on the wait-and-see approach in acute otitis media and in preventing evolution to tracheitis, bronchitis, or rhinosinusitis from nonstreptococcal pharyngitis. Int J Gen Med. 2016;9:409–14.
2. Falagas ME, Mavroudis AD, Vardakas KZ. The antibiotic pipeline for multi-drug resistant gram negative bacteria: what can we expect? Expert Rev Anti-Infect Ther. 2016;14(8):747–63.
3. Wescombe PA, Hale JD, Hen NC, Tagg JR. Developing oral probiotics from Streptococcus salivarius. Future Microbiol. 2012;7(12):1355–71.
4. Borges A, Abreu AC, Dias C, Saavedra MJ, Borges F, Simões M. New perspectives on the use of phytochemicals as an emergent strategy to control bacterial infections including biofilms. Molecules. 2016;21(7):pii:E877.
5. Corbeel L. The 'wait-and-see' approach of acute otitis media. Eur J Pediatr. 2005;164(1):1–2.

6. Brook I. Acute sinusitis. In: Bronze MS, editor. Medscape. Updated: Aug 14, 2023. https://emedicine.medscape.com/article/232670-overview#a4. Accessed online at 10 Dec 2023.
7. Battisti AS, Modi P, Pangia J. Sinusitis. In: StatPearls. Treasure Island: StatPearls Publishing; 2023.
8. Wald ER, DeMuri G. Sinusitis. Long SS, Prober CG, Fischer M, eds. Principles and practice of pediatric infectious disease. 5th ed. Philadelphia: Elsevier; 2018. 230–234.
9. American Academy of Pediatrics - Subcommittee on Management of Sinusitis and Committee on Quality Management. Clinical practice guideline: management of sinusitis. Pediatrics. 2001;108(3):798–808.
10. Brook I. Aerobic and anaerobic bacterial flora of normal maxillary sinuses. Laryngoscope. 1981;91(3):372–6.
11. Su WY, Liu C, Hung SY, Tsai WF. Bacteriological study in chronic maxillary sinusitis. Laryngoscope. 1983;93(7):931–4.
12. Hamilos DL. Clinical manifestations, pathophysiology, and diagnosis of chronic rhinosinusitis. UpToDate. Available at http://www.uptodate.com. Accessed 07 June 2009.
13. Bankova V, de Castro SL, Marcucci MC. Propolis: recent advances in chemistry and plant origin. Apidologie. 2000;31(1):3–15.
14. Burdock GA. Review of the biological properties and toxicity of bee propolis (propolis). Food Chem Toxicol. 1998;36(4):347–63.
15. Marcucci MC. Propolis: chemical composition, biological properties and therapeutic activity. Apidologie. 1995;26(2):83–99.
16. Salatino A, Fernandes-Silva CC, Righi AA, Salatino ML. Propolis research and the chemistry of plant products. Nat Prod Rep. 2011;28(5):925–36.
17. Toreti VC, Sato HH, Pastore GM, Park YK. Recent progress of propolis for its biological and chemical compositions and its botanical origin. Evid Based Complement Alternat Med. 2013;2013:697390.
18. Bankova V. Recent trends and important developments in propolis research. Evid Based Complement Alternat Med. 2005;2(1):29–32.
19. Silici S, Kutluca S. Chemical composition and antibacterial activity of propolis collected by three different races of honeybees in the same region. J Ethnopharmacol. 2005;99(1):69–73.
20. Huang S, Zhang CP, Wang K, Li GQ, Hu FL. Recent advances in the chemical composition of propolis. Molecules. 2014;19(12):19610–32.
21. Nijveldt RJ, van Nood E, van Hoorn DE, Boelens PG, van Norren K, van Leeuwen PA. Flavonoids: a review of probable mechanisms of action and potential applications. Am J Clin Nutr. 2001;74(4):418–25.
22. Dalben-Dota KF, Faria MG, Bruschi ML, Pelloso SM, Lopes-Consolaro ME, Svidzinski TI. Antifungal activity of propolis extract against yeasts isolated from vaginal exudates. J Altern Complement Med. 2010;16(3):285–90.
23. Grange JM, Davey RW. Antibacterial properties of propolis (bee glue). J R Soc Med. 1990;83(3):159–60.
24. Nolkemper S, Reichling J, Sensch KH, Schnitzler P. Mechanism of herpes simplex virus type 2 suppression by propolis extracts. Phytomedicine. 2010;17(2):132–8.
25. Kujumgiev A, Tsvetkova I, Serkedjieva Y, Bankova V, Christov R, Popov S. Antibacterial, antifungal and antiviral activity of propolis of different geographic origin. J Ethnopharmacol. 1999;64(3):235–40.
26. Konishi Y, Hitomi Y, Yoshida M, Yoshioka E. Absorption and bioavailability of artepillin C in rats after oral administration. J Agric Food Chem. 2005;53(26):9928–33.
27. Metzner J, Bekemeier H, Schneidewind EM, Wenzel U. [Pharmacokinetic studies of the propolis constituent pinocembrin in the rat (author's transl)]. Pharmazie. 1979;34(3):185–7. German.
28. Kaur H, Kaur G. A critical appraisal of solubility enhancement techniques of polyphenols. J Pharm (Cairo). 2014;2014:180845.
29. Kidd PM. Bioavailability and activity of phytosome complexes from botanical polyphenols: the silymarin, curcumin, green tea, and grape seed extracts. Altern Med Rev. 2009;14(3):226–46.
30. Voinovich D, Perissutti B, Grassi M, Passerini N, Bigotto A. Solid state mechanochemical activation of Silybum marianum dry extract with betacyclodextrins: characterization and bioavailability of the co-ground systems. J Pharm Sci. 2009;98(11):4119–29.

31. Crişan I, Zaharia CN, Popovici F, et al. Natural propolis extract NIVCRI-SOL in the treatment of acute and chronic rhinopharyngitis in children. Rom J Virol. 1995;46(3–4):115–33.
32. Marchisio P, Esposito S, Bianchini S, et al. Effectiveness of a propolis and zinc solution in preventing acute otitis media in children with a history of recurrent acute otitis media. Int J Immunopathol Pharmacol. 2010;23(2):567–75.
33. Ambardekar RV, Mahadik KR, Paradkar AR, Harsulkar AM. Enhancement of hepatoprotective efficacy of propolis by fabrication of liposomes, as a platform nano-formulation for multi-component natural medicine. Curr Drug Deliv. 2012;9(5):477–86.
34. Fan Y, Ma L, Zhang W, et al. Microemulsion can improve the immune-enhancing activity of propolis flavonoid on immunosuppression and immune response. Int J Biol Macromol. 2014;63:126–32.
35. Božić DD, Ćirković I, Milovanović J, et al. In vitro antibiofilm effect of N-acetyl-L-cysteine/dry propolis extract combination on bacterial pathogens isolated from upper respiratory tract infections. Pharmaceuticals (Basel). 2023;16(11):1604. Published 2023 Nov 14. https://doi.org/10.3390/ph16111604.
36. Žuža O, Minić R, Kotur-Stevuljević J, Žujović D, Đordević B, Ilić A. A combination of N-acetyl cysteine and propolis attenuates oxidative-inflammatory parameters during COPD exacerbation. Eur Rev Med Pharmacol Sci. 2022;26:2467–77.
37. Vekić J, Ivanišević J, Zeljković A, Spasojević-Kalimanovska V, Bogavac-Stanojević N, Mihajlović M, Janać J, Vujˇcić S, Miljković M, Zujović D, et al. Effect of propolis and N-acetylcysteine supplementation on lipoprotein subclasses distribution and paraoxonase 1 activity in subjects with acute respiratory infection. J Med Biochem. 2020;39:467–73.
38. Drago L, Mombelli B, De Vecchi E, Fassina MC, Tocalli L, In Gismondo MR, vitro antimicrobial activity of propolis dry extract. J Chemother. 2000;12:390–5. Erratum in: J. Chemother. 2001, 13, 102.
39. El-Fadaly H, El-Badrawy EEY. Flavonoids of propolis and their antibacterial activities. Pak J Biol Sci. 2001;21:204–7.
40. Stepanović S, Antić N, Dakić I, Švabić-Vlahović M. In vitro antimicrobial activity of propolis and synergism between propolis and antimicrobial drugs. Microbiol Res. 2003;158:353–7.
41. Almuhayawi MS. Propolis as a novel antibacterial agent. Saudi J Biol Sci. 2020;27:3079–86.
42. Lea J, Conlin AE, Sekirov I, Restelli V, Ayakar KG, Turnbull LA, Doyle P, Noble M, Rennie R, Schreiber WE, et al. In vitro efficacy of N-acetylcysteine on bacteria associated with chronic suppurative otitis media. J Otolaryngol Head Neck Surg. 2014;43:20.
43. Domenech M, Garcia E. N-acetyl-L-cysteine and cysteamine as new strategies against mixed biofilms of nonencapsulated Streptococcus pneumoniae and nontypeable Haemophilus influenzae. Antimicrob Agents Chemother. 2017;61:e01992–16.
44. Sempere J, Llamosí M, Román F, Lago D, González-Camacho F, Pérez-García C, Yuste J, Domenech M. Clearance of mixed biofilm of Streptococcus pneumoniae and methicillin-susceptible/resistant Staphylococcus aureus by antioxidants N-acetyl-L-cysteine and cysteamine. Sci Rep. 2022;12:6668.
45. Jun Y, Youn CK, Jo ER, Cho SI. In vitro inhibitory activity of N-acetylcysteine on tympanostomy tube biofilms from methicillin-resistant Staphylococcus aureus and quinolone-resistant Pseudomonas aeruginosa. Int J Pediatr Otorhinolaryngol. 2019;126:109622.
46. Zhao T, Liu Y. N-acetylcysteine inhibits biofilms produced by Pseudomonas aeruginosa. BMC Microbiol. 2010;10:140.
47. Przybyłek I, Karpiński TM. Antibacterial properties of Propolis. Molecules. 2019;24:2047.
48. Magnavacca A, Sangiovanni E, Racagni G, Dell'Agli M. The antiviral and immunomodulatory activities of propolis: an update and future perspectives for respiratory diseases. Med Res Rev. 2022;42:897–945.
49. Wu G, Fang YZ, Yang S, Lupton JR, Turner ND. Glutathione metabolism and its implications for health. J Nutr. 2004;134:489–92.
50. Zullkiflee N, Taha H, Usman A. Propolis: its role and efficacy in human health and diseases. Molecules. 2022;27:6120.

17 Effect of Propolis on Nasal Blockage

17.1 Introduction

The most common manifestation of turbinate dysfunction is nasal congestion, which is also one of the symptoms associated with this condition. In some cases, the symptoms may be mild. In contrast, in others, the congestion may be so severe that the only way to ease it is to overuse topical decongestants such as oxymetazoline or phenylephrine. The fact that the symptoms are not severe is yet another possibility. Quite a few people have tried oral decongestants that are available without a prescription, also known as over-the-counter (OTC) medications, but their results have needed to be consistent. During the management procedure, the two most important processes are identifying the underlying cause of turbinate hypertrophy and the subsequent therapy or correction of the problem following the identification of the cause. The infectious and inflammatory etiologies are encountered the most frequently [1].

17.2 Pathophysiology of Nasal Congestion

Failure of the turbinate to operate correctly can be attributed to several different circumstances. Everything that affects either of these two systems will affect the turbinates and, as a result, the nose [2]. This is because the parasympathetic nervous system is responsible for directing the turbinates and has a highly abundant blood supply.

Patients who are unable to use their nostrils for airflow (for instance, patients who have undergone laryngectomy) or patients who engage in excessive use of topical nasal decongestants (rhinitis medicamentosa) are more likely to develop rhinitis of disuse. The first state is characterized by rebound inflammation, which is the underlying pathophysiology that is being described. This is because the typical

A. E. Tanuğur Samanci et al., *Propolis: Prevention and Healing Effects in Otorhinolaryngology*, Comprehensive ENT,
https://doi.org/10.1007/978-3-031-68546-0_17

nasal airflow does not provide any input when it is present. In the second scenario, the turbinates experience a rebound vasodilation due to topical sympathomimetics [1]. This vasodilation is a manifestation of the reaction.

Like the rest of the upper respiratory tract (URT), the membranes that surround the turbinates are composed of glandular, columnar epithelium that is ciliated and pseudostratified. This is also the case for the remainder of the URT. The mucus is transferred from the nasal cavity to the nasopharynx through the cilia's continual beating. This allows the mucus to be ingested after it has been transported to the nasopharynx. Mucociliary transport requires both the production of mucus and the functioning of cilia to succeed. The nasal passages and paranasal sinuses produce around one quart and a half of mucus on an average school day. There is a possibility that the quantity will more than double with an inflammatory response. Muramidase, immunoglobulin A (IgA), and immunoglobulin E (IgE) are all examples of components that might be present in mucus.

Both the amount of secretions produced by the turbinates and the level of congestion are under the control of the autonomic nervous system and the blood supply. The nose receives its general innervation from the autonomic nervous system, which delivers nasal innervation. At the same time, the parasympathetic nerves are accountable for the delivery of the resting tone and the management of the secretions. The nerve supply originates from the facial nerve, situated at the superior salivary nucleus. The nerve supply then travels through the sphenopalatine ganglion, which distributes the facial nerve. Internal and external carotid artery branches are responsible for supplying blood to the nose. These branches are the source of the blood flow that arrives at the nose. The terminal branches of the internal maxillary artery [1] are responsible for providing the majority of the mucosal surfaces that are located in the nasal cavity.

17.3 Propolis

The compound known as propolis, frequently referred to as "bee glue," is a substance similar to resin and is collected by honeybees from the buds of various plant sources. Honeybees utilize this material to secure honeycombs, smooth out the internal walls, defend the beehive entrance from trespassers, and protect bees from illnesses. Additionally, propolis serves the purpose of better preserving the homeostasis of the environment within the nest. This goal is accomplished by restricting the growth of germs on the walls of the hive, preventing the circulation of unregulated air into the nest, and waterproofing the walls from moisture that comes from the outside. The ultimate product, referred to as raw propolis or propolis in nature, is created by combining the materials gathered with the enzyme α-glycosidase present in the bees' saliva. This enzyme is then added to beeswax after it has been partially digested earlier. Raw propolis comprises 50% plant resins, 30% waxes, 10% essential and aromatic oils, 5% pollens, and 5% other organic substances. These organic substances include elements like vitamins A, C, D, E, and B1, B2, B5, and B6, niacin and folate, and some micro and macro minerals. More than five hundred components have been discovered in propolis originating from various geographical locations [3–8]. These components include phenolic acids, flavonoids (flavones, flavanones, flavanols, dihydro flavanols, and chalcones), terpenes, lignans, amino acids, fatty acids, nutritional vitamins, and minerals. There is a correlation between propolis' chemical qualities and the diverse geographical regions, plant sources, and bee species utilized in propolis' creation [3–8]. Certain studies summarize propolis' chemical composition, considering the geographical region, botanical origin, and bee species stated in the articles. The following is a list of the primary chemical components of propolis that have been confirmed in various percentages: fatty and aliphatic acids (24–26%), flavonoids (18–20%), sugars (15–18%), aromatic acids (5–10%), esters (2–6%), vitamins (2–4%), alcohol and terpenes (2–3.3%), microelements (0.5–2.0%), and other components (21–27%) [6–8].

The propolis has approximately 30 distinct components in total. Calcium, manganese, zinc, copper, silicon, iron, and aluminum are the elements that are typically found in the most incredible abundance [6–8]. Of all the aspects, calcium is the most prevalent. Several vitamins, including vitamins B, C, D, P, and E, and provitamin A (β-carotene), have been proposed as potential components of propolis. There are also trace amounts of enzymes present in propolis, in addition to its vitamins. Several enzymes are included in this category, which are α-amylase, β-amylase, α-lactamase, β-lactamase, maltase, esterase, and transhydrogenase [8]. It has been found that propolis contains enzymes that originate from the glands of bees, and pollen is also responsible for some of the enzymes found in propolis [6–8]. On average, the portion of protein present in EEP is roughly 2.8% [3–8].

On the other hand, the quantity of free amino acids present is relatively low and amounts to approximately 17 [3–8]. Another one of the amino acids, pyroglutamic acid, was found by the bee organism, which is responsible for its discovery. Several polysaccharides in propolis include sucrose, glucose, fructose, rhamnose, ribose, talose, and gulose [3–8]. Moreover, mono- and disaccharides are found in propolis samples. One of the factors that contribute to the existence of different types of propolis is the location of the botanical origin of the propolis, as well as the time of year when it is gathered. According to most studies, there are at least six primary chemical kinds of propolis. These include (1) propolis that is found in Europe, North America, and non-tropical regions of Asia, and its primary source is poplar (Populus spp., most commonly *P. nigra*); (2) propolis that is present in Russia, where birch (Betula verrucosa Ehrh.) is the predominant species; (3) green propolis that is present in Brazil, primarily from Baccharis spp., predominantly *B. dracunculifolia* DC; (4) red propolis, which belonging to the genus Clusia, can be found in Cuba and Venezuela; (5) "Pacific" propolis from Okinawa and Taiwan, for which there is no known plant source; and (6) "Canary" propolis from the Canary Islands, respectively. The resinous exudates produced by the buds of poplar trees (Populus species) are referred to as "poplar propolis," they are distinguished by a chemical composition comparable to that of other substances. The flavonoid aglycones, aromatic acids, and their esters are the fundamental compounds classified as belonging to the phenolic class to which they belong. The prenylated derivatives of p-coumaric acid and o-hydroxy-acetophenone found in Brazilian green (Alecrim) propolis set it apart from standard propolis [8].

In comparison to other varieties of propolis, this one is unique. The chemical components found in Brazilian propolis are not found in propolis from different regions, according to a study that demonstrated this. Because of this distinction, the flavonoid components, diterpenes, and lignans present in American propolis are distinct from those available in European propolis. In comparison to the levels of artepillin C (20.7%), bacharrin (7.5%), and kaempferide (3.6%) that are found in other types of propolis, the levels of these three compounds that are discovered in Brazilian green propolis are substantially more significant. The Clusia nemorosa plant, which belongs to the family Clusiaceae, is Cuba's principal source of red propolis.

On the other hand, the most common source of propolis that bees in Venezuela collect is coming from C. This is nemorosa. This species is known as scrobiculata. In addition to having a high content of polyprenylated benzophenones, Cuban propolis is unique from both European and Brazilian propolis. This is a crucial distinction to make. The chemical compounds known as geranyl flavanones are responsible for distinguishing the properties of propolis produced in the Pacific area. According to [7, 8], these chemicals are also present in propolis that is generated in the African region.

Antibacterial, antioxidant, and immunomodulatory activities are always present in propolis. Additionally, propolis has anti-inflammatory, antiallergic, dermatoprotective, laxative, antidiabetic, antiangiogenic, and anticancer activity. That being said, this holds independent of the specific plant from which it originates or the drug's chemical composition. It is believed that the antibacterial properties of propolis are due to the presence of flavonoids in the substance. These flavonoids include pinocembrin, galangin, pinobanksin, pinobanksin-3-acetate, and caffeic acid ester. Propolis, known to possess potent antioxidant effects, may contain several compounds, including kaempferol, caffeic acid (CA), and phenethyl caffeate, to name a few of the molecules that may be present. It is possible to explain the anti-inflammatory impact by pointing to the presence of active flavonoids, such as quercetin, acacetin, and naringenin, as well as cinnamic acid derivatives, such as baccharin, drupanin, and caffeic acid phenethyl ester (CAPE). These antioxidant flavonoids are responsible for the anti-inflammatory action. CAPE is one of the most critical components of temperate propolis because it exhibits various biological effects. Among the activities included in this category are the suppression of nuclear factor κB (NF-κB), the inhibition of cell proliferation, the induction of cell cycle arrest, and the induction of apoptosis. It was discovered that different components of Brazilian, Cuban, and Mexican propolis exhibit pro- and anti-inflammatory properties depending on the dosage. Each of these components was found to have these effects. These discoveries may prove helpful in the process of developing novel immunomodulatory medications [9].

The concentration of bioactive components in propolis can vary greatly depending on the sample's origin, and these changes may affect the biological activities of the propolis. Since the beginning of time, traditional medicine practitioners have been aware of the healing properties shared by propolis. The effectiveness of propolis as a therapeutic agent has been proven by several studies, including quantitative and qualitative analyses of the expression and degradation of collagen types I and III in the matrix of wounds. Based on these findings, it can be concluded that propolis and its antioxidant and anti-inflammatory properties can trigger re-epithelization. It has been demonstrated that the flavonoids included in propolis can effectively inhibit the production of nucleic acids, the adhesion and formation of biofilms, and the energy metabolism found in bacteria.

In addition, they can impede the development of bacterial cells and cause malfunctions inside the cytoplasm, finally leading to the inactivation of bacterial production and growth. This is accomplished through a variety of mechanisms that involve several cellular and molecular processes that are involved in integrated stages. Some examples of these processes include hemostasis, inflammation, cell proliferation, and tissue remodeling [10, 11]. The process of wound repair and regeneration is speed up due to their ability to modify the production of collagen and simultaneously stimulate skin tissue growth and regeneration.

Propolis can stimulate the expression of genes associated with antioxidants, and it can reduce oxidative stress in wounds. Heme oxygenase-1 (HO-1) and glutamate-cysteine ligase-modifier (GCLM) are examples of genes that fall within this category. Catalytic GCLC subunits are also included. In addition, propolis can boost collagen formation and cell survival in cells exposed to high levels of oxidative stress. Propolis and some of its active components were shown to have a considerable cytostatic impact [11–15] and an anticarcinogenic and antitumor effect [11–15] in both in vitro and in vivo tumor models. This was demonstrated through the use of multiple tumor models. As possible anticancer and anti-inflammatory drugs, honeybee propolis and its contents have shown the most promise [3, 4, 11–16]. These ingredients include CA, CAPE, artepilin C, quercetin, naringenin, resveratrol, galangin, and genistein. It has also been proven to have anti-inflammatory properties. Implementing this technique offers a way for the treatment of cancer and the treatment of a wide range of diseases related to oxidative stress and inflammation, including allergy disorders.

17.4 Nasal Obstruction, Congestion, and Propolis

Suppose the nasal mucosa of the respiratory tract is harmed during a nasal surgical operation, and the mucosa does not recover usually. In that case, revision surgery may be required. In the process of wound healing, which is a highly complex, coordinated, and multi-stage system process, the formation of a clot, an inflammatory reaction, an immune response, and the remodeling and maturation of tissue are all components that are included. Several endogenous and exogenous factors, such as infection, food, systemic parameters, and surgical technique, impacted this process [17, 18]. Patients can recover from nasal surgery more quickly and reduce the number of times they need revision surgery when they receive postoperative care delivered appropriately following the procedure. Within the corpus of research conducted on this subject, a method of treatment considered to be standard has yet to be developed [19].

It has been hypothesized that removing scabs and secretions by using nasal saline irrigation and wound debridement can avoid the formation of scars that would otherwise be present [20]. Following the completion of endonasal treatments, it is common practice to apply topical steroids due to their local anti-inflammatory benefits. Even though the administration of systemic steroids during the postoperative period results in a significantly improved appearance on endoscopic examination, the utilization of these steroids is controversial because they have the potential to cause adverse effects and can only provide a moderate level of relief to the symptoms that the patient is experiencing [19]. Because steroids are used after endonasal treatments due to the anti-inflammatory features that they possess, the idea that a variety of anti-inflammatory medications can be employed for this purpose has evolved. This is because steroids are used after endonasal treatments. Propolis, a traditional medicinal ingredient, has been utilized extensively in treating burns and wounds because of its effectiveness. Several studies have shown that it possesses antibacterial, anti-inflammatory, and antioxidant effects [21]. Propolis has been the subject of a substantial number of studies that have been published in the scientific literature [17, 22, 23]. These studies have focused on the therapeutic benefits of using propolis in treating skin wounds, burns, ulcers, intra-abdominal adhesions, and oral cavity lesions. Propolis can be applied topically or when it is administered systemically.

Justifications for endoscopic nasal surgery include chronic rhinosinusitis, nasal polyposis, tumors in the paranasal region, septal deviation, turbinate surgery, hypophysis tumors, cerebrospinal fluid rhinorrhea, and encephalocele therapy. These are by far the most prevalent justifications for endoscopic nasal surgery. The time it takes for the patient to recover and the number of times they require revision surgery is reduced when postoperative care is delivered appropriately [19]. The administration of antibiotics, local wound debridement, systemic and topical steroids, and nasal saline irrigation techniques are all options that might be considered during the initial stages of postoperative care. Because steroids are used after endonasal treatments due to the anti-inflammatory features that they possess, the idea that a variety of anti-inflammatory medications can be employed for this purpose has evolved. This is because steroids are used after endonasal treatments. Propolis has been used to treat burns and wounds for a long time [21]. This is because it possesses antibacterial, anti-inflammatory, and antioxidant capabilities.

Kavaz and colleagues [17] conducted a study to determine whether propolis had a good impact on the healing process of wounds. Specifically, the researchers wanted to discover whether propolis could reduce inflammation in the nasal mucosa and speed up the process of epithelial closure [17]. Honeybees are the people responsible for gathering propolis, which is a substance that resembles resin. Enzymes produced by bees are necessary for the modification of propolis [24]. It has been hypothesized that honeybees make use of propolis for a variety of reasons, including but not limited to the following: repairing fractures and rips in the hive; preventing the putrefaction of foreign insects that die inside the hive; preserving the warmth of the interior of the hive; and preventing contamination [24]. There have been prior studies that have demonstrated the therapeutic effects of using propolis in the treatment of inflammation-induced arthritis, peritonitis, and pleurisy, as well as in the healing process of fractures, surgical anastomotic lines, and skin and mucosal injuries [22, 25, 26]. Propolis has also been shown to be effective in the treatment of pleurisy.

Propolis has the potential to be utilized in both systemic and local applications. Kilicoglu et al. [27] conducted a study on the effects of systemic propolis on the healing process in the anastomotic zone following colon resection. Both of these effects were investigated. It was proven that propolis offered an early start to angiogenesis, increased and regular collagen production, and quick epithelium regeneration, all of which significantly accelerated wound healing at the surgical site by using propolis. This was in addition to the fact that it possessed beneficial qualities in reducing inflammation.

Propolis was discovered to have a good effect on the healing process according to the findings of an experiment that was carried out by Iyyam Pillai and colleagues [22]. The experiment involved the generation of skin wounds in rats. The effects of this substance were equivalent to those of nitrofurazone, a common medication for treating wounds on the skin. Research was carried out by Temiz and colleagues [25] to investigate the healing process that occurs in the anastomosis zone after resection. In the course of their inquiry, they utilized both local and systemic propolis solutions. During the healing phase of wounds in the anastomosis region, it was discovered that using propolis in both a systemic and local environment positively impacted the healing process. As a result of the findings of the research that came before.

We decided to adopt oral administration for our research because it was the most straightforward method. El-Anwar et al. [28] conducted a study comparable to this one. They wound the nasal mucosa of rats and then fed them oral propolis for 15 days. The researchers discovered that propolis had an anti-inflammatory impact.

References

1. Archer SM. Turbinate dysfunction. In: Meyers AD, editor. Medscape. Updated: Jun 24, 2021. https://emedicine.medscape.com/article/877872-overview#a8. Accessed online at December 10, 2023.
2. Salzano FA, Mora R, Penco S, Traverso D, Gaggero G, Salzano G, et al. Nasal tactile sensitivity in allergic rhinitis. Acta Otolaryngol. 2011;131(6):640–4.
3. Ahangari Z, Naseri M, Vatandoost F. Propolis: chemical composition and its applications in endodontics. Iran Endod J. 2018;13:285–92.
4. Sena-Lopes Â, Bezerra FSB, Das Neves RN, De Pinho RB, Silva MTO, Savegnago L, Collares T, Seixas F, Begnini K, Henriques JAP, et al. Chemical composition, immunostimulatory, cytotoxic and antiparasitic activities of the essential oil from Brazilian red propolis. PLoS One. 2018;13:e0191797.
5. Popova M, Giannopoulou E, Skalicka-Woźniak K, Graikou K, Widelski J, Bankova V, Kalofonos H, Sivolapenko G, Gaweł-Bęben K, Antosiewicz B, et al. Characterization and biological evaluation of propolis from Poland. Molecules. 2017;22:1159.

6. Huang S, Zhang C-P, Wang K, Li G, Hu F-L. Recent advances in the chemical composition of propolis. Molecules. 2014;19:19610–32.
7. Shahinozzaman M, Obanda DN, Tawata S. Chemical composition and pharmacological properties of Macaranga-type Pacific propolis: a review. Phytother Res. 2021;35:207–22.
8. Toreti VC, Sato HH, Pastore GM, Park YK. Recent progress of propolis for its biological and chemical compositions and its botanical origin. Evid Based Complement Alternat Med. 2013;2013:697390.
9. Oršolić N. Allergic inflammation: effect of propolis and its flavonoids. Molecules. 2022;27(19):6694. https://doi.org/10.3390/molecules27196694. Published 2022 Oct 8.
10. Martinotti S, Ranzato E. Propolis: a new frontier for wound healing? Burn Trauma. 2015;3:9.
11. Oršolić N, Bašić I. Cancer chemoprevention by propolis and its polyphenolic compounds in experimental animals. In: Singh VK, Govil JN, Arunachalam C, editors. Recent progress in medicinal plants. Houston: Studium Press LLC.; 2007. p. 55–113.
12. Oršolić N, Jazvinšćak Jembrek M. Molecular and cellular mechanisms of propolis and its polyphenolic compounds against cancer. Int J Mol Sci. 2022;23:10479.
13. Oršolić N, Kunštić M, Kukolj M, Gračan R, Nemrava J. Oxidative stress, polarization of macrophages and tumour angiogenesis: efficacy of caffeic acid. Chem Biol Interact. 2016;256:111–24.
14. Ančić D, Oršolić N, Odeh D, Tomašević M, Pepić I, Ramić S. Resveratrol and its nanocrystals: a promising approach for cancer therapy? Toxicol Appl Pharmacol. 2022;435:115851.
15. Oršolić N, Odeh D, Jembrek MJ, Knežević J, Kučan D. Interactions between cisplatin and quercetin at physiological and hyperthermic conditions on cancer cells in vitro and in vivo. Molecules. 2020;25:3271.
16. Nyman GSA, Tang M, Inerot A, Osmancevic A, Malmberg P, Hagvall L. Contact allergy to beeswax and propolis among patients with cheilitis or facial dermatitis. Contact Dermat. 2019;81:110–6.
17. Kavaz E, Kurnaz SÇ, Güvenç D, Yarım M, Aksoy A. Effects of oral propolis on mucosal wound healing after endoscopic nasal surgery in a rabbit model. Turk Arch Otorhinolaryngol. 2019;57(2):68–74. https://doi.org/10.5152/tao.2019.4164.
18. Watelet JB, Bachert C, Gevaert P, Van Cauwenberge P. Wound healing of the nasal and paranasal mucosa: a review. Am J Rhinol. 2002;16:77–84.
19. Rudmik L, Soler ZM, Orlandi RR, Stewart MG, Bhattacharyya N, Kennedy DW, et al. Early postoperative care following endoscopic sinus surgery: an evidence-based review with recommendations. Int Forum Allergy Rhinol. 2011;1:417–30.
20. Patel ZM, Govindaraj S. The prevention and management of complications in ethmoid sinus surgery. Otolaryngol Clin N Am. 2010;43:855–64.
21. Kumazawa S, Hamasaka T, Nakayama T. Antioxidant activity of propolis of various geographic origins. Food Chem. 2004;84:329–39.
22. Iyyam Pillai S, Palsamy P, Subramanian S, Kandaswamy M. Wound healing properties of Indian propolis studied on excision wound-induced rats. Pharm Biol. 2010;48:1198–206.
23. de Groot AC. Propolis: a review of properties, applications, chemical composition, contact allergy, and other adverse effects. Dermatitis. 2013;24:263–82.
24. Sforcin JM. Propolis and the immune system: a review. J Ethnopharmacol. 2007;113:1–14.
25. Temiz M, Aslan A, Canbolant E, Hakverdi S, Polat G, Uzun S, et al. Effect of propolis on healing in experimental colon anastomosis in rats. Adv Ther. 2008;25:159–67.
26. Hu F, Hepburn HR, Li Y, Chen M, Radloff SE, Daya S. Effects of ethanol and water extracts of propolis (bee glue) on acute inflammatory animal models. J Ethnopharmacol. 2005;100:276–83.
27. Kilicoglu SS, Kilicoglu B, Erdemli E. Ultrastructural view of colon anastomosis under propolis effect by transmission electron microscopy. World J Gastroenterol. 2008;14:4763–70.
28. El-Anwar MW, Abdelmonem S, Abdelsameea AA, AlShawadfy M, El-Kashishy K. The effect of propolis in healing injured nasal mucosa: an experimental study. Int Arch Otorhinolaryngol. 2016;20:222–5.

Effect of Propolis on Allergic Rhinitis 18

18.1 Introduction

Propolis not only possesses antiviral and antibacterial activities, but it also seems to regulate the immunological responses of the hosts in connection to respiratory tract diseases. Propolis and its bioactive component 3,4-dicaffeoylquinic acid stimulate the production of tumor necrosis factor-related apoptosis-inducing ligand (TRAIL), which improves the elimination of the influenza A virus in infected mice [1, 2]. Takeshita et al. [3] showed that propolis can lessen the severity of the sickness caused by tetrabromobisphenol-A in mice infected with RSV. This is achieved by considerably decreasing viral titers and producing interferon-γ (IFN-γ), TNF-α, and IL-6 [3]. Propolis enhances the expression of myxovirus resistance-1 (MX1) and reduces the expression of IFN-β in a model involving the transfection or viral infection of double-stranded RNA [4].

Furthermore, propolis has been demonstrated to stimulate the growth of lymphocytes and increase the concentration of antibodies in the blood after hens are given an avian influenza vaccination [5]. Propolis can increase the reproduction of lymphocytes, the level of antibodies, and the concentration of IgG and IgM in animals with weakened immune systems after being given a vaccine [6]. The positive impact of propolis as an additional treatment in this regard has also been demonstrated in at least two human clinical studies. Permatasari and Hasan [7] showed that propolis enhanced the expression of IFN-γ and the activity of superoxide dismutase (SOD) in patients with multiple-drug resistant (MDR) tuberculosis who were undergoing treatment with anti-MDR-TB drugs. In contrast, the control group experienced a decrease in both of these parameters throughout the study [7]. Furthermore, a survey conducted by Mahani et al. [8] showed that adding propolis to the treatment of tuberculosis (TB) patients resulted in faster effectiveness of anti-TB medications and improved weight gain [1, 8].

A. E. Tanuğur Samanci et al., *Propolis: Prevention and Healing Effects in Otorhinolaryngology*, Comprehensive ENT,
https://doi.org/10.1007/978-3-031-68546-0_18

Propolis can hinder the adhesion of viral or bacterial infections by disrupting the proteins necessary for the pathogens' attachment and penetration into the host cells. Propolis can bind with the host's surface proteins and hinder the interaction between pathogens and the host cells. Furthermore, propolis possesses immunomodulatory properties that help the hosts effectively combat pathogenic infections and their associated pathophysiology. This is achieved by increasing the expression of tumor necrosis factor-related apoptosis-inducing ligand (TRAIL) and myxovirus resistance-1 (MX1), which in turn enhance the elimination of the pathogens. Propolis can increase the reproduction of lymphocytes and promote the function of antioxidant enzymes like supermutase dismutase (SOD). Additionally, it can reduce inflammation by decreasing the expression of TNF-α and IL-6 [1].

18.2 Allergic Inflammation

Allergic inflammation is a type of inflammation that occurs as a result of an allergic reaction. The immune system is a sophisticated network of organs and cells that play a crucial role in preserving the body's internal balance by defending against dangerous microbes and internally developed abnormal cells, such as virus-infected or cancerous cells. Protection against infectious illnesses comprises generic and specialized elements [9, 10]. The adaptive immune response is crucial for maintaining normal health since it offers targeted defense against bacterial, viral, parasitic, and fungal infections. Effector cells of the immune system often eliminate antigens that trigger an inflammatory response, avoiding inflammatory reactions and tissue harm under normal physiological circumstances. Prolonged unregulated inflammation can lead to tissue damage or cellular demise [9].

Inflammation is a reactive reaction to many stimuli and circumstances, such as infection, tissue injury, and cellular stress or dysfunction. The primary attributes of the local inflammatory response are dolor (pain), calor (heat), rubor (redness), tumor (swelling), and function laksa (loss of function). Systemic inflammation can arise in several settings, including severe trauma, chronic illness, or as a reaction to an infection, in which case it is referred to as sepsis [11].

Controlled physiological inflammation is a beneficial and adaptive response that helps defend against infection, promote tissue healing, and facilitate adaptation to stress or the development of "disturbed" homeostasis. However, in the absence of regulation, it can have detrimental effects and present as tissue damage, septic shock, autoimmunity, fibrosis, metaplasia, or disruption of homeostasis, leading to chronic autoinflammatory disorders. Inflammation most likely developed as an adaptive reaction to preserve homeostasis, regardless of origin. The numerous pathological and clinical burdens associated with allergic illness result from the prolonged effects of chronic allergic inflammation at locations with continuous or repeated contact with allergens [12].

An allergy is an exaggerated immune response that occurs when our body is exposed to an antigen for a second time. This immunological response can lead to tissue damage and can result in severe illness. Hypersensitive, also known as hypersensitive reaction or intolerance, refers to an undesired response of the immune system, encompassing allergies and autoimmunity. Allergic responses result in pruritus, discomfort, and the enlargement of body tissues (edema) [13]. Allergic illnesses have the potential to significantly impact the essential functioning of the body and result in psychological issues in patients. They also have a detrimental effect on the patient's quality of life and the broader community. Additionally, allergic diseases can impose a substantial economic cost.

Gell and Coombs divided hypersensitivity responses into four kinds. In summary, the production of IgE antibodies mediates Type 1 hypersensitivity reaction. The reaction frequently manifests as an acute allergic response to food and pollen, medications, bug stings, or severe anaphylactic reactions in those who have already encountered the related allergen. Aside from IgE antibodies, the response is distinguished by mast cell hypersensitivity, helper CD4 T cells (Th2) stimulation, and attraction of eosinophils. Type II hypersensitivity reactions are immune responses that destroy specific tissues in the body. These reactions involve the production of IgM and IgG antibodies that target and attack cells in these tissues. Examples of type II hypersensitivity reactions include autoimmune hemolytic anemia, Hashimoto's thyroiditis, Goodpasture syndrome, and erythrocyte transfusion reactions. The outcome of this response is phagocytosis, namely the stimulation of cytotoxic cells or cell destruction facilitated by complement activation. The complement system activation leads to opsonization, the clumping of red blood cells, cell lysis, and cell death. Type III hypersensitivity reactions are characterized by the involvement of immune complexes, which lead to tissue damage by the deposition of antigen–antibody complexes. Examples of conditions associated with this type of reactions include vasculitides and glomerulonephritis. Activated neutrophils and medium-sized immunocomplexes are crucial in causing damage to blood vessels in many tissues, including the kidneys, heart, arteries, and joints. Type IV hypersensitivity reactions, such as skin tests for tuberculosis and contact dermatitis, are delayed reactions that often occur more than 72 hours after exposure to the allergen. These reactions are caused by sensitized T cells and macrophages. Unlike accurate hypersensitivity responses that happen after sensitization, nonallergic hypersensitivity reactions (also known as pseudoallergies) lead to the activation of mast cells and the release of histamine at the first exposure to a triggering chemical (such as radiocontrast medium) [14].

18.3 Propolis

Propolis and its constituents play a crucial role in safeguarding health, as well as in the prevention and treatment of minor ailments. Propolis is a vital component of (bio)cosmetics and is used as a natural antibiotic for treating ear, throat, and nose infections. Propolis has many applications in several industries, including the food sector, medicine (as an immunomodulator for healing wounds and burns), cosmetics, and hygiene goods. Although propolis has beneficial characteristics, extensive research has shown that it can trigger allergic responses in those susceptible to its components. Multiple patch test investigations have demonstrated varying response levels to propolis and its constituents. European studies have shown a prevalence of propolis sensitivity ranging from 1.2% to 6.6%. In Finland, the prevalence was 0.5% to 1.4% in adults and 2% to 13.7% in children. In Poland, the prevalence was 16.5% in children and 5.4% in young people [15]. Research conducted in Prague reported a prevalence of 4%. The documented allergic responses included contact cheilitis, stomatitis, perioral eczema, labial edema, oral discomfort, peeling of lips, and dyspnea. Several allergens have been identified in propolis, including 3-methyl-2-butenyl caffeate, phenylethyl caffeate, and benzyl caffeate [9].

The compounds present are geranyl caffeate, benzyl alcohol, benzyl cinnamate, methyl cinnamate, ferulic acid, and tectochrysin. Furthermore, propolis has been identified as a common cause of contact sensitivity and should be routinely tested for in children and adolescents before giving it [9].

Propolis consists of around 30 pieces. The elements calcium, manganese, zinc, copper, silicon, iron, and aluminum are found in the highest concentrations, ranging from 16 to 18. Propolis contains various vitamins, such as B vitamins, vitamins C, D, P, and E, and provitamin A (β-carotene). Propolis contains a variety of enzymes, including _amylase, _amylase, _lactamase, _lactamase, maltase, esterase, and transhydrogenase, in addition to vitamins [18]. The enzymes found in propolis originate from the glands of bees, with a portion of them also derived from pollen [16–18]. The typical protein content in EEP is around 2.8% [16–21], with a low concentration of free amino acids. EEP contains around 17 different amino acids [16–21].

Pyroglutamic acid, an amino acid, was identified in bees. Propolis contains a variety of carbohydrates, including polysaccharides, disaccharides, and monosaccharides. These include sucrose, glucose, fructose, rhamnose, ribose, talose, and gulose [16–21]. Propolis can vary in types according to where it comes from and when it is collected. Although there is a wide range of diversity, most studies identify at least six primary chemical types of propolis. These include (1) propolis found in Europe, North America, and non-tropical regions of Asia, which primarily comes from the poplar tree (Populus spp., most commonly *P. nigra*); (2) propolis found in Russia, where the dominant source is the birch tree (Betula verrucosa Ehrh.); (3) green propolis found in Brazil, mainly derived from Baccharis spp., with a predominant species being B. There are several types of propolis found in different regions. One type, called dracunculifolia DC., is found in Brazil. Another type, red propolis, is found in Cuba and Venezuela and comes from Clusia spp. plants. There is also a type called "Pacific" propolis, found in Okinawa and Taiwan, but its plant source has yet to be identified. Lastly, there is "Canary" propolis, which comes from the Canary Islands. The resinous exudates of the buds of poplar trees, known as "poplar propolis," have a consistent chemical makeup. The primary components of poplar propolis are phenolic and comprise flavonoid aglycones, aromatic acids, and their esters. Brazilian green propolis, or Alecrim propolis, is distinguished by prenylated derivatives of p-coumaric acid and o-hydroxy-acetophenone [18]. The chemical components found in Brazilian propolis are not found in propolis from other areas. European and non-European propolis differ regarding their flavonoid components, diterpenes, and lignans. The composition of Brazilian green propolis is characterized by elevated levels of artepillin C (20.7%), bacharrin (7.5%), and kaempferide (3.6%). Clusia nemorosa, a member of the Clusiaceae family, is the primary plant species that produces red propolis in Cuba. In Venezuela, bees predominantly gather propolis from Clusia scrobiculata. Cuban propolis has distinct characteristics compared to both European and Brazilian propolis, and it contains a high concentration of polyprenylated benzophenones. Geranyl flavanones are the distinctive chemicals discovered in propolis produced in the Pacific and African regions [16, 18].

Despite its botanical origin and chemical makeup, propolis consistently exhibits antimicrobial, antioxidant, immunomodulatory, anti-inflammatory, antiallergic, dermato-protective, laxative, antidiabetic, antiangiogenic, and anticancer properties. The antibacterial properties of propolis are ascribed to the existence of flavonoids, including pinocembrin, galangin, pinobanksin, pinobanksin-3-acetate, and caffeic acid ester. Propolis that exhibits potent antioxidant action comprises bioactive components like kaempferol, caffeic acid (CA), and phenethyl caffeate. The anti-inflammatory effects can be attributed to the presence of potent flavonoids such as quercetin, acacetin, and naringenin, as well as cinnamic acid derivatives, including baccharin, drupanin, and caffeic acid phenethyl ester (CAPE). CAPE, a prominent temperate propolis component, possesses many biological properties, including the suppression of nuclear factor _B (NF-_B), the prevention of cellular growth, and the triggering of cell cycle arrest and programmed cell death (apoptosis). The concentration of bioactive compounds in propolis might vary significantly depending on its origin, such as Brazilian, Cuban, or Mexican propolis. These composition variations can impact propolis' biological effects [9].

18.4 Propolis in Allergic Rhinitis

Evidence shows that propolis and its related chemicals, including CAPE, pinocembrin, and chrysin, have efficacy against IgE-mediated allergy in both systemic and local anaphylaxis animal models. Propolis and its bioactive compounds decrease the amount of histamine in the blood by reducing the activity of the histamine H-1 receptor and the release of histamine from mast cells. They also inhibit the activation of NF-κB, the release of platelet-activating factor and cys-leukotrienes, and the expression of TNF-α, IL-1β, and Th2-related cytokines: IL-4, IL-5, IL-6, IL-13. As a result, the IgE antibody reaction is significantly reduced [22–27]. The presentation of allergic symptoms, such as itching, nasal rubbing, sneezing, and watery rhinorrhea, in animal models is significantly reduced when the levels of allergy-related components, pro-inflammatory cytokines, and IgE antibody response are decreased [1, 22, 23, 27].

Allergic rhinitis has a complex pathogenesis. However, it is often initiated by allergen-induced IgE complexes that activate mast cells to produce mediators such as histamine, leukotrienes, and prostaglandins by degranulation. The subsequent release of these mediators leads to the development and activity of inflammatory cytokines and chemokines, ultimately causing allergic rhinitis [28]. Studies have demonstrated that propolis can prevent the release of histamine and block the activity of the histamine receptor H1R. Propolis also inhibits the activation of inflammatory cytokines, including TNF-α, IL-1β, IL-4, IL-6, IL-9, and NF-kB, decreasing the frequency and intensity of allergy symptoms [1].

A comprehensive analysis identified 11 research studies, of which 7 documented adverse effects linked to propolis in treating respiratory tract-related disorders. In a study conducted by Lin et al. [29], a case was reported in which the prolonged inhalation of liquid propolis led to the development of a tumor-like growth in the patient's lungs [29]. In a study conducted by Wu and Hsu [30], a middle-aged woman developed aspiration pneumonia and descending mediastinitis as a result of using a propolis solution for allergy therapy. Menniti-Ippolito et al. [31] undertook surveillance research to evaluate the effectiveness of different types of propolis in treating allergic responses. They documented cases of sudden-onset asthma as a concomitant negative outcome associated with the utilization of propolis [31].

Furthermore, Lobsiger et al. documented a case in 2012 when an older female patient experienced an allergic response that mainly involved the activation of T-cells. This occurrence was recorded after treatment with a propolis solution [32]. Basista and Filipek [33] conducted a questionnaire survey in Poland, finding that between 3.5 and 7.6% of beekeepers experienced allergic responses to propolis. These responses manifested clinically as atopic dermatitis, allergic rhinitis, eczema, and other similar conditions [33]. Zhang and Yan [34] conducted a case study where propolis throat candies were used to treat contact stomatitis caused by allergic responses in the patient [1, 34].

Middleton et al. [35] showed that quercetin effectively suppressed the histamine release from basophils triggered by ragweed antigens. This inhibition occurred in a concentration-dependent manner, with concentrations ranging from 5 to 50 μM. At the highest concentration tested (50 _M), quercetin achieved a remarkable inhibition rate of 80 to 100%. Quercetin significantly suppressed the activation of basophils in the first stage of histamine release, which is not reliant on calcium. Also, it inhibited the second stage, which is unrelated to the antigen and depends on calcium. Based on the information provided, it can be inferred that quercetin does not impact the release of histamine in unstimulated cells. However, it does have an inhibitory effect on histamine release during or after antigen activation. Therefore, it can be concluded that quercetin affects a basophil process that is activated due to antigen activation. Thus, quercetin impacts the calcium channel in an "opened" state. Quercetin is highly secure when used in the treatment of allergic rhinitis. Quercetin possesses several other advantages, such as its antioxidant, anti-inflammatory, and capillary stabilizing properties. Moreover, it exerts a potent inhibitory effect on basophil and mast cell degranulation, as evidenced by studies [36–39]. Basophils have a role in immunological responses.

When mast cells are sensitized by IgE antibodies connected to their cell surface, they forcefully release their granules when exposed to the allergen again. Degranulation necessitates energy and a surge of calcium (Ca2+), leading to the simultaneous discharge of histamine, adenosine triphosphate, and other stored mediators from the granules. During degranulation, mast cells utilize calcium-activated enzymes to construct contractile microtubules. These microtubules then exert force to move the granules toward the cell membrane. As a result, the inflammatory substances contained inside the granules are released outside the cell, triggering an allergic response [35–41]. Quercetin inhibits mast cell degranulation, hence blocking the influx of Ca2+ into the cells. Phospholipase A2 facilitates the release of secondary mediators of inflammation, such as arachidonic acid metabolites, from the cell. Steroids are recognized for their role as anti-inflammatory medicines because they can inhibit phospholipase A2. Quercetin can hinder many stages of the eicosanoid membrane pathway, such as phospholipase A2 and lipoxygenase. Multiple authors have confirmed that quercetin possesses various beneficial effects, including (1) the ability to inhibit mast cell degranulation; (2) the reduction of airway hyperreactivity; (3) the reduction of mucus and collagen production; (4) the reduction of eosinophil and neutrophil recruitment; (5) the reduction of bronchial epithelial cell activation and the expression of MMP-9 and MMP-12; (6) the modulation of Th1/Th2 cytokine production; (7) the demonstration of anti-fibrotic activities; (8) the reduction of collagen deposition by inducing HO-1 upregulation; (9) the decrease in the production of IL-4, IL-5, CCL11, and LTB4, and the increase in IL-4 and IFN- concentration; (10) the decrease in the synthesis of type I and type III collagen; and (11) the downmodulation of P-selectin expression by blocking NF-kB signaling. These effects might be linked to reducing the PI3-kinase, Akt, and NF-kB signaling pathways. Reports indicate that the combination of quercetin and vitamin C can decrease symptoms associated with hay fever [9, 38, 42].

Studies have demonstrated that flavonoids can inhibit enzymes, including cAMP phosphodiesterase and calcium-dependent ATPase, which are responsible for increasing histamine release from mast cells and basophils. Cyclic adenosine monophosphate (cAMP) phosphodiesterase breaks down cAMP; high levels of cAMP prevent the release of histamine from intracellular storage. In addition, calcium-dependent ATPase hydrolyzes ATP to generate energy and assist the transport of Ca2+ across the cell membrane. Elevated levels of intracellular Ca2+ also trigger the release of histamine from cellular storage granules. Quercetin exhibits a high attraction toward mast cells and basophils. It can stabilize membranes and block the release of histamine. Additionally, it can inhibit two enzymes that control the release of leukotrienes, which are known to be involved in asthmatic-type responses [35, 36, 39, 41–44]. Quercetin inhibits allergy symptoms, such as enlarged nasal passages, congestion, sneezing, watery eyes, and irritation in the eyes and nose, by blocking the release of histamines and leukotrienes into the circulation [9].

The antiallergic action of flavonoids, such as luteolin, quercetin, and baicalein, is based on their structure and ability to inhibit various enzymes and processes involved in allergic immune responses. These flavonoids can inhibit enzymes such as hexosaminidase, phospholipase A2, and 5-lipoxygenase, which are critical players in the degranulation process of mast cells. They can also inhibit ATPase, which is responsible for mast cells' histamine secretion. Additionally, flavonoids can inhibit the activation of human basophils by allergens. Furthermore, they can suppress the synthesis and secretion of cytokines such as IL-4, IL-13, CD40 ligand, GM-CSF, IL-6, and TNF, essential for differentiating B cells into IgE-producing cells. Currently, the specific processes via which flavonoids hinder the production and release of histamine in response to the binding of the high-affinity IgE receptor (Fc″RI) are not well understood and require more investigation. Several studies [39, 40, 42, 44–46] have found that flavonoids possess antioxidant and antiallergic qualities that can effectively hinder the production and release of several allergic mediators. These include Th2-type cytokines such as IL-4 and IL-13, as well as the expression of CD40.

IgE is a crucial molecule involved in many interactions between cells. Certain types of cells, such as mast cells and basophils, have a high-affinity immunoglobulin E (IgE) receptor, which, when activated, causes an inflammatory response. B cells require two signals to generate IgE. The initial signal is triggered by the cytokines IL-4 and IL-13. The second signal comes when CD40L, produced on T cells' surface upon exposure to allergens, attaches to CD40 on the surface of B cells. The link between CD40 and CD40L is essential for activating and induction isotype switching in B cells. Upon meeting an allergen, T cells exhibit the expression of CD40L and subsequently interact with CD40 on B cells, monocytes, dendritic cells, and epithelial cells. Polyphenols and flavonoid chemicals modulate the Th1/Th2 equilibrium and hinder the development of antigen-specific IgE antibodies by impacting the synthesis of allergen-IgE complexes and their interaction with receptors (Fc″RI) on mast cells and basophils. Tannins derived from apples can prevent food allergies by promoting an increase in intestine TCR T cells and Th2 cells.

The presence of intraepithelial lymphocytes [40, 46, 47] has been observed.

References

1. Zulhendri F, Perera CO, Tandean S, et al. The potential use of propolis as a primary or an adjunctive therapy in respiratory tract-related diseases and disorders: a systematic scoping review. Biomed Pharmacother. 2022;146:112595.
2. Kuwata K, Takemura T, Urushisaki T, Fukuoka M, Hosokawa-Muto J, Hata T, Okuda Y, Hori S, Tazawa S, Araki Y, Kuwata K. 3,4-dicaffeoylquinic acid, a major constituent of Brazilian propolis, increases TRAIL expression and extends the lifetimes of mice infected with the influenza a virus. Evid-Based Complement Altern Med. 2012;2012:946867. https://doi.org/10.1155/2012/946867.
3. Takeshita T, Watanabe W, Toyama S, Hayashi Y, Honda S, Sakamoto S, Matsuoka S, Yoshida H, Takeda S, Hidaka M, Tsutsumi S, Yasukawa K, Park YK, Kurokawa M. Effect of Brazilian propolis on exacerbation of respiratory syncytial virus infection in mice exposed to tetrabromobisphenol a, a brominated flame retardant. Evid-Based Complement Altern Med. 2013;2013:698206. https://doi.org/10.1155/2013/698206.
4. Hayakari R, Matsumiya T, Xing F, Tayone JCJC, Dempoya J, Tatsuta T, Aizawa-Yashiro T, Imaizumi T, Yoshida H, Satoh K. Effects of Brazilian green propolis on double-stranded RNA-mediated induction of interferon-inducible gene and inhibition of recruitment of polymorphonuclear cells. J Sci Food Agric. 2013;93:646–51. https://doi.org/10.1002/jsfa.5892.
5. Fan Y, Wang D, Liu J, Hu Y, Zhao X, Han G, Nguyen TL, Chang S. Adjuvanticity of epimedium polysaccharide-propolis flavone on inactivated vaccines against AI and ND virus. Int J Biol Macromol. 2012;51:1028–32. https://doi.org/10.1016/j.ijbiomac.2012.08.025.

6. Fan Y, Ma L, Zhang W, Xu Y, Suolangzhaxi ZX, Cui E, Song X. Microemulsion can improve the immune-enhancing activity of propolis flavonoid on immunosuppression and immune response. Int J Biol Macromol. 2014;63:126–32. https://doi.org/10.1016/j.ijbiomac.2013.09.039.
7. Permatasari A, Hasan H. The effect of ethanol extract propolis (EEP) on the level of IFN-F and superoxide dismutase (SOD) activities in patients with MDR tuberculosis. Respirol Conf. 2014:58.
8. Mahani A, Sulaeman A, Anwar F, Damanik MRM, Hardinsyah H, Ploeger A. Efficacy of propolis supplementation to accelerate healing process and body weight recovery of pulmonary tuberculosis patients. J GIZI DAN Pangan. 2018;13:1–10. https://doi.org/10.25182/jgp.2018.13.1.1-10.
9. Oršolić N. Allergic inflammation: effect of propolis and its flavonoids. Molecules. 2022;27(19):6694. https://doi.org/10.3390/molecules27196694. Published 2022 Oct 8.
10. Oršoli'c N, Baši'c I. Immunomodulation by water-soluble derivative of propolis: a factor of antitumor reactivity. J Ethnopharmacol. 2003;84:265–73.
11. Hartupee J, Mann DL. Role of inflammatory cells in fibroblast activation. JMCC. 2016;93:143–8.
12. Haque TT, Frischmeyer-Guerrerio PA. The role of TGF_ and other cytokines in regulating mast cell functions in allergic inflammation. Int J Mol Sci. 2022;23:10864.
13. Nyman GSA, Tang M, Inerot A, Osmancevic A, Malmberg P, Hagvall L. Contact allergy to beeswax and propolis among patients with cheilitis or facial dermatitis. Contact Dermat. 2019;81:110–6.
14. Global Asthma Network. The global asthma report 2018. Auckland: Global Asthma Network; 2018.
15. Suryakanth D, Basavaiah N. Propolis and allergic reactions. J Pharm Bioallied Sci. 2012;4:345.
16. Huang S, Zhang C-P, Wang K, Li G, Hu F-L. Recent advances in the chemical composition of propolis. Molecules. 2014;19:19610–32.
17. Shahinozzaman M, Obanda DN, Tawata S. Chemical composition and pharmacological properties of Macaranga-type Pacific propolis: a review. Phytother Res. 2021;35:207–22.
18. Toreti VC, Sato HH, Pastore GM, Park YK. Recent progress of propolis for its biological and chemical compositions and its botanical origin. Evid Based Complement Alternat Med. 2013;2013:697390.
19. Ahangari Z, Naseri M, Vatandoost F. Propolis: chemical composition and its applications in endodontics. Iran Endod J. 2018;13:285–92.
20. Sena-Lopes Â, Bezerra FSB, Das Neves RN, De Pinho RB, Silva MTO, Savegnago L, Collares T, Seixas F, Begnini K, Henriques JAP, et al. Chemical composition, immunostimulatory, cytotoxic and antiparasitic activities of the essential oil from Brazilian red propolis. PLoS One. 2018;13:e0191797.
21. Popova M, Giannopoulou E, Skalicka-Wo'zniak K, Graikou K, Widelski J, Bankova V, Kalofonos H, Sivolapenko G, Gaweł-Beben K, Antosiewicz B, et al. Characterization and biological evaluation of propolis from Poland. Molecules. 2017;22:1159.
22. Jung WK, Lee DY, Kim JH, Choi I, Park SG, Seo SK, Lee SW, Lee CM, Park YM, Jeon YJ, Lee CH, Jeon BT, Qian ZJ, Kim SK, Choi IW. Anti-inflammatory activity of caffeic acid phenethyl ester (CAPE) extracted from Rhodiola sacra against lipopolysaccharide-induced inflammatory responses in mice. Process Biochem. 2008;43:783–7. https://doi.org/10.1016/j.procbio.2008.03.004.
23. Shinmei Y, Yano H, Kagawa Y, Izawa K, Akagi M, Inoue T, Kamei C. Effect of Brazilian propolis on sneezing and nasal rubbing in experimental allergic rhinitis of mice. Immunopharmacol Immunotoxicol. 2009;31:688–93. https://doi.org/10.3109/08923970903078443.
24. Tani H, Hasumi K, Tatefuji T, Hashimoto K, Koshino H, Takahashi S. Inhibitory activity of Brazilian green propolis components and their derivatives on the release of cys-leukotrienes. Bioorg Med Chem. 2010;18:151–7. https://doi.org/10.1016/j.bmc.2009.11.007.
25. Bae Y, Lee S, Kim SHS-HH. Chrysin suppresses mast cell-mediated allergic inflammation: involvement of calcium, caspase-1 and nuclear factor-κB. Toxicol Appl Pharmacol. 2011;254:56–64. https://doi.org/10.1016/j.taap.2011.04.008.

26. Gu X, Zhang Q, Du Q, Shen H, Zhu Z. Pinocembrin attenuates allergic airway inflammation via inhibition of NF-κB pathway in mice. Int Immunopharmacol. 2017;53:90–5. https://doi.org/10.1016/j.intimp.2017.10.005.
27. Shaha A, Mizuguchi H, Kitamura Y, Fujino H, Yabumoto M, Takeda N, Fukui H. Effect of royal jelly and Brazilian green propolis on the signaling for histamine H1 receptor and interleukin-9 gene expressions responsible for the pathogenesis of the allergic rhinitis. Biol Pharm Bull. 2018;41:1440–7. https://doi.org/10.1248/bpb.b18-00325.
28. Bjermer L, Westman M, Holmström M, Wickman MC. The complex pathophysiology of allergic rhinitis: scientific rationale for the development of an alternative treatment option, allergy, asthma. Clin Immunol. 2019;15:24. https://doi.org/10.1186/s13223-018-0314-1.
29. Lin W-C, Tseng Y-T, Chang Y-L, Lee Y-C. Pulmonary tumour with high carcinoembryonic antigen titre caused by chronic propolis aspiration. Eur Respir J. 2007;30:1227–30. https://doi.org/10.1183/09031936.00141706.
30. Wu J-Y, Hsu N-Y. Propolis-induced descending necrotizing mediastinitis and aspiration pneumonia. Ann Thorac Surg. 2013;95:e87–9. https://doi.org/10.1016/j.athoracsur.2012.09.086.
31. Menniti-Ippolito F, Mazzanti G, Santuccio C, Moro PA, Calapai G, Firenzuoli F, Valeri A, Raschetti R. Surveillance of suspected adverse reactions to natural health products in Italy. Pharmacoepidemiol Drug Saf. 2008;17:626–35.
32. Lobsiger C, Borer-Reinhold M, Weiss M, Muller U, Helbling A. Allergy to propolis: behind the symptoms of an immediate-type reaction a T-cell sensitization may be hiding. Allergologie. 2012;35:209–13. https://doi.org/10.5414/ALX01451.
33. Basista KM, Filipek B. Allergy to propolis in Polish beekeepers. Post DERMATOLOGII I Alergol. 2012;29:440–5. https://doi.org/10.5114/pdia.2012.32391.
34. Zhang W, Yan Z. Allergic contact stomatitis caused by propolis throat candies. Contact Dermat. 2020;83:58–9. https://doi.org/10.1111/cod.13525.
35. Middleton E. Effect of plant flavonoids on immune and inflammatory cell function. Adv Exp Med Biol. 1998;439:75–182.
36. Oršoli'c N, Baši'c I. Polyphenols from propolis and plants in control of allergy and inflammation. Scientific evidence of the use of propolis in ethnomedicine. In: Oršoli'c N, Baši'c I, editors. Ethnopharmacology-review book. Trivandrum: Transworld Research Network; 2008. p. 311–36.
37. Oršoli'c N, Skuri'c J, Điki'c D, Stani'c G. Inhibitory effect of a propolis on Di-n-Propyl Disulfide or n-Hexyl salicilate-induced skin irritation, oxidative stress and inflammatory responses in mice. Fitoterapia. 2014;93:18–30.
38. Shaik Y, Caraffa A, Ronconi G, Lessiani G, Conti P. Impact of polyphenols on mast cells with special emphasis on the effect of quercetin and luteolin. Cent Eur J Immunol. 2018;43:476–81.
39. Weng Z, Zhang B, Asadi S, Sismanopoulos N, Butcher A, Fu X, Theoharides TC. Quercetin is more effective than cromolyn in blocking human mast cell cytokine release and inhibits contact dermatitis and photosensitivity in humans. PLoS One. 2012;7:e33805.
40. Kawai M, Hirano T, Higa S, Arimitsu J, Maruta M, Kuwahara Y, Tanaka T. Flavonoids and related compounds as anti-allergic substances. Allergology Int. 2007;56:113–23.
41. Guan Y, Shen H, Shen J, Jia Y, Dong X, Jin Y, Xie Q. Anti-allergic activities of 5,7-dimethoxy-3,4′-dihydroxyflavone via inhalation in rat allergic models. Eur J Pharmacol. 2019;848:55–61.
42. Mlcek J, Jurikova T, Skrovankova S, Sochor J. Quercetin and its anti-allergic immune response. Molecules. 2016;21:623.
43. Chitranshi N, Verma N, Saad S, Gupta G, Hansbro PM, Oliver BG, Madheswaran T, Dua K, Chellappan DK. Unravelling the therapeutic potential of nano-delivered functional foods in chronic respiratory diseases. Nutrients. 2022;14:3828.
44. Jafarinia M, Sadat HM, Kasiri N, Fazel N, Fathi F, Ganjalikhani HM, Eskandari N. Quercetin with the potential effect on allergic diseases. Allergy Asthma Clin Immunol. 2020;16:36.
45. Ding S, Jiang H, Fang J. Regulation of immune function by polyphenols. J Immunol Res. 2018;2018:1264074.

46. Park H-H, Lee S, Son H-Y, Park S-B, Kim M-S, Choi E-J, Kim S-H. Flavonoids inhibit histamine release and expression of proinflammatory cytokines in mast cells. Arch Pharm Res. 2008;31:1303–11.
47. Hirano T, Higa S, Arimitsu J, Naka T, Shima Y, Ohshima S, Tanaka T. Flavonoids such as luteolin, fisetin and apigenin are inhibitors of Interleukin-4 and interleukin-13 production by activated human basophils. Int Arch Allergy Immunol. 2004;134:135–40.

Effects of Propolis on Asthma

19

19.1 Introduction

Allergens are foreign substances to the body and trigger an inflammatory response through IgE-mediated pathways. Those genetically predisposed to atopic dermatitis, a condition in which even low levels of exposure to environmental triggers cause the production of IgE antibodies, are more likely to have sensitization than the general population. Variations in living standards and exposure to different germs and viruses may explain why allergic sensitization is lower in Eastern Europe than in the West [1]. The genesis and triggers of allergies have been associated with both genetic and environmental variables, such as air pollution, housing conditions, and other lifestyle factors [2]. According to Humbert et al. [3], who speculated that immunologic variables significantly impact both types of asthma, there are more parallels than differences between atopic and non-atopic asthma.

Recent studies have shown that diet significantly affects allergy sensitization, particularly the quantity and quality of dietary fat [4], which are staples in the average Western diet [5–7]. According to the hygiene hypothesis, lowering infectious stresses in early childhood leads to fewer allergies and longer life expectancy. Increased synthesis of allergen-specific IgE and eosinophilic inflammation are caused by the secretion of Th2 cytokines (IL-4, IL-5, and IL-13) either during the fetus' intrauterine life or in the early phase of the newborn's underdeveloped immune system postnatally. Conversely, viral infections—and maybe other intracellular organisms—influence Th1 response development by triggering the release of cytokines similar to Th1, such as IL-12 and IFN, and downregulating Th2 responses. Atopic sensitization and clinical illnesses, including asthma, allergic rhinitis, and eczema, are more common when people do not get enough exposure to germs and have a lower Th1 response, as demonstrated by the hygiene hypothesis. How microbial exposure is evolving, with the decrease.

A. E. Tanuğur Samanci et al., *Propolis: Prevention and Healing Effects in Otorhinolaryngology*, Comprehensive ENT,
https://doi.org/10.1007/978-3-031-68546-0_19

The immune system may take longer to mature in response to some viral illnesses, delaying the onset of well-balanced immunological responses [8].

19.2 Propolis

The flavonoids in propolis have a long history of usage in traditional medicine, exhibiting anti-inflammatory, antifungal, anticoagulant, antiretroviral, antiallergic, and anticancer properties. For a very long time, propolis has been utilized in folk medicine. Plaque aggregation, rat paw edema, adjuvant-induced arthritis, eicosanoid synthesis, cytokine production, and other mediators necessary for managing allergic illnesses are all inhibited by propolis, which is why it has an anti-inflammatory effect. The radioprotective properties of propolis help it ward off both UV radiation and DNA damage caused by gamma radiation. This is how propolis shields the skin from many harmful effects, including skin cancer [9, 10] and the signs of aging (wrinkles, scaling, dryness, dilated blood vessels, and collagen loss). Not only can propolis promote wound healing, but it also can trigger the creation of type I and III collagen, which aids in wound matrix breakdown as well. Propolis facilitates the proliferation, differentiation, and migration of human keratinocytes and includes many chemicals that hasten the skin's healing process, including increasing its tensile strength and flexibility. Wound healing may benefit from these characteristics and metabolic alterations in propolis, which may encourage re-epithelization. Notably, there are several benefits to using propolis as a dressing for wound healing, including its low cost, safety, and absence of discomfort during application. It also helps avoid infections, promotes rapid wound healing, requires few dressing changes during recovery, and does not develop scar tissue. There has been a new "back to nature" trend among modern people, and they are looking for medical natural goods, especially those made from plants and bees, that may help with inflammation and allergies. Clinical and laboratory studies on phytochemicals, propolis, and the flavonoids and other antioxidants they contain have shown promise in treating and preventing various disorders, including allergies. In this review, we will go over what is currently known about the effects of propolis' polyphenolic and flavonoid components on the management of allergy diseases and potential antiallergic reaction mechanisms, as well as the mechanisms by which these components generate sensitivities and inflammation [8].

Bees gather a resin-like substance called propolis from the buds of different plants. They utilize this substance to plug cracks in honeycombs, smooth down the inside walls, guard the entrance of their hive against invaders, and even defend themselves from diseases. By inhibiting the growth of germs on the hive walls, sealing the walls from external moisture, and restricting uncontrolled airflow into the nest, propolis also helps with better maintenance of the homeostasis of the nest environment. Raw propolis, also known as propolis in nature, is made when beeswax is combined with the materials that have been gathered and the enzyme, glycosidase, which is found in bees' saliva.

Half of the raw propolis is plant resins, a third is waxed, 10% is essential and aromatic oils, 5% is pollen, and 5% is other organic substances like niacin, folate, and various micro and macro minerals. The remaining 5% comprises various vitamins and other organic compounds. Around 500 different components are found in propolis, originating from various parts of the world. These include phenolic acids, flavonoids (including chalcones, dihydroflavonols, and flavones), terpenes, lignans, amino acids, fatty acids, vitamins, and minerals [11–16].

The variety of propolis' chemical properties is correlated with the variety of its plant sources, bee species, and geographical locations. Several articles have provided a synopsis of the chemical makeup of propolis, broken down by region, botanical source, and species of bee [11–16]. With varying percentages of confirmation, the following chemical components of propolis have been identified: fatty and aliphatic acids (24–26%), sugars (15–18%), aromatic acids (5–10%), esters (2–6%), vitamins (2–4%), alcohol and terpenes (2–3.3%), microelements (0.5–2.0%), and others (21–27%) [8, 14–16].

19.3 Allergy and Immunology

As a broad concept, "sensitivity" can encompass anything from actual allergies to reactions that do not impact the immune system (and so are not considered allergies) to reactions for which the underlying cause is unknown. The degree to which an allergen can trigger a Th2-cell response—the synthesis of IgE by B cells through the promotion of immunoglobulin class-switch recombination—is a measure of the allergen's sensitivity. Host genotype, allergen type, environmental allergen concentration, exposure route, presence of other agents that may enhance sensitization, and myeloid and plasmacytoid DC subpopulation characteristics all influence the likelihood of developing clinically significant sensitization. Some forms of sensitivity that aren't allergic are known as intolerances, and they can be brought on by chemicals in food, water, medicine, cosmetics, perfumes, fabrics, construction materials, and plastics; enzyme deficiencies; drug-like chemical reactions; to psychological associations; and poisons. To give just two examples of intolerances, there is lactose intolerance, which occurs when the digestive enzyme lactase is not present, and there is phenylketonuria, which is a metabolic condition that runs in families and is caused by a lack of the enzyme, phenylalanine hydroxylase in the liver. It takes a lot of time, effort, and the assistance of many specialists to pinpoint food allergies and other sensitivities [8].

One category of food allergies is known as immune-mediated reactions, while another is known as non-immune-mediated reactions. In contrast to food intolerance, which produces antibodies against specific food proteins, immune-mediated reactions to food can be mediated by IgE antibodies or other immunological routes. There is no production of IgE antibodies, which would indicate the onset of an allergic reaction. During the first phase, IgA antibodies are produced. Subsequently, IgG antibodies are produced after various stimulations. Also included in the category of food intolerances are responses that are not mediated by the immune system but rather by enzyme deficits, pharmacological reactions, or other unknown mechanisms. In youngsters (those between the ages of 0 and 17), food allergies can seriously affect their health. 32 million people in the United States are allergic to some food. According to studies published in 2018 and 2019, 8.2 million people are milk allergic, 6.1 million are peanut allergic, 3.9 million are egg allergic, 2.6 million are fish allergic, 2.6 million are wheat food allergic, 2.4 million are soy allergic, and 2.6 million are fish allergic. In industrialized nations, 3–8% of kids and 1–3% of adults suffer from food allergies linked to IgE. From an estimated 3% of the global population in 1960 to an estimated 7% in 2018, the prevalence of food allergies has risen dramatically. Roughly 7.6% of American children are believed to suffer from food allergies, with 40% afflicted with more than one [17]. The fact that the food we consume daily contains allergen-promoting and antiallergic nutrients suggests that we can control our allergies by making different food choices [18]. Omega-3 polyunsaturated fatty acids+ (PUFAs), probiotics, selenium, copper, zinc, and magnesium are among the minerals and vitamins that have antiallergic effects; in contrast, omega-6 PUFAs are known to promote allergic inflammation through their role as precursors to leukotriene C4 [8].

When exposed to allergens, B cells produce IgE immunoglobulins. Interleukin (IL)-4 and IL-13 are two of the most important cytokines during B cells' transition from IgG to IgE production. When immunoglobulin E (IgE) binds to its high-affinity receptor, Fc" RI, it triggers the release of mediators from mast cells. People who are allergic already have their mast cell surface IgE receptors linked to allergen-specific IgE. Mast cell activation is primarily mediated by Fc" RI, toll-like, complement, and IgG receptors FcRI (CD64) and FcRII (CD32) [19]. Intracellular signaling processes lead to the release of essential biologically active products, such as (1) mediators stored in primary cytoplasmic granules and (2) mediators formed from lipids and newly synthesized cytokines, chemokines, growth factors, and other products, when bivalent or multivalent allergens cross-link adjacent IgE molecules. An "immediate hypersensitivity reaction" happens when a mediator is involved in an allergic reaction. There are genes that code for the total IgE response or the functions of IgE receptors; these genes are involved in different aspects of the immune response and inflammation. Some genes are involved in the specific immune response, such as HLA-D, TCR, CD14, toll-like receptor, STAT6, and the differentiation of T-helper 1 (Th1) cells. Other genes, such as TNF-, IFN-, and IL-3, are involved in the inflammatory process [3, 19, 20].

In acute and chronic inflammation, the IgE/allergen cross-linking event is triggered by two-phase responses. The initial step of an allergic reaction is the release of mediators like histamine, interleukins, serotonin, and Hagemann's factor from basophils and mast cells, which is triggered by calcium, the major switch in the cascade reaction. Allergenic (inflammatory) reactions, including the widening of blood vessels, heightened permeability of blood vessels, and increased migration of other inflammatory cells, are caused by chemical mediators released into the bloodstream. In the second part of the reaction, lipid mediators are synthesized. This is achieved by phospholipase A2 converting phospholipids to arachidonic acid and then by leukotrienes (LT), platelet activation factor (PAF), and prostaglandins (PG) from arachidonic acid [3, 19, 20]. The production of prostaglandin D2, inflammatory cells, vascular smooth muscles, connective tissue, and metabolic by-products LTD4 and LTE4, as well as LTB4 and LTC4 itself, continues the inflammatory cascade. In addition to TNF-_, IL-4, IL-5, and IL-13, mast cells produce many other cytokines, further enhancing inflammation [3, 21]. In the latter stages of inflammation, when mast cells entice leukocytes—particularly Th2 cells and eosinophils—through the production and control of adhesion molecules on blood vessel endothelial cells, their numbers grow. Local antigen-presenting cells (APCs) in the airways deliver allergens, which reactivate Th2 memory cells, generating cytokines (IL-4, IL-5, and IL-13) that trigger an inflammatory response. The allergen does not possess the properties that cause allergic rhinitis; rather, the symptoms are brought about by lipid mediators that have already developed on the upper respiratory tract mucous membrane. An individual's susceptibility to allergens varies from case to case; these reactions are influenced by factors such as heredity, environment, and degree of exposure [3, 19–21].

19.4 Propolis in Asthma

Animal studies and in vitro investigations have shown that propolis can lessen the frequency and intensity of asthma attacks. The bioactive component CAPE found in propolis has decreased the expression of IL-5, IL-10, IL-12 p40, and IL-12 p70 indicators associated with the inflammatory signaling pathway and asthma. CAPE also prevents human CD4+ T cell proliferation, Akt activation, and the phosphorylation of inhibitor of κB kinase (IKK)α/IKKβ, IκBα, and NF-κB in human CD4+ T cells [22–24]. The level of white blood cell and polymorphonuclear cell infiltrates, α-SMA, MMP-9, MDA, ROS, IgE, IgG1, TNF-α, and Th1- and Th2-related cytokines including IFN-γ, IL-5, IL-6, and IL-10 is considerably reduced in animal models when propolis and its bioactive components like CAPE and tectochrysin are used [25–28]. In addition to downregulating the Th2 immune response, propolis increases the expression of glutathione-S-transferase, Treg differentiation, and polymorphonuclear myeloid-derived suppressor cells (PMN-MDSC) [29, 30]. In asthma-induced mice, symptoms such as pulmonary inflammation, airway hyperresponsiveness, infiltration of eosinophils, and epithelium mucus formation are reduced by modulating these pro-inflammatory and antioxidant biochemical indicators [25, 26, 31]. Numerous human clinical trials have shown promising outcomes in lowering inflammation-related illnesses such as asthma, COPD, and bronchitis when administered as a main treatment with propolis and its bioactive components. A study by Khayyal et al. [32] demonstrated that taking a milk formula supplemented with propolis greatly diminished the intensity and frequency of asthma attacks throughout the night. Leukotrienes, prostaglandins F2a and E2, IL-6, IL-8, TNF-α, and ICAM-1 were some of the inflammatory markers that decreased in correlation with the decrease in asthma attacks [32]. Patients with chronic obstructive pulmonary disease (COPD), asthma, and bronchitis reported dramatically improved quality of life and less sputum production after using a proprietary combination of propolis and N-acetylcysteine [33–35]. Studies including juvenile pulmonology patients and older adults with chronic obstructive pulmonary disease (COPD) found that propolis had a favorable effect [22, 36, 37].

Activating dendritic cells, which in turn encourages the formation and proliferation of T-helper cells (Th1, Th2, Th9, and Th17), is the typical starting point for asthma attacks caused by allergens. After that, these T-helper cells encourage the production of chemokines and cytokines involved in inflammation. The result is a cascade of events that involves the airway smooth muscle cells undergoing epithelial–mesenchymal transition and eosinophilic and neutrophilic inflammation [38]. Asthma episodes are reduced by propolis because it increases the number of CD4+Foxp3+ regulatory T cells and decreases the expression of CD4+ T cells. In addition, propolis suppresses the production of inflammatory cytokines and chemokines like TNF-α, IL-5, IL-6, IL-8, IL-10, NF-kB, IFN-γ, PGF2a, and PGE2. Additionally, by reducing the expression of TGF-1β, ICAM-1, α-SMA, MMP-9, IgE, and IgG1, propolis reduces inflammations of neutrophils and eosinophils as well as an epithelial–mesenchymal transition [22].

Flavonoids stop naïve CD4+ T cells from transforming into effector T cells by blocking the activation of the aryl hydrocarbon receptor (AhR) and NF-B caused by the IL-4-induced signal transduction. One of the many aromatic environmental contaminants, AhR, mediates the biological and toxic effects of dioxins and other similar pollutants [39]. The activation of AhR was significantly inhibited by flavonoids, apigenin, luteolin, baicalein, quercetin, kaempferol, and myricetin, with an EC70 value ranging from 1.9 to 5.1 _M, which is 70% of the peak response to dioxin (2,3,7,8-tetrachlorodibenzo-p-dioxin, or TCDD). Isoflavones like daidzein and resveratrol (a stilbene) and flavanones like naringenin and flavones like baicalein, on the other hand, showed strong AhR activation. Thanks to the cytosolic AhR/nuclear factor erythroid 2-related factor 2 (Nrf2) pathway, flavonoids boost levels of antioxidant enzymes, including peroxiredoxin, heme oxygenase-1, glutathione peroxidase, catalase, and superoxide dismutase [40]. Inflammasome activation can be inhibited by propolis and its flavonoids through oxidative stress reduction, which in turn inhibits the NLRP3 gene family [41–43].

References

1. Oršoli'c N, Baši'c I. Immunomodulation by water-soluble derivative of propolis: a factor of antitumor reactivity. J Ethnopharmacol. 2003;84:265–73.
2. Hartupee J, Mann DL. Role of inflammatory cells in fibroblast activation. JMCC. 2016;93:143–8.
3. Haque TT, Frischmeyer-Guerrerio PA. The role of TGF_ and other cytokines in regulating mast cell functions in allergic inflammation. Int J Mol Sci. 2022;23:10864.
4. Bloomfield SF, Rook GA, Scott EA, Shanahan F, Stanwell-Smith R, Turner P. Time to abandon the hygiene hypothesis: new perspectives on allergic disease, the human microbiome, infectious disease prevention and the role of targeted hygiene. Perspect Public Health. 2016;136:213–24.
5. Nyman GSA, Tang M, Inerot A, Osmancevic A, Malmberg P, Hagvall L. Contact allergy to beeswax and propolis among patients with cheilitis or facial dermatitis. Contact Dermat. 2019;81:110–6.

6. Global Asthma Network. The global asthma report 2018. Global Asthma Network: Auckland, New Zealand; 2018.
7. Suryakanth D, Basavaiah N. Propolis and allergic reactions. J Pharm Bioallied Sci. 2012;4:345.
8. Oršolić N. Allergic inflammation: effect of propolis and its flavonoids. Molecules. 2022;27(19):6694. https://doi.org/10.3390/molecules27196694. Published 2022 Oct 8.
9. Benkovi'c V, Orsoli'c N, Kneževi'c AH, Rami'c S, Điki'c D, Baši'c I, Kopjar N. Evaluation of the radioprotective effects of propolis and flavonoids in gamma-irradiated mice: the alkaline comet assay study. Biol Pharm Bull. 2008;31:167–72.
10. Oršoli'c N, Baši'c I. Antitumor, hematostimulative and radioprotective action of water-soluble derivative of propolis (WSDP). Biomed Pharmacother. 2005;59:561–70.
11. Ahangari Z, Naseri M, Vatandoost F. Propolis: chemical composition and its applications in endodontics. Iran Endod J. 2018;13:285–92.
12. Sena-Lopes Â, Bezerra FSB, Das Neves RN, De Pinho RB, Silva MTO, Savegnago L, Collares T, Seixas F, Begnini K, Henriques JAP, et al. Chemical composition, immunostimulatory, cytotoxic and antiparasitic activities of the essential oil from Brazilian red propolis. PLoS One. 2018;13:e0191797.
13. Popova M, Giannopoulou E, Skalicka-Wo'zniak K, Graikou K, Widelski J, Bankova V, Kalofonos H, Sivolapenko G, Gaweł-Beben K, Antosiewicz B, et al. Characterization and biological evaluation of propolis from Poland. Molecules. 2017;22:1159.
14. Huang S, Zhang C-P, Wang K, Li G, Hu F-L. Recent advances in the chemical composition of propolis. Molecules. 2014;19:19610–32.
15. Shahinozzaman M, Obanda DN, Tawata S. Chemical composition and pharmacological properties of Macaranga-type Pacific propolis: a review. Phytother Res. 2021;35:207–22.
16. Toreti VC, Sato HH, Pastore GM, Park YK. Recent progress of propolis for its biological and chemical compositions and its botanical origin. Evid Based Complement Alternat Med. 2013;2013:697390.
17. Kim EH, Burks AW. Food allergy immunotherapy: Oral immunotherapy and epicutaneous immunotherapy. Allergy. 2020;75:1337–46.
18. Chitranshi N, Verma N, Saad S, Gupta G, Hansbro PM, Oliver BG, Madheswaran T, Dua K, Chellappan DK. Unravelling the therapeutic potential of Nano-delivered functional foods in chronic respiratory diseases. Nutrients. 2022;14:3828.
19. González-de-Olano D, Álvarez-Twose I. Mast cells as key players in allergy and inflammation. J Investig Allergol Clin Immunol. 2018;28:365–78.
20. Yu W, Freeland DMH, Nadeau KC. Food allergy: immune mechanisms, diagnosis and immunotherapy. Nat Rev Immunol. 2016;16:751–65.
21. Amin K. The role of mast cells in allergic inflammation. Respir Med. 2012;106:9–14.
22. Zulhendri F, Perera CO, Tandean S, et al. The potential use of propolis as a primary or an adjunctive therapy in respiratory tract-related diseases and disorders: a systematic scoping review. Biomed Pharmacother. 2022;146:112595.
23. Wang L-C, Lin Y-L, Liang Y-C, Yang Y-H, Lee J-H, Yu H-H, Wu W-M, Chiang B-L. The effect of caffeic acid phenethyl ester on the functions of human monocyte-derived dendritic cells. BMC Immunol. 2009;10:39. https://doi.org/10.1186/1471-2172-10-39.
24. Sy LB, Yang LK, Chiu CJ, Wu W-M. The immunoregulatory effects of caffeic acid phenethyl ester on the cytokine secretion of peripheral blood mononuclear cells from asthmatic children. Pediatr Neonatol. 2011;52:327–31. https://doi.org/10.1016/j.pedneo.2011.08.005.
25. Sy LB, Wu Y-L, Chiang B-L, Wang Y-H, Wu W-M. Propolis extracts exhibit an immunoregulatory activity in an OVA-sensitized airway inflammatory animal model. Int Immunopharmacol. 2006;6:1053–60. https://doi.org/10.1016/j.intimp.2006.01.015.
26. Jung W-K, Lee D-Y, Choi YH, Yea SS, Choi I-W, Park S-G, Seo S-K, Lee S-W, Lee C-M, Kim S-K, Jeon Y-J, Choi I-W. Caffeic acid phenethyl ester attenuates allergic airway inflammation and hyperresponsiveness in murine model of ovalbumin-induced asthma. Life Sci. 2008;82:797–805. https://doi.org/10.1016/j.lfs.2008.01.014.
27. De Farias JHCD, Reis AS, Araújo MAR, Araújo MJAM, Assunção AKM, Farias JCD, Fialho EMS, Silva LA, Costa GC, Guerra RNM, Ribeiro MNS, Do Nascimento FRF. Effects

of stingless bee propolis on experimental asthma. Evid-Based Complement Altern Med. 2014;2014:951478. https://doi.org/10.1155/2014/951478.
28. Fang L, Yan Y, Xu ZX, He ZP, Zhou ST, Jiang X, Wu F, Yuan XL, Zhang T, Yu DN. Tectochrysin ameliorates murine allergic airway inflammation by suppressing Th2 response and oxidative stress. Eur J Pharm. 2021;902:174100. https://doi.org/10.1016/j.ejphar.2021.174100.
29. Jabir FA, Al Ali AS. Biochemical study and gene expression of Glutathione-S-transferase (GST) in induced asthma in rat. Orient J Chem. 2015;31:1587–94. https://doi.org/10.13005/ojc/310337.
30. Pineros A, de Lima M, Rodrigues T, Gembre A, Bertolini T, Fonseca M, Berretta A, Ramalho L, Cunha F, Hori J, Bonato V. Green propolis increases myeloid suppressor cells and CD4+Foxp3+ cells and reduces Th2 inflammation in the lungs after allergen exposure. J Ethnopharmacol. 2020;252:112496. https://doi.org/10.1016/j.jep.2019.112496.
31. Ma Y, Zhang J-X, Liu Y-N, Ge A, Gu H, Zha W-J, Zeng X-N, Huang M. Caffeic acid phenethyl ester alleviates asthma by regulating the airway microenvironment via the ROS-responsive MAPK/Akt pathway. Free Radic Biol Med. 2016;101:163–75. https://doi.org/10.1016/j.freeradbiomed.2016.09.012.
32. Khayyal MT, El-Ghazaly MA, El-Khatib AS, Hatem AM, De Vries PJF, El-Shafei S, Khattab MM. A clinical pharmacological study of the potential beneficial effects of a propolis food product as an adjuvant in asthmatic patients. Fundam Clin Pharmacol. 2003;17:93–102. https://doi.org/10.1046/j.1472206.2003.00117.x.
33. Zujovic D. The randomized, double-blind, placebo-controlled study of efficacy and safety of propolis and N-acetylcysteine compared to placebo in adults in acute condition with sputum production. Am J Respir Crit Care Med. 2017;195:A2675.
34. Zujovic D, Zugic V. The randomized, double-blind, placebo-controlled study of efficacy and safety of propolis and n-acetylcysteine compared to placebo in adults in acute condition with sputum production. Am J Respir Crit Care Med. 2018;197:A3196. http://www.embase.com/search/results?subaction=viewrecord&from=export&id=L622969973
35. Zujovic D, Zuza O, Djordjevic B. Assessment of the quality of life of patients with acute bronchitis on the propolis with N-acetylcysteine versus N-acetylcysteine. Am J Respir Crit Care Med. 2020;201:A7773–A777. https://doi.org/10.1164/ajrccm-conference.2020.201.1_meetingabstracts.a7773.
36. Hirayama F, Lee AH, Binns CW, Taniguchi H. Dietary supplementation by Japanese patients with chronic obstructive pulmonary disease. Complement Ther Med. 2009;17:37–43. https://doi.org/10.1016/j.ctim.2008.02.007.
37. Živanović S, Pavlovi'c D, Stojanovi'c N, Veljkovi'c M. Attitudes to and prevalence of bee product usage in pediatric pulmonology patients. Eur J Integr Med. 2019;27:1–6. https://doi.org/10.1016/j.eujim.2019.02.001.
38. Kudo M, Ishigatsubo Y, Aoki I. Pathology of asthma. Front Microbiol. 2013;4:263. https://doi.org/10.3389/fmicb.2013.00263.
39. Amakura Y, Tsutsumi T, Sasaki K, Nakamura M, Yoshida T. Maitani, T. Influence of food polyphenols on aryl hydrocarbon. receptor-signaling pathway estimated by in vitro bioassay. Phytochemistry. 2008;69:3117–30.
40. Zhang H, Tsao R. Dietary polyphenols, oxidative stress and antioxidant and anti-inflammatory effects. Curr Opin Food Sci. 2016;8:33–42.
41. Chih-Yu H, Lan-Hui L, Koteswara RY, Tz-Chuen J, Yu-Shin N, Yue-Wen C, Kuo-Feng H. Mechanistic insight into the attenuation of gouty inflammation by Taiwanese green propolis via inhibition of the NLRP3 inflammasome. J Cell Physiol. 2018;234:4081–94.
42. Lee H, Yang G, Kim N, Jeong S, Jung Y, Choi JY, Park HH, Young JL. Targeting ASC in NLRP3 inflammasome by caffeic acid phenethyl ester: a novel strategy to treat acute gout. Sci Rep. 2016;6:38622.
43. Roy S, Manna K, Jha T, Saha KD. Chrysin-loaded PLGA attenuates OVA-induced allergic asthma by modulating TLR/NF-_B/NLRP3 axis. Nanomed Nanotechnol Biol Med. 2020;30:102292.

Propolis in the Treatment of Nasal Skin Lesions

20

20.1 Introduction

Many branches of medicine treat skin conditions that manifest on the nose. When people experience skin lesions on the nose, they often seek the advice of dermatologists, otorhinolaryngologists, primary care physicians, and general plastic and dermatologic surgeons. Skin lesions on the face and head are common in dermatologic surgeons' daily practice, and this article is part two of a review series covering this topic. When assessing skin diseases on the nose or planning the reconstruction of surgical defects, it is essential to consider the nose skin's special anatomical and histological features. Areas of the skin that are thinner, less sebaceous, and more pliable include the dorsum, columella, and sidewalls. There is thicker, more sebaceous, adhesive, and less flexible skin around the nasal tip and alae [1].

One of the most harmful types of light for the skin in this area, ultraviolet (UV) light, is a known carcinogen, and the exposed face is a prime example. This explains why the skin of the nose is so often affected by cancer, even though it is the most common site for skin cancer in the human body. This has also contributed to the idea that the face is like a "sun terrace," with the forehead, ears, and nose being the parts most directly exposed to the sun. Because of this, people are subjected to more ultraviolet light, which includes the potentially cancerous UVB spectrum (290–320 nm), which has been identified as one of the most potent skin carcinogens. The production of dimeric photoproducts between neighboring pyrimidine bases is a common mechanism for UVB-induced DNA damage. Mutations caused by ultraviolet radiation often affect the tumor suppressor gene p53. In addition, ultraviolet A light causes skin cancer by producing highly reactive free radicals that damage DNA. In addition to its carcinogenic effects, ultraviolet A light causes skin to age more quickly by damaging collagen [1].

Inflammation begins as soon as the immune system identifies *P. acnes*. When *P. acnes* causes severe inflammation, the immune system may respond by producing

A. E. Tanuğur Samanci et al., *Propolis: Prevention and Healing Effects in Otorhinolaryngology*, Comprehensive ENT,
https://doi.org/10.1007/978-3-031-68546-0_20

chemostatic agents such as macrophages, neutrophils, and lymphocytes. Research has demonstrated that reactive oxygen species (ROS) produced by neutrophils damage the follicular epithelium, leading to inflammation in acne [2, 3]. Managing and curing existing lesions, minimizing scarring, shortening the duration of the illness, and reducing morbidity are the primary goals of acne treatment. Isotretinoin, tretinoin, adapalene, tazarotene, spironolactone, cyproterone acetate, doxycycline, minocycline, benzoyl peroxide, and other chemicals are available for both topical and systemic use in the treatment of acne [4, 5].

The cosmetic industry has invested significantly in propolis for acne treatment, particularly in cosmeceuticals. Dermo-cosmetics containing up to 4% propolis can effectively prevent and treat acne vulgaris [6, 7] thanks to its anti-inflammatory, antibacterial, healing, and immunomodulatory properties.

20.2 Anatomy of the Skin

The skin is the main interface between the outside world and the human body, covering every surface externally. As a barrier, it shields inside tissues from pathogens, excessive heat or cold, harmful chemicals, and ultraviolet (UV) radiation. Aside from these critical roles, the skin regulates temperature, controls insensible fluid loss, and monitors the immune system [8].

Subcutaneous adipose tissue (panniculus adiposus) supports the integuments' two interdependent layers, the dermis and the epidermis. The surface ectoderm is the main source of the epidermis, but it is also colonized by cells from the neural crest that contain pigment, cells from the bone marrow that process antigens, and cells from the neural crest that sense pressure. Dermis components include fibroblasts, sensory structures, elastic fibers, blood vessels, and collagen, mostly produced from mesoderm [9].

The multi-layered skin is there from birth, yet it is a living organ that changes constantly as we age, losing its outer layers and gaining new ones. Different parts of the body, different sexes, and different ages have different skin thicknesses. Dermal thickness is the primary variable here; epidermal thickness, on the other hand, is rather stable between individuals and throughout different body parts. The palms and soles of the feet have the thickest skin at 1.5 mm, whereas the eyelids and post-auricular region have the thinnest skin at 0.05 mm [8].

Male skin is noticeably thicker than female skin in every part of the body. Skin starts thin in children and gradually thickens until it starts to thin again in the 40s or 50s. This thinning is mostly a dermal alteration, accompanied by the loss of ground material, epithelial appendages, and elastic fibers [10].

Due to its lack of blood vessels, the epidermis must rely on the dermis underneath it to transport nutrients and remove waste products through the dermo-epidermal junction. As they advance from deeper to more superficial layers, keratinocytes in various stages of development make up the bulk of the stratified squamous epithelium known as the epidermis. The layers that make up the epidermis are stratum spinosum, stratum granulosum, stratum corneum, and stratum germinativum [8].

20.2.1 Layers of Skin

The dermis' principal role is supporting and sustaining the epidermis. The dermis has two layers: the more intricate papillary dermis and the deeper reticular dermis. The thinner papillary dermis is less densely packed with collagen, elastic and reticular fibers, and capillaries. Coarse bundles of collagen fibers organized in parallel layers to the surface, bigger blood vessels, and densely interwoven elastic fibers comprise the reticular dermis, a thicker layer of connective tissue [8].

Additional components of the reticular layer include epidermal appendages, lymphatics, nerve terminals, mast cells, and fibroblasts. Glycoproteins, chondroitin sulfates, and mucopolysaccharides (mostly hyaluronic acid) comprise the gel-like ground substance surrounding the dermal components. Additional padding for the skin is provided by the subcutaneous layer, the panniculus adiposus, which borders the extremely uneven deep dermal surface [8–10].

20.3 Moisturizing

The primary goal of skin care was identified as moisturizing. Among the many claims made by cosmetics companies, "moisturizing" is the most common. While the term "moisturizer" is not universally agreed upon, most people understand it to mean a product that, when applied topically, helps alleviate dry skin. Since Blank's groundbreaking work, much information on elements that moisturize the stratum corneum (SC) has been uncovered. The SC is a complex structure that consists of a continuous matrix of specialized lipids (mortar) and noncontinuous, proteinaceous, terminally differentiated keratinocytes or corneocytes (bricks). Corneocytes are empty cells that lack cytoplasm and intracellular organelles. They comprise a keratin matrix held together by disulfide bonds and enclosed in a cornified cell envelope, a protein membrane [11, 12]. The transglutaminase family, which includes at least two members, crosslinks the specialized proteins that comprise the envelope. Desquamation breaks down the structure of other specific proteins, which hold the corneocytes together. Water is an important component of this structure, affecting skin elasticity, tensile strength, barrier properties, and overall look. Natural moisturizing factor (NMF) binds water in the SC, and intercellular lamellar lipids offer a barrier to water loss. When all of these things are in harmony, the skin stays healthy [11, 12].

Presently, humectants—hygroscopic substances—are applied topically to the stratum corneum (SC) to enhance its water-holding ability. Some components of NMF, such as lactic acid and urea, are also utilized in moisturizers; these substances have an action similar to that of NMF. As an additional tactic, occlusive agents—oily substances that are insoluble in water—can be applied to the skin surface to collect water in the SC. To prevent surface evaporation, oily substances act similarly to the skin's natural lipid bilayers (petrolatum) [11].

When applied to the skin, the formulation will turn tacky because the necessary quantities of occlusive agents are often somewhat high. When occlusive agents are emulsified with hygroscopic agents, the final product may have less of the agent's occlusive power. Although humectants are typically used to make skin more moisturizing, there are few situations in which they might cause water loss from the skin. A humectant's ability to absorb water reduces water activity coefficient. If the water in skin tissue does not have a lower water activity than the surrounding humectant-water blend, water molecules will not be transferred to the skin. Cosmetic chemists should exercise caution when choosing the humectant for their formulations to avoid interfering with the enzyme-controlled natural desquamatory process. Because of this, glycerin is often the humectant that is used for moisturizing purposes. The formulation needs to undergo suitable clinical testing to guarantee it will be an efficient moisturizer, as aqueous humectant blends plasticize skin. Hydrophilic polymers in more modern formulations may act as humectants and aid skin smoothing [13, 14].

Formulators are aware of potential factors impacting epidermal health, including hydrolysis and oxidation reactions of intracorneal lipid components, enzymatic reliance on NMF production, and environmental fluctuations. Glycerin-based moisturizers have the disadvantage of not being good solvents for cosmetic lipids. To get the most out of a formulation that calls for a lipophilic cosmetic active component, the formulator needs to rely on their expertise and experience [11].

20.4 UVA Protection

Medical professionals specializing in skin care mostly use photoprotection as a prophylactic measure. Sun protection is ideal. However, many people can only live partially indoors due to their jobs or hobbies that require them to be outside. A reasonable middle ground in this regard is the consistent application of sunscreens. Sunscreens protect animals from developing squamous cell carcinomas. Sunscreens lessen the risk of actinic keratoses, solar elastosis, and squamous cell carcinoma in people when used regularly [14–16]. Applying sunscreen regularly may also lower the incidence of melanoma [17]. Sunscreen, particularly those with higher UVA blocking capabilities, may protect against drug photosensitization and photoinduced or photo-aggravated dermatoses [14].

The key metric of the SPF test, erythema, is a basic biological goal. Subclinical damage (sunburn cell development) without apparent erythema was observed in a sunscreen with an SPF of 15 compared to one with an SPF of 30 [15]. The SPF 30 product offered a far higher level of protection. A formulation with an SPF of 15 may cause additional subclinical harm. UVA protection isn't great with any sunscreen, but it improves with a higher SPF, especially in the shorter UVA range or UVA II (320–340 nm). Under real-world situations, sun protection factors (SPFs) of 100 or higher have been demonstrated to have an even greater impact on preventing sunburn [11]. On the other hand, according to FDA Proposed Order OTC00000 [14], there is a dearth of scientific data demonstrating additional meaningful clinical advantages above this level. Hence, products with SPF values of 60 or higher should be marketed as SPF 60+ at most.

Sunscreens are great at blocking out UVB rays but don't do much against UVA rays, especially UVA I. Some have questioned whether higher SPF creams adequately protect against UVA radiation, even though they allow people to spend more time in the sun without burning. Indeed, people who only use sunscreens to shield themselves from the sun could be exposing themselves to more UVA radiation over time [6].

When it comes to determining the most accurate way to measure UVA protection, opinions vary. Several approaches have been suggested. Direct UVA erythema, persistent pigment darkening, and psoralen photosensitization have all been used to build in vivo approaches [6].

Depending on the patient's condition and skin type, each approach has its own set of advantages and disadvantages. In Europe, they now use an in vitro approach that uses transmittance via a thin film as a substrate. An in vitro test called the Critical Wavelength Method is also used in the FDA Proposed Final Rule (2019). The wavelength at which 90% of the total UV absorption lies is called the critical wavelength (CW). The characteristics of a "broad spectrum" sunscreen include an absorption coefficient (CW) of at least 370 nm and an average UVA/UV ratio of 0.70 or higher. The active ingredient in the mix should be either avobenzone or an inorganic particle sunscreen if UV radiation protection into the UVA I range is required [6].

20.5 Propolis in Skincare

There has been a recent uptick in the usage of botanical antiaging creams. In addition to their strong antioxidant capabilities, many extracts contain components that have photoprotective or synergistic effects when combined with sunscreens. Interest has been piqued in using natural extracts in sunscreens and other cosmetics to prevent skin disorders [12, 13].

People all around the globe swear by propolis extract for its purported health benefits and illness-prevention properties. Important polyphenols and flavonoids in propolis have an absorption spectrum that can be employed as a UV radiation screen, limiting skin penetration and the resulting inflammation, oxidative stress, and DNA-damaging effects [13]. Their antioxidant and anti-inflammatory properties mitigate or postpone the negative effects of free radicals (singlet oxygen and hydroxyl free radicals) generated by ultraviolet light [14]. As more people learned about the sun's detrimental effects, the search for sun protection products became even more intense. Sunburn, skin aging, and cancer are all possible outcomes of prolonged skin exposure to UV radiation [12].

Because of its strong chemical affinity with propolis, ethanol is the solvent of choice for many techniques used to extract propolis worldwide. Solvents like water, methanol, chloroform, or ethylic ether can also be suggested for extracting propolis components [15, 16]. Ethanol extraction also removes waxes and other organic residues [17].

We were unable to find any studies that assessed the cytotoxicity and microbial activity of ethanol extracts of Brazilian red propolis (EEPV) in sunscreens at a concentration that would enhance the sun protection of the formulation under investigation, even though numerous studies have already been conducted on EEPV for sun protection. Keeping in mind the significance of cytotoxic characterization for a skin-contact product and its antimicrobial capabilities, these tests were conducted in this study to gain a better grasp of the sunscreen produced. These biological results were obtained by a cell viability assay using MTT and pertain to the cytotoxic profile of EEPV in both immune system cells and cells found in the epidermal leaflet. Nosocomial infections caused by Gram-positive bacteria, including *Staphylococcus aureus* and *Staphylococcus epidermidis*, common in healthcare settings, were also tested for propolis' antimicrobial properties. Furthermore, we confirmed that the propolis extract suggested here possesses significant anti-inflammatory characteristics for creating skin-application formulations by evaluating nitric oxide generation in macrophage cells [12].

Propolis' antiviral, antibacterial, antifungal, anti-inflammatory, immunoregulatory, antioxidant, and wound-healing characteristics are just a few documented actions. The antioxidant and anti-inflammatory properties of propolis have recently come to attention due to its possible use in the cosmetics and pharmaceutical sectors.

The primary polyphenolic chemicals in propolis have strong antioxidant properties and work well as sunscreens that block UVB and UVA rays. An evaluation of the ethanolic red propolis extracts (EEPV) using qualitative phytochemical methods revealed the presence of flavonoids and terpenoids in concentrations of 70% at room temperature and 70% when heated. The antioxidant activity was demonstrated by a 50% reduction of DPPH at 17 and 12 g/mL, respectively, when extracted at room and high temperatures [12].

20.6 Anti-inflammatory Activities of Propolis

The antibacterial action of propolis extract against *P. acnes* has been shown in in vitro tests at concentrations of 10%, 5%, 2.5%, 1.25%, and 0.625%. This action is likely due to propolis' flavones and p-coumaric acid derivatives. As a bonus, propolis has anti-inflammatory and healing properties, making it a great supplement to acne treatments.8 Recent years have seen a proliferation of research highlighting the anti-inflammatory properties of isoflavonoids and their actions. In acute and chronic inflammation, neovestitol significantly decreases neutrophil and leukocyte migration. Also, neovestitol pretreatment lowers IL-6 levels and suppresses proinflammatory cytokine production. Hence, neovestitol may have anti-inflammatory effects [18–24].

20.7 Propolis in Nasal Skin Lesion Treatment

Different forms of acne treatment are reserved for various stages of the condition. A topical treatment may be more effective and have fewer side effects than a systemic therapy, which can improve certain areas of symptomatology and reduce undesirable skin reactions. This is important even after a systemic treatment is set up. Most patients initially try topical therapy for mild to moderate comedonal or papulopustular acne [25, 26].

The majority of people who suffer from acne vulgaris are young people, making it the most common skin illness. Hyperkeratinization of the follicles, hyperplasia of the sebaceous glands, hypercolonization of bacteria, immunological responses, and inflammatory processes are all factors in the development of this disease [27, 28]. Whether systemic medication is also utilized, topical treatments are commonly used to treat acne. Benzoyl peroxide, retinoids, azelaic acid, keratolytic agents, and antibiotics are widely used. Antibiotic therapy is the current standard of care for *P. acnes* [28]. Still, people are increasingly looking for alternatives, focusing on natural products, due to synthetic antibiotics' side effects and bacterial resistance [27].

For this reason, propolis plays a significant role in acne vulgaris treatments. Thanks to its anti-inflammatory and antibacterial activities, it significantly reduces seborrhea and oiliness excess of the skin with high tolerability [29]. It also reduces non-inflammatory lesions. Dermatology products that target acne vulgaris and other skin disorders are being developed using their anti-inflammatory and antibacterial capabilities [29, 30].

Much work goes into developing safer cosmetic formulas that are less harsh and toxic than the medications used to treat acne but still get the job done [6, 27]. Cream formulations, procedures, masks, lotions, soaps, and sprays were among the goods mentioned in the reports included in this study. Some of the most popular topical medications are antibiotics, retinoids, azelaic acid, keratolytic, alpha-hydroxy acids, and benzoyl peroxide [28]. Traditional acne treatments, including antibiotics that kill *P. acnes*, are losing their efficacy due to antibiotic resistance. As an alternative to antibiotics, many natural compounds are recognized to have inherent antibacterial action [29]. Forty individuals with face acne vulgaris were studied by Ali et al. [29] to determine the bacteriological and clinical effectiveness of applying propolis extracts topically. Group I patients were given a topical solution of ethanolic propolis extract as treatment, whereas group II patients served as controls and received simply an ethanol solution. The patients were randomly assigned to each group. Treatment of acne vulgaris, particularly seborrhea, and oiliness, using a topical ethanolic propolis extract showed highly significant clinical efficacy in this investigation. According to bacteriological tests, the ethanolic propolis extract topical solution showed a strong antimicrobial effect against aerobic and anaerobic gram-positive bacteria, including *Staphylococcus epidermidis* and *Propionibacterium acnes*. The remedy was safe, had little side effects, and worked as advertised.

Stingless bees make honey, wax, pollen, propolis, and cerumen. Although honeybees build their nests primarily or only from wax, stingless bees often use plant gums, resins, or dirt [31, 32]. Toothpaste, mouthwashes, lotions, drops, nutritional supplements, antipyretic, antiseptic, and wound-healing treatments have used propolis for millennia. Additionally, it is employed in the treatment of burns, acne, neurodermatitis, herpes simplex and genitals, and fungal infections of the eyes and vagina [33]. We isolated active chemicals for antioxidant, anti-inflammatory, and anti-acne from *T. biroi* propolis extracts because no prior research has reported the evaluation of this plant's propolis in anti-acne products [1].

Topical agents such as retinoids, azelaic acid, antibiotics, keratolytics, and alpha-hydroxy acids are the most commonly utilized. The conventional acne treatment—antibiotics that inhibit *P. acnes*—is losing efficacy as antibiotic-resistant strains of *S. epidermidis* and other coagulase-negative staphylococci emerge [34, 35].

Research has shown that propolis has potent antibacterial properties; mainly, it is more effective against Gram-positive bacteria than Gram-negative ones [36]. The synergistic action of the several chemicals in propolis, including flavonoids, caffeic acid, benzoic acid, and cinnamic acid, may be responsible for these antimicrobial benefits. These chemicals likely disrupt microbial activity and structure by acting on their membranes or cell walls [37]. Some antibacterial agents have been found to work in synergy with propolis [38]. Propolis has bacteriostatic and, at higher concentrations, bactericidal antibacterial properties [39]. Paradoxically, the high concentration of polyphenol chemicals in propolis explains why it has anti-inflammatory effects in both short-term and long-term inflammation [40]. There has been no evidence that it effectively treats acne. To lessen the adverse effects noted by other writers, we included 10% propolis in our preparation [25, 41].

The reason why the sebum normalizing activity has been researched is because several chemicals found primarily on propolis, like tannin, isoflavones, and chalcone, have been found to effectively inhibit 5-α reductase enzymes in laboratory tests [42].

Several compounds are isolated from *T. biroi* propolis, some of which have biological activity and others do not. These include sulabiroins A, (2S)-5,7-dihydroxy-4′-methoxy-8-prenylflavanone acid, broussoflavonol F [43] which inhibits the activity of the SARS-CoV-2 protease, sulabiroins B, such as sulabiroins A, (2S)-5,7- dihydroxy-4′-methoxy-8-prenylflavanone acid and broussoflavonol F [43] as an inhibitor of SARS-CoV-2 protease activity; sulabiroins A, sulabiroins B, 2′,3′-dihydro-3′- hydroxypapuanic acid, ( )- papuanic acid, ( )-isocalolongic acid, isopapuanic acid, isocalopolyanic acid, glyasperin A, broussoflavonol F, (2S)-5,7-dihydroxy-4′-methoxy-8- prenylflavanone, isorhamnetin, (1′S)-2-trans, 4-trans-abscisic acid, and (1′S)-2-cis,4-trans-abscisic acid [44] as inhibitors of XO activity; calophylloidic acid A for antibacterial activity against *Staphylococcus aureus* and *Escherichia coli* [45]; 4-(4′-hydroxy-3′-methoxyphenyl)-3,5,7- trihydroxycoumarin, sulawesins A and sulawesins B [46] as inhibitors of XO activity; glyasperin A, propolin E and propolin A [47] for cytotoxicity in breast (MCF-7) and colon (HT-29 and HCT-116) cancer cells; pinobanksin-5,7-dimethyl ether, artepillin C, luteolin-5-methyl ether, pinobanskin-3-0 (butyrate or isobutyrate) and kaempferide [48]; propolin A, propolin E, propolin H, and glyasperin A [1, 49].

References

1. Sand M, Sand D, Thrandorf C, Paech V, Altmeyer P, Bechara FG. Cutaneous lesions of the nose. Head Face Med. 2010;4(6):7. https://doi.org/10.1186/1746-160X-6-7. PMID: 20525327; PMCID: PMC2903548.
2. Arung ET, Syafrizal KIW, et al. Antioxidant, anti-inflammatory and anti-acne activities of stingless bee (*Tetragonula biroi*) propolis. Fitoterapia. 2023;164:105375. https://doi.org/10.1016/j.fitote.2022.105375.
3. Akamatsu H, Horio T, Hattori K. Increased hydrogen peroxide generation by neutrophils from patients with acne inflammation. Int J Dermatol. 2003;42(5):366–9.
4. Lavers I. Diagnosis and management of acne vulgaris. Nurse Prescrib. 2014;12(7):330–6.
5. Olutunmbi Y, Paley K, English JC. Adolescent female acne: etiology and management. J Pediatr Adolesc Gynecol. 2008;21(4):171–6.
6. Matsuchita HLP, Matsuchita ASP. Uso da Própolis na Prevenção e Tratamento da Acne Vulgar. Uniciências. 2015;18(01):19–23.
7. Rao J. Acne vulgaris. In: James WD, editor. Medscape. Updated: Aug 27, 2020. https://emedicine.medscape.com/article/1069804-overview Accessed online at December 10, 2023.
8. Dawson AL, Dellavalle RP. Acne vulgaris. BMJ. 2013;8(346):f2634.
9. Thiboutot D, Gollnick H, Bettoli V, Dréno B, Kang S, Leyden JJ, et al. New insights into the management of acne: an update from the Global Alliance to Improve Outcomes in Acne group. J Am Acad Dermatol. 2009 May;60(5 Suppl):S1–50.
10. Goulden V, McGeown CH, Cunliffe WJ. The familial risk of adult acne: a comparison between first-degree relatives of affected and unaffected individuals. Br J Dermatol. 1999 Aug;141(2):297–300.
11. Kellett SC, Gawkrodger DJ. The psychological and emotional impact of acne and the effect of treatment with isotretinoin. Br J Dermatol. 1999 Feb;140(2):273–82.
12. Kelhälä HL, Fyhrquist N, Palatsi R, et al. Isotretinoin treatment reduces acne lesions but not directly lesional acne inflammation. Exp Dermatol. 2016 Jun;25(6):477–8.
13. Saluja SS, Walker ML, Summers EM, Tristani-Firouzi P, Smart DR. Safety of non-ablative fractional laser for acne scars within 1 month after treatment with oral isotretinoin: a randomized split-face controlled trial. Lasers Surg Med. 2017 Dec;49(10):886–90.
14. Jeremy AH, Holland DB, Roberts SG, Thomson KF, Cunliffe WJ. Inflammatory events are involved in acne lesion initiation. J Invest Dermatol. 2003 Jul;121(1):20–7.
15. Norris JF, Cunliffe WJ. A histological and immunocytochemical study of early acne lesions. Br J Dermatol. 1988;118(5):651–9.
16. Kim J, Ochoa MT, Krutzik SR, et al. Activation of toll-like receptor 2 in acne triggers inflammatory cytokine responses. J Immunol. 2002;169(3):1535–41.
17. Webster GF. Inflammatory acne represents hypersensitivity to *Propionibacterium acnes*. Dermatology. 1998;196(1):80–1.
18. Pochi PE, Strauss JS. Sebaceous gland activity in black skin. Dermatol Clin. 1988;6(3):349–51.
19. Lucky AW, Biro FM, Simbartl LA, Morrison JA, Sorg NW. Predictors of severity of acne vulgaris in young adolescent girls: results of a five-year longitudinal study. J Pediatr. 1997 Jan;130(1):30–9.
20. Baek JH, Ahn SM, Choi KM, Jung MK, Shin MK, Koh JS. Analysis of comedone, sebum and porphyrin on the face and body for comedogenicity assay. Skin Res Technol. 2016 May;22(2):164–9.
21. Trivedi NR, Cong Z, Nelson AM, Albert AJ, Rosamilia LL, Sivarajah S, et al. Peroxisome proliferator-activated receptors increase human sebum production. J Invest Dermatol. 2006 Sep;126(9):2002–9.
22. Smith TM, Cong Z, Gilliland KL, Clawson GA, Thiboutot DM. Insulin-like growth factor-1 induces lipid production in human SEB-1 sebocytes via sterol response element-binding protein-1. J Invest Dermatol. 2006 Jun;126(6):1226–32.

23. Zouboulis CC, Böhm M. Neuroendocrine regulation of sebocytes—a pathogenetic link between stress and acne. Exp Dermatol. 2004;13(Suppl 4):31–5.
24. Franchin M, Colón DF, Cunha MG, Castanheira FVS, Saraiva ALL, Bueno-Silva B, et al. Neovestitol, an isoflavonoid isolated from Brazilian red propolis, reduces acute and chronic inflammation: involvement of nitric oxide and IL-6. Sci Rep. 2016;6:36401.
25. Mazzarello V, Donadu MG, Ferrari M, Piga G, Usai D, Zanetti S, Sotgiu MA. Treatment of acne with a combination of propolis, tea tree oil, and *Aloe vera* compared to erythromycin cream: two double-blind investigations. Clin Pharmacol. 2018;13(10):175–81. https://doi.org/10.2147/CPAA.S180474. PMID: 30588129; PMCID: PMC6298394.
26. Krautheim A, Gollnick HP. Acne: topical treatment. Clin Dermatol. 2004;22(5):398–407.
27. Barbosa V, Scheiffer GFC, Cardozo AGL, Pietruchinski E, Santos CZ, Silveira D, et al. Avaliação da atividade antibacteriana do óleo essencial de Rosmarinus officinalis L. e tintura de própolis frente à bactéria causadora da acne *Propionibacterium acnes*. Revista Brasileira De Plantas Medicinais. 2014;16(2):169–73.
28. Mazzarello V, Donadu MG, Ferrari M, Piga G, Usai D, Zanetti S, et al. Treatment of acne with a combination of propolis, tea tree oil and *Aloe vera* compared to erythromycin cream: two double-blind investigations. Clin Pharmacol. 2018;10:175–81.
29. Ali BMM, Ghoname NF, Hodeib AA, Elbadawy MA. Significance of topical propolis in the treatment of facial acne vulgaris. Egypt J Dermatol Venerol. 2015;35(1):29–36.
30. Barros KBNT, Neto EMR, Fonteles MMF. Propolis and its cosmetic applications: a technological prospection. J Young Pharm. 2019;11(4):350–2.
31. Heard T. The role of stingless bees in crop pollination. Annu Rev Entomol. 1999;44:183–206.
32. Popova M, Trusheva B, Bankova V. Propolis of stingless bees: a phytochemist's guide through the jungle of tropical biodiversity. Phytomedicine. 2021;86:153098.
33. Mohd K, Mat Nafi N, Shafiqha A, Khadar A, Badiazaman AA, Badiazaman M, Annisava A, Mohd K. Propolis: traditional uses, phytochemical composition and pharmacological properties. Int J Eng Technol. 2018;7:78–82.
34. Ross JI, Snelling AM, Carnegie E, et al. Antibiotic-resistant acne: lessons from Europe. Br J Dermatol. 2003;148(3):467–78. [PubMed] [Google Scholar].
35. Humphrey S. Antibiotic resistance in acne treatment. Skin Therapy Lett. 2012;17(9):1–3.
36. Grange JM, Davey RW. Antibacterial properties of propolis (bee glue). J R Soc Med. 1990;83(3):159–60.
37. Scazzocchio F, D'Auria FD, Alessandrini D, Pantanella F. Multifactorial aspects of antimicrobial activity of propolis. Microbiol Res. 2006;161(4):327–33.
38. Fernandes Júnior A, Balestrin EC, Betoni JE, Orsi RO, da Cunha ML, Montelli AC. Propolis: anti-*Staphylococcus aureus* activity and synergism with antimicrobial drugs. Mem Inst Oswaldo Cruz. 2005;100(5):563–6.
39. Drago L, Mombelli B, de Vecchi E, Fassina MC, Tocalli L, Gismondo MR. In vitro antimicrobial activity of propolis dry extract. J Chemother. 2000;12(5):390–5.
40. Martinotti S, Ranzato E. Propolis: a new frontier for wound healing? Burns Trauma. 2015;3:9.
41. Menniti-Ippolito F, Mazzanti G, Vitalone A, Firenzuoli F, Santuccio C. Surveillance of suspected adverse reactions to natural health products: the case of propolis. Drug Saf. 2008;31(5):419–23.
42. Liu J, Ando R, Shimizu K, et al. Steroid 5α-reductase inhibitory activity of condensed tannins from woody plants. J Wood Sci. 2008;54(1):68–75.
43. Dewi LIA, Sahlan M, Pratami D, Agus A, Agussalim A, Sabir A. Identifying propolis compounds potential to be covid-19 therapies by targeting sars-cov-2 main protease. Int J Appl Pharm. 2021;13:103–10.
44. Miyata R, Sahlan M, Ishikawa Y, Hashimoto H, Honda S, Kumazawa S. Propolis components and biological activities from stingless bees collected on South Sulawesi, Indonesia, HAYATI. J Biosci. 2020;27:82.
45. Mizuno S, Miyata R, Mukaide K, Honda S, Sukito A, Sahlan M, Taniguchi T, Kumazawa S. New compound from the plant origin of propolis from Lombok, Indonesia and its antibacterial activity. Results Chem. 2022;4:100276.

46. Miyata R, Sahlan M, Ishikawa Y, Hashimoto H, Honda S, Kumazawa S. Propolis components from stingless bees collected on South Sulawesi, Indonesia, and their xanthine oxidase inhibitory activity. J Nat Prod. 2019;82(2):205–10.
47. De Los Reyes M, Oyong G, Ebajo V Jr, Shen C-C, Ragasa C. Cytotoxic prenylflavanones from Philippine stingless bee (*Tetragonula biroi* Friese) nests. Asian J Chem. 2017;29.
48. Alvarez P, Cruz M, Micor J, Fajardo A, Cervancia C, Hizon-Fradejas APE. Identification of flavonoids and phenolic compounds in propolis from stingless bee (*Tetragonula biroi* Friese) nest and extracts from five tree sources using tandem liquid chromatography—mass spectroscopy. Philippine Entomol. 2013;24:91–9.
49. Ragasa CY, Galian RAF, Ebajo VD, Aguda RM, Cervancia CR, Shen C-C. Propolins and glyasperin a from stingless bee nests. Rev Bras. 2015;25(2):177–9.

Oral Hygiene by Adding Propolis to Toothpaste

21

21.1 Introduction

One of the causes of dysbiosis, an imbalance of the oral microbiota, is inadequate dental hygiene. Oral disorders are caused by dysbiosis [1, 2] since studies have revealed a restricted quantity of harmful bacteria at a healthy host site. A biofilm is formed when harmful bacteria increase too much, that condition is known as microbial dysbiosis [3]. If you have dysbiosis and biofilms are creating in your mouth, it makes sense to employ mechanical or chemical methods, like toothpaste and mouthwash, to eliminate or significantly lower the population of these bacteria [4, 5]. Perceived benefits and persistent advertising and marketing have contributed to the widespread use of mouthwash and toothpaste [4–6]. The fact that they are so popular shows that people are looking for ways to improve their health, whether through diet or medication [7]. Marketers may be unable to promise that their toothpaste can kill bacteria, yet it doesn't stop many people from buying and using the goods [1, 8].

North American consumers can choose from various toothpaste and mouthwashes with unique formula, texture, and flavor. Stannous fluoride, one of the most popular chemicals, has proven to be a potent antibacterial agent after years of study. A more modern development is the introduction of herbal remedies that contain naturally occurring substances with antibacterial solid characteristics, such as mentha, guarana, eucalyptus extract, mastic, Arab acacia, and miswak. Propolis is one of these natural chemicals; it is an essential substance for avoiding oral illnesses and has found its way into several dentifrices, mouthwashes, and toothpaste [6, 9–11].

A. E. Tanuğur Samanci et al., *Propolis: Prevention and Healing Effects in Otorhinolaryngology*, Comprehensive ENT,
https://doi.org/10.1007/978-3-031-68546-0_21

21.2 Propolis in Toothpaste

From Hellenistic ancient Greece comes the phrase "propolis," which can indicate either "suburb/bee glue" or "defense of the city" [12, 13]. At least 300 BC, the Egyptians, Persians, Greeks, and Romans began using propolis [14, 15]. In addition to its use in mummification, the Egyptians applied it topically to wounds, cuts, ulcers, and other skin conditions. The majority of its users were in Eastern Europe (Russia), where it was known as "Russian penicillin" [13], and in the Renaissance, old wisdom and medical practice rediscovered propolis' rising use. Scientific investigation into propolis began in the nineteenth century with distillation, and the first substantial chemical investigation began with fractionation in the early twentieth century [13, 14].

The main functions of propolis for bees include sealing holes and smoothing walls, protecting colonies from outsiders, and maintaining a constant temperature and humidity [16, 17]. Bees glean it from floral, leaf, bud, shoot, stem, fruit resins, and droppings. It is produced by combining it with bee saliva [17–19]. Plant resins comprise around 60% of propolis, with pollens and wax making up 30%. Essential oils and polyphenols are more examples of organic components [20, 21]. Propolis is thought to primarily contain significant compounds such as flavonoids, phenolic acids, and terpenoids with biological activity [17, 19, 22, 23]. According to Okińczyc et al. [23], the quantity of polyphenols and volatile components is primarily responsible for propolis' medicinal effects. Propolis also contains vitamins (B1, B2, B3, and B6), sugar, enzymes, fatty acids, zinc, and iron [24–26].

According to recent research, emerging evidence suggests that propolis has various biological functions. It should be noted that toxicological testing of crude propolis samples should be conducted before using these materials to make nutritional supplements and therapeutic goods [26]. A product containing propolis is not harmful. About 70 milligrams per day, or 1.4 milligrams per kilogram, is the safe human dosage [27]. There has been a recent uptick in using beekeeping goods in alternative medicine. Several disorders can be effectively treated with propolis extracts [28]. Propolis can perform a vast array of biological functions. They have a wide range of uses, including those of anesthetic, anticancer, immune-stimulating, cytostatic, hepatoprotective, spasmolytic, choleric, astringent, anti-inflammatory, antiviral, antiprotozoal, and antioxidant [17, 29–32].

These days, people think the propolis you get is mainly determined by the plant you get it from. As a result of the plant's naturally occurring biologically active compounds, propolis and its medicinal formulations may be more easily identified. Because Apis mellifera tends to gather bud exudates of poplar trees, the most common propolis collected from non-tropical Asia, New Zealand, Africa, and Europe has chemical characteristics typical of poplar trees, such as a high flavonoid content (including flavone content) and low concentrations of phenol and ester [18, 23]. In the temperate zone, propolis mostly comes from the bud exudates of Populus trees, specifically *P. nigra* (black poplar) and, to a lesser extent, P. tremula L. (aspen), as stated by Bankova et al. [35] and Okińczyc et al. [23]. This propolis was dubbed European propolis by the writers. Typical poplar phenolics in European propolis include flavones, flavanones, and esters of substituted cinnamic acids [23, 33–35]. Propolis can occasionally be found in white birch (Betula verrucosa) trees [23, 34]. Mixed varieties of propolis, such as aspen-birch-poplar, aspen-poplar-aspen, etc., are also known [23].

As evidence of propolis' beneficial effects on health, research has demonstrated that it can cure gingivitis and oral ulcers in many patients [36–38]. Internally, it kills Gram-positive cocci, facultative anaerobes, and *Streptococcus mutans*. Additionally, propolis' capacity to eliminate periodontal bacteria may have substantial therapeutic utility, according to several studies [39–41]. Toothpaste and mouthwash containing propolis have been introduced by numerous companies to combat gingivitis and tooth decay, capitalizing on this enormous potential [11]. In addition to aiding in removing and preventing biofilm, various types of toothpaste, dentifrices, and mouthwashes containing propolis have demonstrated excellent anti-inflammatory properties [1, 42].

The beneficial effects of propolis on gum health, oral cleanliness, and eliminating harmful germs are noticeable. One possible explanation for propolis' various beneficial effects is its rich chemical composition [6]. Research has demonstrated that propolis can effectively combat certain mouth bacteria. Some propolis components exhibit bacteriostatic activity, while others have bacteriocidal capabilities against different oral species, according to research by Yoshimasu et al. [41]. This includes Porphyromonas gingivalis. You can see why propolis is good for your teeth and gums because it has anti-inflammatory, antibacterial, antifungal, antiviral, anticancer, and immunomodulatory properties [1, 43].

Rihar et al. [44] tested the antimicrobial properties of propolis-infused toothpaste, which has dual uses as both a dental therapy and an endodontic medicine. The water-soluble propolis extract was used to make the propolis toothpaste. In addition to calcium hydroxide, two commercial and two medicinal toothpastes were tested, which served as a control. Propolis toothpaste targets a few germs: *S. aureus*, *M. luteus*, *E. coli*, *Pseudomonas aeruginosa*, and yeast *Candida albicans*. The effectiveness of the resazurin dye in inhibiting bacterial and yeast development was tested. When resazurin turns pink instead of blue, it means that the growth of bacteria and yeast has been inhibited. We found the MIC (Minimum Inhibitory Concentration) by finding the highest dilution at which either no color change or minimal change happened. The seventh hole, for instance, now has a blue hue instead of pink. They found that when comparing MIC values between medical and propolis toothpaste, the former was 4.53 to 25.0 times more effective. The corresponding frequencies for *Staphylococcus aureus*, *Staphylococcus mutans*, *Escherichia coli*, *Pseudomonas aeruginosa*, and yeast *Candida albicans* were 10.51, 9.33, 25.0, 4.53, and 9.33, respectively. The effectiveness of propolis toothpaste was 0.74 to 18.73 times higher than that of commercial toothpaste. I counted 6.03 for *Staphylococcus aureus*, 1.26 for *Staphylococcus mutans*, 4.13 for *Escherichia coli*, 0.74 for *Pseudomonas aeruginosa*, and 18.73 for yeast *Candida albicans* [44].

There was a statistically significant difference in dental plaque scores between the control and treatment groups, suggesting that propolis-containing toothpaste may have a beneficial effect. Brushing with this toothpaste resulted in lower dental plaque scores than the control group. A decrease in dental plaque scores may suggest that plaque is being inhibited [45].

Forty individuals with long-term periodontitis were split into two treatment groups at random. Twenty participants were in the control group; they underwent scaling, root planing, and gingival irrigation with physiological saline. Twenty participants served as the control group; they underwent scaling and root planing at the treatment areas before receiving ethanolic propolis extract subgingivally. Study findings demonstrated that Spanish propolis extract significantly reduced bacterial counts one-month following periodontal therapy, explicitly targeting *Porphyromonas gingivalis* and *Tannerella forsythensis*. The results indicate that ethanolic propolis extract can be used as a preventative measure or a treatment for periodontal illnesses. It improves clinical parameters, decreases gingival bleeding, and lowers counts of bacteria that cause periodontitis. A potential strategy for avoiding microbial resistance and other side effects in periodontal therapy is the subgingival administration of ethanolic propolis extract [46]. As a component in oral health care products, propolis showed promise due to its antibacterial and anti-biofilm actions [12].

Bhat et al. [47] demonstrated that propolis can decrease the buildup of dental biofilm. Out of the three groups of 30 healthy students, the one using the Forever Bright (propolis-containing) tooth gel had a considerably lower mean modified gingival marginal plaque index (MGMPI) score than the other two. One of the main risk factors for poor oral health is biofilm accumulation; this double-blind, randomized investigation showed that tooth gels or toothpaste containing propolis could lower the rate of biofilm accumulation [11, 47, 48]. The results of the research carried out by Ercan et al. [10] and Skaba et al. [11] are comparable to this discovery made by Bhat et al. [47].

It was discovered that propolis inhibits the growth of certain organisms in addition to reducing biofilm. Research on the impact of a propolis-containing dentifrice on *Streptococcus mutans* was carried out by Mohsin et al. [49]. A statistically significant decrease in *S. mutans* was observed by the third and fourth weeks of the study. The 30 male participants ranged in age from 7 to 12, making the study's sample small and non-generalizable, but these findings lend credence to propolis' potential in bacterial biofilm reduction. Similar results were reported by Skaba et al. [11] using a sample size of 32 consumers, 15 of whom were male and 17 of whom were female. *Streptococcus mutans*, Streptococcus sobrinus, and Streptococcus cricetus, glucosyltransferase activity inhibition was found to be an in vivo and in vitro property of propolis [11].

In addition to Candida spp. [11, 42, 51], *Lactobacillus rhamnosus* [50], Actinomyces spp. [47], and Capnocytophaga spp. [47] propolis is effective against other infections. Results from the study by Machorowska-Pieniazek et al. [51] are noteworthy since they found that propolis effectively decreased the number of two facultative anaerobic bacteria (Actinomyces spp. and Capnocytophaga spp.) in their samples. The odd absence of *Streptococcus mutans* from this investigation should be noted. In the early stages of tooth caries production, prior research has indicated that Streptococcus spp. and Actinomyces spp. Coexist and play a significant role [52, 53]. All 41 participants with non-syndromic cleft lip and palate who participated in the study had fixed orthodontic equipment, so it is probable that this conclusion was due to the study population [51]. It is well-documented that orthodontic appliances change the oral environment, leading to unusual bacteria [54, 55]. However, propolis decreased the amount of these microorganisms [1].

Compared to a triple antibiotic paste—a combination of doxycycline 100 mg, ground metronidazole 500 mg, and ciprofloxacin 250 mg—propolis was just as effective in disinfecting the regenerative endodontic treatment area. In dogs, using propolis as a stopper for the root canal caused the roots and dentin to grow longer and thicker, but the apical diameter shrank, just like with mineral trioxide aggregates, following the revascularization of dead, immature permanent teeth. The decrease in microbial populations within the root canal contributes to this effect. The Egyptian propolis originated in the area of El Monofia. A 1:1 ratio of powdered, frozen propolis to 96% ethanol was used for dissolving it. After two weeks of incubation at 30 °C, the mixture was filtered. After filtering, the mixture was heated to 30 °C and left to concentrate for 6 hours. The density of the final propolis extract was 150 mg/mL. The propolis orifice stopper added 1–2 drops of glycerin to the 150 mg final propolis extract. The ingredients were combined until a thick paste was formed, which could be used to seal off holes [56].

The intracanal administration of AH plus in conjunction with propolis showed encouraging results for improving the sealer-dentin interfacial bond strength, according to Üstün et al. Forty human maxillary central incisors that had just been extracted and had fully developed apices and straight canals were utilized in the study [57].

References

1. Saeed MA, Khabeer A, Faridi MA, Makhdoom G. Effectiveness of propolis in maintaining oral health: a scoping review. Can J Dent Hyg. 2021;55(3):167–76. Published 2021 Oct 1
2. Marsh PD, Head DA, Devine DA. Ecological approaches to oral biofilms: control without killing. Caries Res. 2015;49(Suppl 1):46–54.
3. Marcotte H, Lavoie MC. Oral microbial ecology and the role of salivary immunoglobulin A. Microbiol Mol Biol Rev. 1998;62(1):71–109.
4. Pannuti CM, Mattos JP, Ranoya PN, Jesus AM, Lotufo RF, Romito GA. Clinical effect of a herbal dentifrice on the control of plaque and gingivitis: a double-blind study. Pesqui Odontol Bras. 2003;17(4):314–8.
5. Sgan-Cohen HD, Vered Y. Plaque removal and oral health promotion potential for the elmex interX medium toothbrush: clinical efficacy and safety evaluation. J Clin Dent. 2003;14(3):70–3.
6. Smolarek PC, Esmerino LA, Chibinski AC, Bortoluzzi MC, Dos Santos EB, Junior VAK. In vitro antimicrobial evaluation of toothpaste with natural compounds. Eur J Dent. 2015;9(4):580–6.
7. Annunziata A, Pascale P. Consumers' behaviours and attitudes toward healthy food products: The case of organic and functional foods. Paper presented at the European Association of Agricultural Economists (113th Seminar), September 3–6, 2009, Chania, Crete, Greece.

8. Maturo A. Medicalization: current concept and future directions in a bionic society. Mens Sana Monogr. 2012;10(1):122–33.
9. Netto CA, Marcucci MC, Paulino N, Anido-Anido A, Amore R, de Mendonça S, et al. Effects of typified propolis on mutans streptococci and lactobacilli: a randomized clinical trial. Braz Dent Sci. 2013;16(2):31–6.
10. Ercan N, Erdemir EO, Ozkan SY, Hendek MK. The comparative effect of propolis in two different vehicles—mouthwash and chewing gum—on plaque accumulation and gingival inflammation. Eur J Dent. 2015;9(2):272–6.
11. Skaba D, Morawiec T, Tanasiewicz M, Mertas A, Bobela E, Szliszka E, et al. Influence of the toothpaste with Brazilian ethanol extract propolis on the oral cavity health. Evid Based Complement Alternat Med. 2013;2013:215391.
12. Wieczorek PP, Hudz N, Yezerska O, Horčinová-Sedláčková V, Shanaida M, Korytniuk O, Jasicka-Misiak I. Chemical variability and pharmacological potential of propolis as a source for the development of new pharmaceutical products. Molecules. 2022;27(5):1600.
13. Kuropatnicki AK, Szliszka E, Krol W. Historical aspects of propolis research in modern times. Evid Based Complement Alternat Med. 2013;2013:964149. https://doi.org/10.1155/2013/964149.
14. Anjum SI, Ullah A, Khan KA, Attaullah M, Khan H, Ali H, Bashir MA, Tahir M, Ansari MJ, Ghramh HA, et al. Composition and functional properties of propolis (bee glue): a review. Saudi J Biol Sci. 2019;26:1695–703. https://doi.org/10.1016/j.sjbs.2018.08.013. [PMC free article].
15. Bakdash A, Almohammadi OH, Taha NA, Abu-Rumman A, Kumar S. Chemical composition of propolis from the Baha region in Saudi Arabia. Czech J Food Sci. 2018;36:109–18.
16. Kiziltas H, Erkan C. The effects of different beehives on propolis production and quality. Food Sci Technol. 2020;41:877–83. https://doi.org/10.1590/fst.20120.
17. Neto MSR, Tintino SR, Silva AR, Costa MS, Boligon AA, Matias EEF, Balbino VQ, Menezes IRA, Coutinho HDM. Seasonal variation of Brazilian red propolis: antibacterial activity, synergistic effect and phytochemical screening. Food Chem Toxicol. 2017;107:572–80. https://doi.org/10.1016/j.fct.2017.03.052.
18. Ahangari Z, Naseri M, Vatandoost F. Propolis: chemical composition and its applications in endodontics. Iran Endod J. 2018;13:285–92. https://doi.org/10.22037/iej.v13i3.20994.
19. Tran VH, Duke RK, Abu-Mellal A, Duke CC. Propolis with high flavonoid content collected by honey bees from *Acacia paradoxa*. Phytochemistry. 2012;81:126–32. https://doi.org/10.1016/j.phytochem.2012.06.002.
20. Huang S, Zhang CP, Wang K, Li GQ, Hu FL. Recent advances in the chemical composition of propolis. Molecules. 2014;19:19610–32. https://doi.org/10.3390/molecules191219610.
21. Santos LM, Fonseca MS, Sokolonski AR, Deegan KR, Araújo RP, UmszaGuez MA, Barbosa JD, Portela RD, Machado BA. Propolis: types, composition, biological activities, and veterinary product patent prospecting. J Sci Food Agric. 2020;100:136982. https://doi.org/10.1002/jsfa.10024.
22. Ikeda NY, Ambrosio CMS, Miano AC, Rosalen PL, Gloria EM, Alencar SM. Essential oils extracted from organic propolis residues: an exploratory analysis of their antibacterial and antioxidant properties and volatile profile. Molecules. 2021;26:4694. https://doi.org/10.3390/molecules26154694.
23. Okińczyc P, Szumny A, Szperlik J, Kulma A, Franiczek R, Żbikowska B, Krzyżanowska B, Sroka Z. Profile of polyphenolic and essential oil composition of Polish propolis, black poplar and aspens buds. Molecules. 2018;23:1262. https://doi.org/10.3390/molecules23061262.
24. Farre R, Frasquet I, Sanchez A. Propolis and human health. Ars Pharm. 2004;45:21–43.
25. Rebiai A, Belfar ML, Mesbahi MA, Nani S, Tliba A, Ghamem AD, Chouikh A. Fatty acid composition of Algerian propolis. J Fundam Appl Sci. 2017;9:656–71.
26. Roman A, Popiela-Pleban E. Contamination of propolis used as a dietary supplement. Potravin Slovak J Food Sci. 2012;6:50–2. https://doi.org/10.5219/184.

27. Wang JW, Chen SS, Zhang YM, Guan J, Su GY, Ding M, Li W, Zhao YQ. Anti-inflammatory and analgesic activity based on polymorphism of cedrol in mice. Environ Toxicol Pharmacol. 2019;68:13–8. https://doi.org/10.1016/j.etap.2019.02.005.
28. Pasupuleti VR, Sammugam L, Ramesh N, Gan SH. Honey, propolis, and royal jelly: a comprehensive review of their biological actions and health benefits. Oxidative Med Cell Longev. 2017;2017:1259510. https://doi.org/10.1155/2017/1259510.
29. Hudz N, Korytniuk O, Yezerska O, Motyka O, Turkina V, Korytniuk R, Wieczorek PP. Evaluation of the total flavonoid content and antimicrobial activity of the tinctures of propolis of Ukrainian origin. Acta Pol Pharm Drug Res. 2020;77:897–907. https://doi.org/10.32383/appdr/131651.
30. Burdock GA. Review of the biological properties and toxicity of bee propolis (propolis). Food Chem Toxicology. 1998;36:347–63. https://doi.org/10.1016/S0278-6915(97)00145-2.
31. Fokt H, Pereira A, Ferreira AM, Cunha A, Aguiar C. How do bees prevent hive infection? The antimicrobial properties of propolis. Curr Res Technol Educ Appl Microbiol Biotechnol. 2010;1:481–93.
32. Özkirim A, Çelemli ÖG, Schiesser A, Charistos L, Hatjina F. A comparison of the activities of Greek and Turkish propolis against *Paenibacillus larvae*. J Apic Res. 2014;53:528–36. https://doi.org/10.3896/IBRA.1.53.5.01.
33. Bankova VS, De Castro SL, Marcucci MC. Propolis: recent advances in chemistry and plant origin. Apidologie. 2000;31:3–15. https://doi.org/10.1051/apido:2000102.
34. Graikou K, Popova M, Gortzi O, Bankova V, Chinou I. Characterization and biological evaluation of selected Mediterranean propolis samples. Is it a new type? LWT–Food Sci Technol. 2016;65:261–7. https://doi.org/10.1016/j.lwt.2015.08.025.
35. Bankova V, Popova M, Trusheva B. Propolis volatile compounds: chemical diversity and biological activity: a review. Chem Cent J. 2014;8:28. https://doi.org/10.1186/1752-153X-8-28.
36. Miguel MG, Antunes MD. Is propolis safe as an alternative medicine? J Pharm Bioallied Sci. 2011;3(4):479–95.
37. Dodwad V, Kukreja BJ. Propolis mouthwash: a new beginning. J Indian Soc Periodontol. 2011;15(2):121–5.
38. Mossalayi MD, Rambert J, Renouf E, Micouleau M, Merillon JM. Grape polyphenols and propolis mixture inhibits inflammatory mediator release from human leukocytes and reduces clinical scores in experimental arthritis. Phytomedicine. 2014;21(3):290–7.
39. Furtado Junior JHC, Valadas LAR, Fonseca SGDC, Lobo PDL, Calixto LHM, Lima AGF, et al. Clinical and microbiological evaluation of Brazilian red propolis containing-dentifrice in orthodontic patients: a randomized clinical trial. Evid Based Complement Alterna Med. 2020;2020:8532701.
40. Gebara EC, Lima LA, Mayer M. Propolis antimicrobial activity against periodontopathic bacteria. Braz J Microbiol. 2002;33(4):365–9.
41. Yoshimasu Y, Ikeda T, Sakai N, Yagi A, Hirayama S, Morinaga Y, et al. Rapid bactericidal action of propolis against *Porphyromonas gingivalis*. J Dent Res. 2018;97(8):928–36.
42. Morawiec T, Dziedzic A, Niedzielska I, Mertas A, Tanasiewicz M, Skaba D, et al. The biological activity of propolis-containing toothpaste on oral health environment in patients who underwent implant-supported prosthodontic rehabilitation. Evid Based Complement Alternat Med. 2013;2013:704947.
43. Antonio AG, Maia LC, Vianna RBC, Quintanilha LELP. Preventive strategies in oral health promotion. Ciênc Saúde Colet. 2005;10:279–86.
44. Rihar K, Exel DG, Pereyra A, Kopınč R, Filipič B. Toothpaste with propolis "Apident" shows antimicrobial activity in vitro. J Apither Nat/Apiterapi ve Doğa Dergisi. 2018;1(3):31.
45. Listyasari NA, Santoso O. Inhibition of dental plaque formation by toothpaste containing propolis. Dent J (Maj Kedokt Gigi). 2012;45:208–11. https://doi.org/10.20473/j.djmkg.v45.ı4.p208-211.
46. Lisbona-González MJ, Muñoz-Soto E, Reyes-Botella C, Olmedo-Gaya MV, Diaz-Castro J, Moreno-Fernandez J. Study of the antimicrobial effect of an ethanolic extract of propolis in periodontal disease. Appl Sci. 2021;11:7463. https://doi.org/10.3390/app11167463.

47. Bhat N, Bapat S, Asawa K, Tak M, Chaturvedi P, Gupta VV, et al. The antiplaque efficacy of propolis-based herbal toothpaste: a crossover clinical study. J Nat Sci Biol Med. 2015;6(2):364–8.
48. Wiatrak K, Morawiec T, Rój R, Mertas A, Machorowska-Pieniazek A, Kosnacki P, et al. Oral health of patients treated with acrylic partial dentures using a toothpaste containing bee product. Evid Based Complement Alternat Med. 2017;2017:4034179.
49. Mohsin S, Manohar B, Rajesh S, Asif Y. The effects of a dentifrice containing propolis on Mutans streptococci: a clinicomicrobiological study. Ethiop J Health Sci. 2015;25(1):9–16.
50. Valones MA, Higino JS, Souza PR, Crovella S, Caldas AFJ, Carvalho AA. Dentifrice containing extract of *Rosmarinus officinalis* Linn.: an antimicrobial evaluation. Braz Dent J. 2016;27(5):497–501.
51. Machorowska-Pieniazek A, Morawiec T, Mertas A, Tanasiewicz M, Dziedzic A, Krol W. Influence of propolis on hygiene, gingival condition, and oral microflora in patients with cleft lip and palate treated with fixed orthodontic appliances. Evid Based Complement Alternat Med. 2013;2013:183915.
52. Aas JA, Griffen AL, Dardis SR, Lee AM, Olsen I, Dewhirst FE, et al. Bacteria of dental caries in primary and permanent teeth in children and young adults. J Clin Microbiol. 2008;46(4):1407–17.
53. Perdikogianni H, Papaioannou W, Nakou M, Oulis C, Papagiannoulis L. Periodontal and microbiological parameters in children and adolescents with cleft lip and/or palate. Int J Paediatr Dent. 2009;19(6):455–67.
54. Petti S, Barbato E, Simonetti D'AA. Effect of orthodontic therapy with fixed and removable appliances on oral microbiota: a six-month longitudinal study. New Microbiol. 1997;20(1):55–62.
55. Ristic M, Vlahovic Svabic M, Sasic M, Zelic O. Clinical and microbiological effects of fixed orthodontic appliances on periodontal tissues in adolescents. Orthod Craniofac Res. 2007;10(4):187–95.
56. El-Tayeb MM, Abu-Seida AM, El Ashry SH, El-Hady SA. Evaluation of antibacterial activity of propolis on regenerative potential of necrotic immature permanent teeth in dogs. BMC Oral Health. 2019;19:174. https://doi.org/10.1186/s12903-019-0835-0.
57. Üstün Y, Arslan S, Aslan T. Effects of calcium hydroxide and propolis intracanal medicaments on bond strength of resin-based endodontic sealer as assessed by push-out test. Dent Mater J. 2013;32:913–9. https://doi.org/10.4012/dmj.2013-094.

Anatolian Propolis: What Are the Different Features?

22

22.1 Introduction

The pharmaceutical sector can benefit from the ethnopharmacological approach with chemical and biological technologies. Among these methods is apitherapy, which involves administering medicinal doses of substances derived from bees and hives (Figs. 22.1 and 22.2). One of the most well-known bee products is propolis. Season, geographical origin, the kind of bees that collect it, and native or endemic plants all have a role in how propolis' chemical makeup changes [1].

This chapter aims to review the different features of Anatolian propolis.

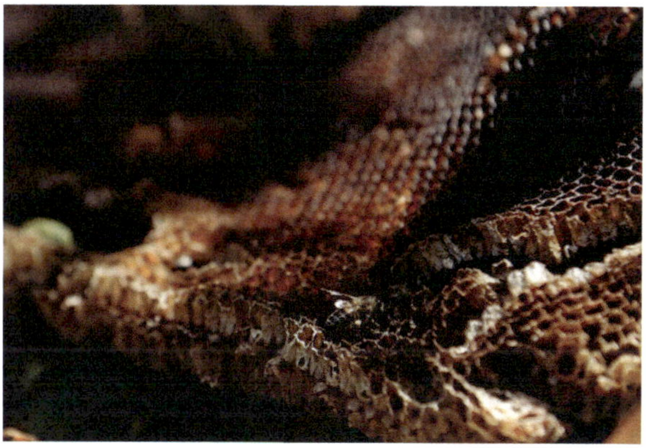

Fig. 22.1 Black honeycomb (Karadeniz region). (*Courtesy of* **Taylan Samancı**)

A. E. Tanuğur Samanci et al., *Propolis: Prevention and Healing Effects in Otorhinolaryngology*, Comprehensive ENT,
https://doi.org/10.1007/978-3-031-68546-0_22

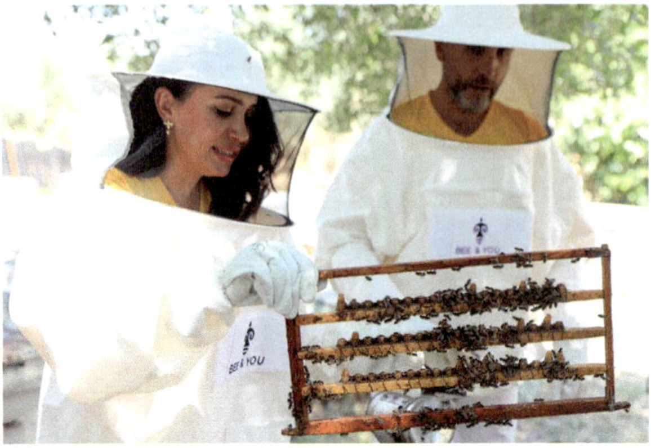

Fig. 22.2 Royal jelly production (queen cells). (*Courtesy of* **Taylan Samancı**)

22.2 Propolis: Overview

Honeybees collect the resinous primary material for propolis from their colonies. Bees collect propolis from various plant materials, such as tree trunks, leaves, and bark. They then combine it with other secretions and store it in their hive. Regarding chemistry, biology, and physical health, honeybees gain from propolis [2]. The substances' antibacterial, antiviral, antioxidant, and antitumoral characteristics are its most highly valued uses. Numerous traditional and alternative medical practices use propolis due to its biological properties [3]. Propolis has shown numerous physiologically active properties in the last 30 years of pharmacological and biochemical study, including antibacterial, antiviral, anti-inflammatory, antitumoral, hepatoprotective, and neuroprotective activities [4].

The specific composition and bioactive characteristics of propolis depend on the local flora from which it is obtained [2, 5, 6]. Half of the propolis is resin and balsam, one-third is wax, and the remaining one-third consists of aromatic compounds and essential oils. The volatile molecules and polyphenols found in propolis' balsamic portion are its active components; the substance contains about 300 different organic compounds. You can use water, glycol, or vegetable oils to a lesser degree, but 60–70% ethanol is the ideal solvent for propolis extraction [7].

In one study, researchers looked at various solvents and concentrations to see which would work best for extracting bioactive compounds from Turkish propolis. They found that 70% glycol at 10% and 15% concentrations produced water-soluble extracts, while 70% ethanol at 20% and 30% concentrations extracted the same compounds. Our goals in conducting this analysis were to compare and contrast these extracts' dry matter, total phenolic, total flavonoid, and antioxidant capacities. Noteworthy variations were seen throughout the concentrations; the 30% ethanol extract exhibited the highest levels of bioactive components, indicating that higher ethanol concentrations enable the extraction of beneficial propolis compounds. This work not only highlighted the importance of solvent concentration and choice in efficiently extracting the critical components of propolis [8], but it also paved the way for standardizing these techniques to assure consistent quality in propolis-based products.

Propolis extracts are available in many different forms, including drops, sprays, tablets, pastilles, and more. If you want high-quality propolis, look for samples rich in polyphenols and flavonoids [7]. Diets high in polyphenols, the largest class of phytochemicals, have been associated with many health benefits. Scientific studies have shown that consuming foods rich in polyphenols can reduce the risk of developing degenerative diseases such as cancer, heart disease, and neurological disorders [3, 9].

One potent ingredient is propolis, which has inherent antimicrobial and antiviral properties [10]. Multiple studies have shown that propolis has antiviral characteristics that can fight against many RNA and DNA viruses. Herpes simplex virus (HSV), avian reovirus, para-influenza, influenza A and B, adenovirus, bovine rotavirus, pseudorabies virus, and Newcastle virus disease are all examples of viruses in this category [11, 12]. The possible antiviral benefits of propolis against coronaviruses were not investigated until 1990. Of the five flavonoids in propolis—chrysin, kaempferol, acacetin, and galangin—only quercetin demonstrated dosage-dependent antiviral activity in one in vitro study [13].

The most critical pharmacologically active components of propolis are flavonoids, which include aromatics, phenolics, flavones, flavonols, and flavonones. Flavonoids are thought to be responsible for most of propolis' biological activity. This mixture of natural compounds with antibacterial properties is flavanone pinocembrin, flavonol galangin, and caffeic acid phenethyl ester. Inhibiting bacterial RNA-polymerase is probably the basis of their activity [14].

According to Marcucci [15], there are three sources for the compounds found in raw, unprocessed propolis (propolis resin): metabolites generated by bees, plant exudates that bees collect, and components added during propolis synthesis. The specific ingredients in raw propolis vary based on their origin. Fifty percent resin and vegetable balsam, 30% wax, 10% aromatic and essential oils, 5% pollen, and 5% other components, like organic waste, make up a typical composition [16, 17].

Poplar buds (Populus spp.) are the likely source of most propolis. These buds are native to temperate zones (e.g., Asia, Europe, and North America) and include several flavonoids, aromatic acids, esters, and phenolic chemicals [7].

22.3 Anatolian Propolis

Anatolian propolis samples vary in origin and a few additional characteristics. In four samples of Anatolian propolis, flavonoids including pinocembrin, pinostrobin, isalpinin, pinobanksin, quercetin, naringenin, galangin, and chrysin were the primary components. Despite coming from various parts of Anatolia, all propolis samples tested positive for antibacterial activity against yeasts and Gram-positive bacteria. Because of its antimicrobial solid action against oral disease-causing microbes such as *Streptococcus mutans*, *Streptococcus sobrinus*, and *Candida albicans*, propolis helps protect teeth from caries [18].

The antibacterial activity and chemical compositions of four distinct Anatolian propolis samples were examined in the investigation by Uzel et al. [18]. Their phytogeographical regions were as follows: European-Siberian (Bursa-Orhangazi), Irano-Turanian (Ankara-Mamak), and European-Siberian (Trabzon). Antimicrobial screening revealed that propolis samples from Bursa exhibited significantly more vigorous antifungal activity than propolis samples from other Anatolian regions ($p < 0.05$). There is hope for the prevention of dental caries and other oral disorders by the use of propolis, as samples from Anatolian trees have been found to suppress the growth of oral pathogens like *Streptococcus mutans*, *Streptococcus sobrinus*, *Enterococcus faecalis*, and *Candida albicans*.

Among the four samples of Anatolian propolis, the flavonoids pinocembrin, pinostrobin, isalpinin, pinobanksin, quercetin, naringenin, galangin, and chrysin made up the bulk [18]. These findings are consistent with those of other writers; for example, Kujumgiev et al. [19] identified flavonoids and phenolic acid esters as the primary components of propolis samples from Bulgaria. Pinocembrin and galangin were identified as the primary active components in the antibacterial action of two Italian propolis samples against *Streptococcus pyogenes*, according to Bosio et al. [20].

There are three distinct phytogeographic regions within Anatolia, defined by their location: (i) Europe-Siberia in the north, (ii) the Mediterranean in the west and south, and (iii) Iran-Turan in the center and southeast [21]. Around 11,000 infrageneric taxa are in the Anatolian force, with about a third being endemic [22]. A wide variety of plants in Anatolia provide honeybees with propolis, including chestnut, willow, juniper, pine, oak, apple, poplar, birch, linden, hazelnut, and rhododendron varieties. The color of the propolis species can range from yellow to brownish-red, brown, grayish-brown, or gray-black; the exact shade depends on the botanical species [22–24].

The many forms of propolis are described in the literature in various ways. As an example, propolis from Brazil [25, 26], Poland [27], Chile [28], Azerbaijan [29], and Venezuela [30], among others is typically designated for the place of production. Anatolian propolis is the name given to a propolis that originated in Anatolia because the region is geographically different. The botanical source of the pollen is another possible naming convention for propolis. The dominance of the pollen spectrum in naming propolis is also significant. It goes by various names, including chestnut, linden, oak, willow, etc., depending on the plant species that produces the most pollen. Each of the seven geographical regions comprising the Anatolian region has its unique climate and set of features. The areas around the Black Sea, Marmara, and Aegean are known for their thriving beekeeping industries. The antioxidant capabilities, phenolic composition, humidity, balsam, total polyphenolic content (TPC), total flavonoid content (TFC), and regional fingerprint of Anatolian propolis were examined and compared in depth in this work [31].

22.4 Content of Anatolian Propolis

Anatolian propolis is composed of a diverse array of plant types, including Pinaceae, Quercus spp., Castanea sativa, Helianthus annuus, Asteraceae, Apiaceae, Cistaceae, Campanula spp., Fabaceae, Salix spp., Brassicaceae, Platanus spp., Centaurea spp., and several others. Various tree pollens were found, including those from Populus, Tilia, Onobrychis, Juniperus, Acer, Anthemis, and Poaceae. The presence of these pollens in propolis samples is a consequence of their geographical and botanical characteristics; nonetheless, melissopalynological data do not allow for an exact determination of the botanical origin of propolis. On average, 38% of Anatolian propolis contained balsamic chemicals, while 26% contained wax substances. Balsam concentration in propolis is proportional to polyphenol concentration. The TPC is the single most critical metric for evaluating propolis quality. The average amount of polyphenols in Anatolian propolis is 15%, with around 3% of that amount being flavonoids [31].

The phenolic content of Anatolian propolis varied among the regions of Central Anatolia, Southeast Anatolia, and Eastern Anatolia. Still, it was consistent among the Marmara, Black Sea, and Aegean regions. The presence of chrysin and pinocembrin in Anatolian propolis made it stand apart. There was no significant variation between the seven areas of Anatolian propolis, which were found to have a high phenolic content containing components such as caffeic acid, caffeic acid phenethyl ester (CAPE), chrysin, pinocembrin, and cinnamic acid [31].

In a comprehensive study aimed at standardizing propolis based on its antioxidant properties, 23 propolis samples from various regions of Turkey were analyzed using high-performance liquid chromatography (HPLC). The study quantified total flavonoids and phenolics and evaluated each sample's antioxidant capacity (CUPRAC). Results showed significant variation, with total flavonoid content ranging from 21.28 to 152.56 mg CE/g and total phenolic content from 34.53 to 259.4 mg GAE/g. Antioxidant capacities varied between 95.35 and 710.43 mg TE/g. Key bioactive components such as quercetin, galangin, apigenin, pinocembrin, and various phenolic acids were also quantitatively profiled, revealing diverse concentrations across the samples. Multidimensional scaling analysis highlighted the regional differences in antioxidant properties. This study significantly advances the efforts toward national and international standardization of propolis by establishing a detailed profile of its bioactive compounds and antioxidant activity [32].

22.5 Health Benefits of Anatolian Propolis

22.5.1 The Antiviral Properties of Anatolian Propolis on COVID-19

Due to its possible antiviral qualities against SARS-CoV-2, the virus that causes COVID-19, Anatolian propolis has garnered a lot of interest in scientific studies. Research has concentrated on its high phenolic and flavonoid content, investigating its potential use in adjuvant and preventive medicine. Pinocembrin, caffeic acid, and p-coumaric acid are among the substances that have been the focus of molecular study. These compounds can suppress the virus by binding to the spike S1 protein and ACE-2 receptor, as demonstrated by molecular docking studies, HPLC-UV, and in vitro ELISA testing [4]. Studies on the effectiveness of flavonoids in vitro have shown that they can stop the SARS-CoV-2 virus from attaching to the ACE-2 receptor, which prevents the virus from infecting host cells [33]. Propolis has demonstrated encouraging outcomes in clinical settings. A case study detailed how a COVID-19 patient quickly weaned off mechanical ventilation in the ICU after seeing a considerable improvement in respiratory function after ingesting 30% propolis extract [34]. In addition, a study on propolis use as a preventative measure among healthcare professionals showed that propolis consumers had a much lower infection rate than the control group [35]. These results highlight the potential of Anatolian propolis in creating antiviral therapies and COVID-19 prevention strategies, calling for more research.

22.5.2 The Antimicrobial Effect of Anatolian Propolis

Research on the antibacterial properties of Anatolian propolis has shown that it is precious for various medical uses, particularly in dental hygiene, gut health, and wound healing.

22.5.2.1 Wound Healing

A critical randomized controlled experiment evaluated the effectiveness of 15% Anatolian propolis extract in treating pilonidal sinus wounds. Thirty-three patients were involved in the trial; they were split into two groups: an experimental group that received the propolis treatment and a control group that did not. Records made on three critical postoperative days—the 7th, 14th, and 28th—showed that the propolis-treated group's wound healing was noticeably quicker. The propolis extract's antibacterial, antioxidant, and anti-inflammatory qualities are responsible for this accelerated healing process, underscoring the extract's medicinal advantages in promoting efficient wound care [36].

22.5.2.2 Dental Health

Thirty percent Anatolian propolis extract was found to be effective as an antibacterial agent against a range of oral infections, including *Candida albicans* and *Staphylococcus aureus*, in a study. The study compared the effectiveness of propolis with other common dentin disinfectants by assigning 75 molars to various treatment groups. The outcomes verified that propolis extract functions similarly to well-known antibacterial agents, offering a feasible natural substitute for maintaining oral health and preventing infections in dental offices [37].

All of these studies show how Anatolian propolis' broad-spectrum antimicrobial qualities can be used in medical treatment and preventive care. These include improving wound healing, fighting bacteria that cause stomach ulcers, and protecting oral health.

22.5.3 The Positive Effect of Anatolian Propolis on Nasal Health

Recent investigations have explored Anatolian propolis' therapeutic potential in managing allergic rhinitis, focusing on its safety and efficacy when applied topically as a nasal spray. In one study, 0.3% Anatolian propolis nasal spray was used to cultured nasal epithelial cells, and the cells were then incubated for a full day. The results showed that Anatolian propolis did not cause any harmful effects on the nasal epithelial cells, even at high concentrations, maintaining the morphology and survival of the cells. This can validate the use of Anatolian propolis in treating inflammatory sinonasal disorders like acute and chronic rhinosinusitis and implies that it is safe for topical administration. The study also detected a slight increase in primary cells, which might help with the healing processes needed after septal operations and in epistaxis cases [38].

Expanding upon these results, a more extensive, multicenter observational trial evaluated how a propolis-containing nasal spray affected people with allergic rhinitis symptoms. The trial involved 10,000 patients and assessed the efficacy of applying the propolis nasal spray three times a day for three weeks. The outcomes showed a significant decrease in symptoms and improved quality of life and ear, nose, and throat examination scores, including reduced concha color and edema. Additionally, there was a significant improvement in nasal discharge, sneezing, itching, and congestion [39].

All of this research points to Anatolian propolis' effectiveness in reducing allergic rhinitis symptoms and suggests it is safe to apply topically in nasal applications. Propolis spray is a potential choice to supplement current treatments for allergic rhinitis because it improves nasal health and general quality of life. Scientists recommend including it in more comprehensive treatment plans, highlighting its potential as a helpful addition to the treatment of nasal allergies [38, 39].

References

1. Sönmez E. Investigation of chemical content and antimicrobial activities of different plant sources of Anatolian propolis samples. U Arı D/U Bee J. 2023;23(1):37–48. https://doi.org/10.31467/uluaricilik.1208667.
2. Bankova V, Bertelli D, Borba R, Conti BJ, da Silva Cunha IB, et al. Standard methods for Apis mellifera propolis research. J Apic Res. 2019;58(2):1–49. https://doi.org/10.1080/00218839.2016.1222661.
3. Pasupuleti VR, Sammugam L, Ramesh N, Gan SH. Honey, propolis, and royal jelly: a comprehensive review of their biological actions and health benefits. Oxidative Med Cell Longev. 2017;2017:1259510. https://doi.org/10.1155/2017/1259510.
4. Güler Hİ, Ay Şal F, Can Z, Kara Y, Yildiz O, Belduz AO, Çanakçı S, Kolaylı S. Targeting CoV-2 spike RBD and ACE-2 interaction with flavonoids of Anatolian propolis by in silico and

in vitro studies in terms of possible COVID-19 therapeutics. Turk J Biol. 2021;45(4):530–48. https://doi.org/10.3906/biy-2104-5. PMID: 34803452; PMCID: PMC8576337.
5. Aliyazıcıoglu R, Sahin H, Erturk O, Ulusoy E, Kolaylı S. Properties of phenolic composition and biological activity of propolis from Turkey. Int J Food Prop. 2013;16:277–87. https://doi.org/10.1080/10942912.2010.551312.
6. Kiziltas H, Erkan C (2020). The effects of different beehives on propolis production and quality. Food Sci Technol. Ahead of Print. https://doi.org/10.1590/fst.20120.
7. Oroian M, Ursachi F, Dranca F. Influence of ultrasonic amplitude, temperature, time and solvent concentration on bioactive compounds extraction from propolis. Ultrason Sonochem. 2020;64:105021. https://doi.org/10.1016/j.ultsonch.2020.105021.
8. Characterization of propolis extracts prepared using different solvents at the different concentrations. Progr Nutr [Internet]. 2021 Oct. 7 [cited 2024 Jun. 21];23(3):e2021108. Available from: https://www.mattioli1885journals.com/index.php/progressinnutrition/article/view/10795. Accessed online at June 22nd, 2024.
9. Characterization of propolis extracts prepared using different solvents at the different concentrations. Progr Nutr [Internet]. 2021 Oct. 7 [cited 2024 Apr. 15];23(3):e2021108. Available at: www.mattioli1885journals.com/index.php/progressinnutrition/article/view/10795
10. Przybyłek I, Karpiński TM. Antibacterial properties of propolis. Molecules. 2019;24(11):2047. https://doi.org/10.3390/molecules24112047.
11. Bankova V, Galabov AS, Antonova D, Vilhelmova N, Di Perri B. Chemical composition of propolis extract ACF® and activity against herpes simplex virus. Phytomedicine. 2014;21(11):1432–8. https://doi.org/10.1016/j.phymed.2014.04.026.
12. Bachevski D, Damevska K, Simeonovski V, Dimova V. Back to the basics: propolis and COVID-19. Dermatol Ther. 2020;33(4):e13780. https://doi.org/10.1111/dth.13780.
13. Debiaggi M, Tateo F, Pagani L, Luini M, et al. Effects of propolis flavonoids on virus infectivity and replication. Microbiologica. 1990;13(3):207–13.
14. Takaisi-Kikuni NB, Schilcher H. Electron microscopic and microcalorimetric investigations of the possible mechanism of the antibacterial action of a defined propolis provenance. Planta Med. 1994;60:222–7.
15. Marcucci MC. Propolis: chemical composition, biological properties and therapeutic activity. Apidologie. 1995;26:83–99.
16. Monti M, Berti E, Carminati G, Cusini M. Occupational and cosmetic dermatitis from propolis. Contact Derm. 1983;9:163.
17. Cirasino L, Pisati A, Fasani F. Contact dermatitis from propolis. Contact Derm. 1987;16:110–1.
18. Uzel A, Sorkun K, Onçağ O, Cogŭlu D, Gençay O, Salih B. Chemical compositions and antimicrobial activities of four different Anatolian propolis samples. Microbiol Res. 2005;160(2):189–95. https://doi.org/10.1016/j.micres.2005.01.002. PMID: 15881836
19. Kujumgiev A, Tsvetkova I, Serkedjieva Y, Bankova VS, Christov R, Popov S. Antibacterial, antifungal and antiviral activity of propolis of different geographic origin. J Ethnopharmacol. 1999;64:235–40.
20. Bosio K, Avanzini C, D'Avolio A, Ozino O, Savoia D. In vitro activity of propolis against *Streptococcus pyogenes*. Lett Appl Microbiol. 2000;31:174–7.
21. Aghanabati SA. A brief review of the geology of West Asia. Ancient West Asian Civilization. 2017:39–50.
22. Guzelmeric E, Ristivojević P, Trifković J, Dastan T, Yilmaz O, Cengiz O. Authentication of Turkish propolis through HPTLC fingerprints combined with multivariate analysis and palynological data and their comparative antioxidant activity. LWT. 2018;87:23–32.
23. Değirmencioğlu HT, Güzelmeriç E, Yüksel PI, Kırmızıbekmez H, Deniz İ, Yeşilada E. A new type of Anatolian propolis: evaluation of its chemical composition, activity profile and botanical origin. Chem Biodivers. 2019;16(12):e1900492.
24. Barth OM. Palynological analysis of geopropolis samples obtained from six species of Meliponinae in the campus of the universite de Ribeirão Preto, USP, Brazil. Apiacta. 2006;41(2):71–85.

25. Freires IA, de Alencar SM, Rosalen PL. A pharmacological perspective on the use of Brazilian red propolis and its isolated compounds against human diseases. Euro J Med Chem. 2016;110:267–79.
26. Svečnjak L, Marijanović Z, Okińczyc P, Marek Kuś P, Jerković I. Mediterranean propolis from the Adriatic Sea islands as a source of natural antioxidants: comprehensive chemical biodiversity determined by GC-MS, FTIR-ATR, UHPLC-DAD-QqTOFMS DPPH and FRAP assay. Antioxidants. 2020;9(4):337.
27. Popova M, Trusheva B, Bankova V. Content of biologically active compounds in Bulgarian propolis: a basis for its standardization. Bulgarian Chem Com. 2017;49:115–20.
28. Barrientos L, Herrera CL, Montenegro G, Ortega X, Veloz J, Alvear M. Chemical and botanical characterization of Chilean propolis and biological activity on cariogenic bacteria *Streptococcus mutans* and *Streptococcus sobrinus*. Braz J Microbiol. 2013;44:577–85.
29. Degirmenci A, Can Z, Boyraci GM, Yildiz O, Asadov E, Kolayli S. Honeys from some different regions of Azerbaijan: bioactive characteristics based on phenolic profile and antioxidant activity. J Apicul Res. 2020;59(4):390–7.
30. Mohtar LG, Messina GA, Bertolino FA, Pereira SV, Raba J, Nazareno MA. Comparative study of different methodologies for the determination the antioxidant activity of Venezuelan propolis. Microchem J. 2020;158:105244.
31. Kolaylı S, Birinci C, Kara Y, Ozkok A, Tanugur Samancı AE, Sahin H, Yildiz O. A melissopalynological and chemical characterization of Anatolian propolis and an assessment of its antioxidant potential. Eur Food Res Technol. 2023;249:1213–33.
32. Ozkok A, Keskin M, Tanuğur Samancı AE, Yorulmaz Onder E, Takma C. Determination of antioxidant activity and phenolic compounds for basic standardization of Turkish propolis. Appl Biol Chem. 2021;64(1):37.
33. Guler HI, Tatar G, Yildiz O, Belduz AO, Kolayli S. Investigation of potential inhibitor properties of ethanolic propolis extracts against ACE-II receptors for COVID-19 treatment by molecular docking study. Arch Microbiol. 2021;203(6):3557–64.
34. Zorlu D. Covid-19 and Anatolian propolis: a case report. Acta Medica Mediterranea. 2021;37:1229.
35. Guler E, Bilir O, Osman Kocak A, Atas I, Tanugur Samanci AE. The prophylactic efficacy of Anatolian propolis in individuals at high risk of COVID-19. Eur Rev Med Pharmacol Sci. 2022;26(2 Suppl):53–60.
36. Kubat M, Karabulut Z, Şengül S. Effect of propolis on wound healing in sacrococcygeal pilonidal disease: a randomized controlled clinical trial. Pak J Pharm Sci. 2021;34(3(Supplementary)):1063–7.
37. Kalay TS, Kara Y, Karaoglu SA, Kolayli S. Evaluation of stabilized chlorine dioxide in terms of antimicrobial activity and dentin bond strength. Comb Chem High Throughput Screen. 2022;25(9):1427–36.
38. Tanugur Samanci AE, Bayar Muluk N, Vejselova Sezer C, Kutlu HM, Topsakal V, Cingi C. Efficacy and toxicity of Anatolian propolis on healthy nasal epithelial cells. Eur Rev Med Pharmacol Sci. 2022;26(2 Suppl):103–11.
39. Cingi C, Bayar Muluk N, Çukurova İ, Dündar R, Osma U, Bal C, Zirek A, Budak A, Seyed Resuli A, Selimoğlu A, Tanuğur Samancı AE, Karaoğullarından A, Yılmaz B, Arslan B, Sizer B, Cihan C, Koca ÇF, Avcı D, Aydenizöz D, Ünver E, Alaskarov E, Gülmez E, Gündoğan F, Günay G, Çetiner H, Güngör H, Salcan İ, Gündoğan ME, Akbay MÖ, Akdağ M, Kaplama ME, Yaşar M, Koparal M, Kar M, Altıntaş M, Torun MT, Bozan N, Sarı N, Susaman N, Küçük N, Erdoğan O, Gül O, Sancaklı Ö, Kundi P, Budak RO, Karaman S, Taşar S, Demir S, Belli Ş, Yağcı T, Bilici T, Çelik T, YSS Y, Atayoglu AT, Irkan RK, Zorlu D, Can D. Effects of Anatolian propolis and hypertonic saline combination nasal spray on allergic rhinitis symptoms: a prospective, multicenter study. Ear Nose Throat J. 2024;103(4):NP190–8.

GPSR Compliance

The European Union's (EU) General Product Safety Regulation (GPSR) is a set of rules that requires consumer products to be safe and our obligations to ensure this.

If you have any concerns about our products, you can contact us on ProductSafety@springernature.com

In case Publisher is established outside the EU, the EU authorized representative is:

Springer Nature Customer Service Center GmbH
Europaplatz 3
69115 Heidelberg, Germany

Batch number: 10732044

Printed by Printforce, the Netherlands